Handbook of Quality Management in Behavioral Health

Issues in the Practice of Psychology

SERIES EDITOR:

George Stricker, *Derner Institute of Advanced Psychological Studies, Adelphi University, Garden City, New York*

HANDBOOK OF QUALITY MANAGEMENT IN BEHAVIORAL HEALTH
Edited by George Stricker, Warwick G. Troy, and Sharon A. Shueman

PSYCHOTHERAPY AND BUDDHISM: Toward an Integration
Jeffrey B. Rubin

A Continuation Order Plan is available for this series. A continuation order will bring delivery of each new volume immediately upon publication. Volumes are billed only upon actual shipment. For further information please contact the publisher.

Handbook of Quality Management in Behavioral Health

GEORGE STRICKER
Adelphi University
Garden City, New York

WARWICK G. TROY
University of Southern California
Los Angeles, California

SHARON A. SHUEMAN
Shueman Troy Associates
Pasadena, California

KLUWER ACADEMIC/PLENUM PUBLISHERS
NEW YORK, BOSTON, DORDRECHT, LONDON, MOSCOW

Library of Congress Cataloging-in-Publication Data

Handbook of quality management in behavioral health / [edited by] George Stricker, Warwick G. Troy, Sharon A. Shueman.
p. cm. -- (Issues in the practice of psychology)
Includes bibliographical references and index.
ISBN 0-306-46149-8
1. Mental health services--Quality control. 2. Mental health services--United States--Quality control. I. Stricker, George. II. Troy, Warwick G. III. Shueman, Sharon A. IV. Series.

RA790.5 .H33 1999
362.2'068'5--dc21

99-047994

ISBN: 0-306-46149-8

233 Spring Street, New York, N.Y. 10013

10 9 8 7 6 5 4 3 2 1

A C.I.P. record for this book is available from the Library of Congress

Printed in the United States of America

Contributors

DANIEL J. ABRAHAMSON Traumatic Stress Institute, South Windsor, Connecticut 06074-1369

KATHY ALLEN Student Health Service, University of California Davis, Davis, California 95616

STEPHEN L. BAIR University of Alabama at Birmingham, Birmingham, Alabama 35294-0018

SHEILA BALER Menninger Care Systems, Plano, Texas 75093

BARRY BLACKWELL Department of Psychiatry, University of Wisconsin Medical School, Milwaukee, Wisconsin 53211

WILLIAM L. CLAIBORN Alexandria Community Services Board, Alexandria, Virginia 22314

EDWARD COHEN United Behavioral Health, Oakland, California 94612

PATRICK H. DeLEON American Psychological Association, Washington, DC 20002-4242

PAUL A. ECKERT Office of Senator Breaux, Washington, DC 20510

KATHLEEN EILERS Milwaukee County Mental Health Division, Milwaukee, Wisconsin 53226

JUDITH EMERSON Portland Veterans Administration Medical Center, Portland, Oregon 97207

G. R. FORD University of Alabama at Birmingham, Birmingham, Alabama 35294-0018

NANCY K. GILMORE-LEE Office of Senator Inouye, Washington, DC 20510

JUDY E. HALL National Register of Health Service Providers in Psychology, Washington, DC 20005

SHIRLEY ANN HIGUCHI American Psychological Association, Washington, DC 20002-4242

JONATHAN C. HUEFNER Magellan Behavioral Health, Salt Lake City, Utah 84070

CHERIE JONES American Psychological Association, Washington, DC 20002-4242

MICHAEL JOSPE California School of Professional Psychology, Alhambra, California 91803

MICHAEL J. LAMBERT Department of Psychology, Brigham Young University, Provo, Utah 84602

NANCY E. LANE Massachusetts Behavioral Health Partnership, Boston, Massachusetts 02110

STEPHEN LONG Los Angeles, California 90048

MAUREEN MANGOTICH Pfizer Health Solutions, Santa Monica, California 90404

A. THOMAS McLELLAN Department of Psychiatry, University of Pennsylvania, Philadelphia, Pennsylvania 19104

RON L. MEREDITH University of Alabama at Birmingham, Birmingham, Alabama 35294-0018

RICHARD J. MORRIS School Psychology Program, University of Arizona, Tucson, Arizona 85719

YVONNE P. MORRIS Tucson, Arizona 85718

SUSAN J. PENNER Department of Nursing, Holy Names College, Oakland, California 94619

STEPHEN A. RAGUSEA Child, Adult, and Family Psychological Center, State College, Pennsylvania 16801

CURTIS W. REISINGER Department of Psychiatry, Hackensack University Medical Center, Hackensack, New Jersey, 07601 and Department of Psychiatry, UMDNJ-New Jersey Medical School, Newark, New Jersey 07103

DON ROBINSON, JR. Merck-Medco Managed Care, Montvale, New Jersey 07645

KAREN W. SAAKVITNE Traumatic Stress Institute, South Windsor, Connecticut 06074-1369

STEVEN S. SHARFSTEIN Sheppard Pratt Health System, Baltimore, Maryland 21204, and Department of Psychiatry, University of Maryland, Baltimore, Maryland 21201

SHARON A. SHUEMAN Shueman Troy Associates, Pasadena, California 91106

ANNE M. STOLINE Women's Psychiatry Unit, Mercy Medical Center, Baltimore, Maryland 21202

GEORGE STRICKER The Derner Institute, Adelphi University, Garden City, New York 11530

WARWICK G. TROY Department of Family Medicine, University of Southern California, Los Angeles, California 90033

MARGARET WALKOVER California Mental Health Directors Association, Sacramento, California 95814

DAVID A. YOUNG Pathmakers, Berkeley, California 94705

DAVID A. ZANIS Department of Psychiatry, University of Pennsylvania, Philadelphia, Pennsylvania 19104

Preface

The reader familiar with *Quality Assurance in Mental Health* (1988) will note that this second edition is written in a way that is less technical and academically focused than the previous edition. The new orientation of this handbook is intended to make its contents available to a wider audience than might have been true for the first edition. In the years since 1988, quality management has evolved from an activity delegated to specialists—academics, researchers, program evaluators, and "the nurses on the Quality Assurance Committee"—to an activity that is now considered *everyone's business.*

For the first time in history, behavioral health providers are expected to understand and participate in activities intended to assess and improve the quality of services that they provide, whether as a solo practitioner or as part of an organized delivery setting. Employers and other purchasers of care are also required to understand issues related to quality of care, since they are increasingly in the position of eliciting specific performance outcomes from the managed care organizations with which they contract. Finally, the increasing empowerment of consumers and their families and carers brings with it an expectation that these stakeholders will be involved in defining and assessing quality of the services they receive.

This edition of the handbook, then, is addressed not only to quality assurance professionals, but also to those who might be considered stakeholders in the delivery of accountable behavioral health services. The volume is designed as a general resource in the field of behavioral health quality management for a diverse group of readers including graduate and undergraduate students in the behavioral health professions, payers and purchasers, administrators within managed care organizations, public sector service system planners and managers, providers and provider groups across the disciplinary spectrum, applied health services researchers and program evaluators, faculty associated with professional education and training programs, health plan executives, representatives of consumer and carer organizations, and policy analysts and developers.

We are, as editors, very aware of the latent pitfalls associated with targeting such a heterogeneous group of readers. Frankly, we saw no other way. Some measured acquaintance with the concepts and technologies of this ever-changing field is now required by more and more people. Further, the imperatives of an essentially chaotic professional world are such as to shift to an earlier time in one's professional life an initial exposure to issues of quality and the assessment and management of its technologies. This field can no longer claim to be esoteric; for providers and service systems to think otherwise puts them, in our judgment, significantly at risk. Consumers inevitably suffer the consequences of this lack of professional preparedness.

George Stricker
Warwick G. Troy
Sharon A. Shueman

Contents

PART I THE CHANGING CONTEXT FOR QUALITY MANAGEMENT IN BEHAVIORAL HEALTH

PART II TOOLS FOR QUALITY MANAGEMENT

I

THE CHANGING CONTEXT FOR QUALITY MANAGEMENT IN BEHAVIORAL HEALTH

1

The Changing Health Services Environment and Its Impact on Quality Management in Behavioral Health

WARWICK G. TROY AND SHARON A. SHUEMAN

Almost a decade has passed since the first edition of this handbook appeared. For those of us involved in health services, this decade truly has been a professional lifetime. The climate of rapid and pervasive change in health services prevailing during this period has been no less revolutionary in those aspects of service delivery related to quality management. Indeed, it is these developments—in the structure of health services financing and organization—that have impelled the changes in approaches to quality management in the past 10 years.

Differences in the wording of the title from the first to the second edition of this volume are indicative of the scope of the changes. Quality assurance has become "quality management," and mental health has become "behavioral health." These differences are neither semantic nor cosmetic. They are reflections of a manifest change—if not a revolution—in ways of conceptualizing, assessing, and managing quality on the one hand and in the changing role and status of mental health and substance abuse services within health care on the other.

The changes also reflect larger socioeconomic shifts that have been occurring within the United States and, to a somewhat lesser extent, in much of the industrialized world. These include demands for increased accountability and efficiency, the advent of more participatory models of organizational structure and function, and the emergence of a more sophisticated and discriminating market for health services, a market previously imperfectly understood by consumers themselves and the third-party entities who most often purchased health services.

Probably the single-most significant dynamic in the evolution of health services is the advent of for-profit health care corporations, specifically large, publicly held companies. (This phenomenon has been referred to as the "corporatization" of American health care.) One may argue the wisdom of allowing stockholders to profit from a "commodity" such as health care that is commonly regarded as a general entitle-

WARWICK G. TROY • Department of Family Medicine, University of Southern California, Los Angeles, California 90033. SHARON A. SHUEMAN • Shueman Troy Associates, Pasadena, California 91106.

Handbook of Quality Management in Behavioral Health, edited by Stricker *et al.* Kluwer Academic / Plenum Publishers, New York, 2000.

ment. At the same time, there is no doubt that the demand for accountability inherent in for-profit environments and the financial capital made available through these corporations for development activities have been two of the most significant factors in shaping the health care system in the last decade. These factors have been potentiated by demands for accountability increasingly stemming from the purchaser (primarily large employers) and consumer communities.

It is the thesis of this chapter that rather than having an adverse impact on the quality of behavioral health services (as is stoutly maintained by the organized mental health professions), the contextual changes discussed here have induced a fresh set of contingencies associated with the planning and delivery of services that are ultimately conducive to more effective management of service quality and, it is to be hoped, associated with improved health outcomes for consumers. These contingencies include:

1. Demands for true integrated systems characterized by interdisciplinary and interprofessional collaboration and respect; interdependence of system elements critical to quality; a shift in emphasis from single episodes to overall continuity of care; and an enhanced role for population-based services planning.
2. Increasing demands on the provider community to accept financial risk and a corresponding decreased emphasis on the (micro) management role of the managed care entity.
3. Explicit emphasis on accountability to multiple stakeholders, including consumers and purchasers.
4. Explicit acknowledgment of accountability for vulnerable populations.
5. Service quality increasingly defined by desired outcomes.
6. An enhanced and central role for sophisticated information management systems for services monitoring and quality management purposes.
7. Expanded access to services made possible by increased use of (lower cost) alternative treatment modalities.
8. Routine use of empirically derived treatment protocols and guidelines.

The rapid penetration of managed care in the health care "marketplace" (itself a relatively new and conjectural concept) and the corresponding rapid change in the ways (behavioral) health services are organized, staffed, and delivered caught the behavioral health provider community (long grown used to the practitioner-friendly, fee-for-service payment model) very much unaware. Providers found themselves unprepared to meet the demands of the new managed systems. Their knowledge and skills as well as their attitudes and values by and large were incompatible with these demands. More importantly perhaps, these rapid changes also exceeded the capacity of service systems themselves to conduct business in ways appropriate to the changing imperatives of an inordinately competitive and essentially chaotic world.

THE STRUCTURE OF SERVICE DELIVERY

A major potential threat to service quality is deficiencies in structural aspects of services organization and delivery. While structural issues tend to be most obviously associated with organized care settings, for example, facilities, it is nonetheless meaningful to identify structural aspects of a solo practice, for example, the presence of operational links with community-based services; use of external specialists as consultants in care planning and delivery; the nature of the office's client flow system, client tracking, and other follow-up procedures; the availability and nature (including language) of information routinely provided to clients by print or other media; and the way emergency or other on-call arrangements are organized. To be sure, while in the case of a solo practice structural deficiencies such as these may be considered as inadequacies of the provider (who both embodies and is directly responsible for the solo practice's system of care), they are more usefully considered structural faults of a solo "system."

As we shall see, as managed care penetration comes to affect the majority of independent providers, such structural inadequacies as we have identified pose an increasingly large threat to the quality of behavioral health. With respect to organized care settings, entities in which the structural dimension of quality has historically played such a visible role, the very survival of these organizations, involved as they are in a competitive maelstrom, is predicated on the extent to which effective solutions to the myriad threats to quality can be found and sustained. Managed care then has come to pose a set of curiously urgent challenges in the form of a set of essentially nonnegotiable imperatives to large care systems and "independent" practitioners alike. And since the large systems must still rely on the (erstwhile) independent provider for the delivery of care, these two very different systems of care are putative partners (whether they care to be or not) in a strange and (to both) profoundly disturbing dance. [It is worth noting in this regard that one particular challenge to managed care organizations (MCOs) that by and large has not been well handled by the industry is that of provider relations: working constructively and effectively with providers who are part of MCO system operations.]

In summary, threats to the quality of behavioral health care are myriad, highly enduring, and extremely resistant to amelioration, significantly due to the entrenched, guild-oriented commitments of the professional organizations. The two major sources of these threats are: (1) prevailing deficiencies in the professional competencies of providers, particularly in view of the new and emerging challenges associated with the context of health care; and (2) significant structural inadequacies in the ways in which behavioral health services are planned, provided, and managed. It is obvious that these two categories are not mutually exclusive; the former surely affects the latter.

The continued prevalence of these two monolithic threats to quality is due largely to the relative ignorance of payers–purchasers of behavioral health services about what constitutes quality and how it may be measured on the one hand and an inadequately informed and empowered consumer community that itself lacks developed awareness of what characteristics of behavioral health services are associated with better outcomes and what members can do to increase the probability of their provider consultatively working with them in using such approaches on the other. Again, these are endemic problems that are only likely to be ameliorated in the longer term by the incorporation of strategic educational approaches targeted at payers and consumers. As MCOs and large multidisciplinary provider groups continue to seek competitive advantage by highlighting quality assessment and management initiatives, structural threats to quality will diminish, although competitive advantage itself depends on the capacity of the public and private purchasing communities to exercise fine discrimination among plans and vendors on the basis of quality.*

BACKGROUND: THE FEE-FOR-SERVICE HEALTH SERVICES ENVIRONMENT

The fee-for-service health care environment that was the dominant model in the United States through the mid-1980s was characterized by the relatively unfettered authority of independent service providers, commonly solo practitioners. They were subject to few calls for accountability from payers or consumers. Further, since providers themselves only minimally understood the concept of accountability to a third party, independent practitioners put little effort into developing technologies for self-monitoring and reporting, either for the improvement of services quality within their practice or for reporting to an external (third) party.

The Demand for Accountability

Historically, in behavioral health care there has not been a clear and effective demand for accountability from payers or from consumers. As discussed above, payers, typically insurance companies, have been generally poorly informed about behavioral health services. Further, under traditional indemnity financing arrangements there was little real incentive for these payers to concern themselves with either services costs or efficacy. If claims costs rose, the third parties merely raised premiums for employers in subsequent contract years. Nor did employers and other purchasers possess any sophistication at all about behavioral health services.† Since such services accounted for a relatively small portion of the health care dollar, payers and purchasers were little exercised in mind about cost-effectiveness issues.

A majority of consumers lacked not only the conceptual framework essential to an understanding of accountability issues but also the kind of empowerment that might have allowed them to express clear expectations for behavioral health services and their outcomes. The mystique surrounding these services was difficult for consumers to penetrate, and behavioral health professionals, in common with their counterparts in general health care, saw no need or had no incentive consistently to adhere to consumerist tenets of service planning and provision.

In the mind of providers, to demystify was potentially to limit the expression of the "art" of their profession; to talk about measurable or observable outcomes was to misunderstand the true purpose of psychotherapy. As a consequence, patients typically received the services practitioners wanted to provide, and desired outcome was defined not by the patient but by the practitioner, often in vague terms that allowed the practitioner to be the ultimate arbiter of the success of the treatment plan.

Many providers not only dismissed the need for accountability to an external entity but also regarded some strategies implemented in the interest of accountability

*Some argue that national credentialing organizations will play increasingly important roles in helping both consumers and payers better discriminate better from poorer quality health service organizations.

†Nonetheless, third-party payers, as well as other stakeholders, including the federal government, had long cast a jaundiced eye on mental health services in view of the historic incapacity of mental health services, as delivered, to be subject to cost-effectiveness questions (see Wells & Brook, 1988).

as potentially damaging to the therapeutic process. For example, many behavioral health professionals believed that the very act of monitoring or measuring any aspect of the therapeutic process violated confidentiality, precluded effective relationship building, and consequently threatened the translation of therapeutic goals. Though claiming a sense of accountability to their individual patients, providers in general were poorly equipped to respond constructively to the challenges of care systems or the cost accountability yet to be routinely required by payers. In many cases this was because they practiced independently, outside of any organized service delivery setting, and more frequently alone. Their primary concern was doing the best they could, as they understood it, for their patients. They had neither awareness nor a sense of responsibility for a covered population and no incentive to ensure that available funds were allocated appropriately and equitably across a large group of beneficiaries.

A Technology of Accountability

Historically, the level of sophistication of quality assessment and improvement activities associated with health services delivery has been low. Certainly, sophisticated methods existed, but they were most often used in the context of large-scale research and evaluation activities, almost always in academic settings frequently funded by the government or private foundations. The research program of Brook and his colleagues at the Rand Corporation is a good example of such activities (see, for example, Brook, McGlynn, & Cleary, 1996).

One reason for the low level of utilization of a developed technology for ensuring and improving service quality within many health care environments was a prevailing lack of financial and human resources to design and implement models of quality assessment and management. A second and perhaps more important reason was that particularly within many behavioral health service delivery settings a climate supportive of accountability and its mechanisms was rare indeed. In those instances where a commitment of sorts to the assessment of aspects of service quality did prevail, such assessment, together with any attempts at system improvement, was invariably marginalized within the service organization itself. Quality assurance responsibilities were most often delegated to a small group of individuals (e.g., a quality assurance or quality management committee) isolated from service delivery, usually underresourced, possessing little or no authority, and whose activities were seen as severely peripheral to the central purpose of the organization. Probably the most significant factors related to the consistent failure of such individuals to achieve measurable change in quality was the power differential between those who "did" quality assurance (i.e., nurses) and those who were the subject of evaluation and requests for corrective actions (i.e., doctors). To make matters worse, quality assurance staff were seen as the creators of the standards against which performance was measured rather than as reflections of values of the organization as a whole. In other words, these staff were seen as the single stakeholder whose values determined how standards were set and otherwise what was done in the name of quality assessment and improvement within the organization.

Within this kind of context, the mainstay of quality assessment was the medical record audit conducted by quality management staff, usually nurses, and overseen by a quality assurance committee. Audits were intrinsically episodic, they could focus only retrospectively on service patterns (process of care), and their scope was typically limited, both in terms of the number of episodes of care they could examine and the complexity and range of clinical issues they could investigate. Quality improvement activities growing out of quality assessment were most frequently requests from quality assurance staff to medical staff for correction of deficiencies, and these requests more often than not went unanswered.

THE CHANGING HEALTH SERVICES MARKETPLACE

During the 1970s and 1980s, inflation in health care costs accelerated, with the percentage increases in some cases being significantly greater in the field of behavioral health. At the same time, articles proliferated in the popular press describing apparent outrageous abuses in behavioral health services, most notably in inpatient treatment of alcohol and substance abuse and residential treatment of children and adolescence. From the payers' perspective, they were paying more and more for services the quality of which was highly suspect. (For some employers behavioral health services consumed as much as 25% of the total health care dollar, with the vast proportion being consumed by inpatient and residential treatment services of doubtful effectiveness.)

During these years, a number of entrepreneurial health services professionals recognized a potential market for organizations willing to and capable of introducing accountability mechanisms into the unstructured morass of health services and provide some assurance to payers that they were getting appropriate value for the money they spent purchasing behavioral health services for consumers (usually employed). These emerging efforts built on the rather primitive utilization review activities mandated by previous federal government efforts to evaluate health services, namely, the professional standards review organizations (PSRO), funded by the Health Care Financing Administration, and the mental health review programs of the Civilian Health and Medical Program of the Uniformed Services (CHAMPUS), funded by the Department of Defense (Wells & Brook, 1988).

The primary goal of these early review organizations was to impose monitoring and reporting requirements on networks consisting primarily of independent practitioners and facilities providing services to beneficiaries covered by a private group health plan. These requirements were intended to create service systems from these networks and increase accountability for the services they provided. The principal function of the earliest models was to determine that services were necessary and appropriate for the problem being treated. This function was very similar to that of the PSRO and CHAMPUS review programs, although the methodologies were somewhat more advanced. The companies evolved, however, developing increasingly sophisticated methods of monitoring and reporting that allowed them increasing control over service costs and quality.

CREATING SYSTEMS OF CARE

With the exception of the early staff model health maintenance organizations (HMOs) such as Kaiser-Permanente, Ross-Loos, and Group Health of the Puget Sound, health services in this country have traditionally been delivered using a fragmented, unorganized network of facilities, programs, and practitioners. As a result of the demands for accountability, however, systems of care are rapidly becoming the dominant mode of health services delivery in the United States. Currently, these systems most often take the form of MCOs, which have evolved from the early review organizations described above. MCOs selectively contract with a loosely organized network of facilities, integrated practice groups, and individual practitioners to provide a comprehensive set of services to defined populations. They typically require providers to participate in a variety of clinical and utilization management activities (e.g., case management, outcomes assessment, patient surveys) intended to ensure that services provided through the MCO are necessary, appropriate, and of reasonable quality. MCOs function as intermediaries between the purchasers of care (employers, labor trusts, etc.) and providers and in essence construct a "virtual" service system with policies and procedures to guide the professional activity of providers and structures to conduct effective quality assessment and improvement activities (Shueman, Troy, & Mayhugh, 1994).

While this more recent phase in the evolution in health services has been largely the result of private sector MCO development, integrated provider groups themselves are increasingly organizing in an attempt to present to payers accountable systems of service delivery without acceding to the control of the MCOs. Health care professionals have grown increasingly frustrated with MCOs, the accountability requirements they impose, and the control of services that they (are felt to) usurp. In response, these professionals have begun to create their own organizations that not only have many of the attributes of the MCOs but also return responsibility for decisions about utilization of resources to those persons directly involved in service planning and delivery. In order to function effectively, however, these organizations must themselves be able to demonstrate that resources are utilized appropriately and that services they deliver satisfy explicit standards of quality.

It should be noted that just as providers have begun to realize the need to develop the structures and procedures of accountability in order to reclaim control of services delivery and management, so too have MCOs come to realize the weaknesses inherent in the systems they have implemented to micromanage services. They actively encourage provider groups to organize, take responsibility for aspects of utilization and quality management, and assume financial risk.

Typically, provider-based organizations, as single entities representing a large number of providers and facilities, may contract with MCOs. A few are large enough and have developed the necessary technical capabilities to bypass MCOs and contract directly with employers and other purchasers, offering the buyer many of the accountability features common to MCOs without the additional administrative layer (and cost) associated with the MCO.

It is only since providers have become organized into integrated systems of care, whether through MCOs or provider-based organizations, that the potential has existed within behavioral health for realizing operational accountability to purchasers of health services. Accountability is defined in this context as the capacity to demonstrate that financial resources available to the organizational entity charged with managing behavioral health care are being used so as to maximize their value to the population of consumers being served.

The Influence of Purchasers in Defining Quality

Purchasers, primarily employers, union trusts, and purchasing coalitions, have become significant forces in shaping foci and nature of quality management. They are concerned about the entire population on whose behalf they purchase behavioral health care; specifically that every person in need has access to appropriate services, that the services provided benefit the user, and that the user is satisfied with those services. Purchasers require that the MCO or provider-based organization routinely provide them with utilization, cost, and outcome data that are understandable to the layperson and demonstrate access, appropriateness, and effectiveness of care as well as patient satisfaction.

Purchasers have not been totally accepting, however, of the types of data mentioned above as evidence of quality of the service system. They have heard the charges of providers and consumers—that MCOs actually sacrifice quality in the interest cost-cutting and their own profits—and have begun to ask questions about the quality of the system (the MCO) that is itself intended to assure quality. They have increasingly turned to a national accrediting organization, the National Committee for Quality Assurance (NCQA), to provide them with data demonstrating that the MCOs themselves possess the structures and processes necessary to ensure the quality of the services they provide. The NCQA accreditation is rapidly becoming the standard set by the marketplace for MCOs, whether medical–surgical HMOs or behavioral health organizations. Further, the NCQA has recently announced plans to include provider-based organizations in their accreditation program.

THE TRANSFORMATION OF QUALITY MANAGEMENT

Due to the contextual changes in health services delivery, approaches to assessing and improving the quality of behavioral health services have developed significantly over the last decade. The most significant change, however, has been a normative one: Activities related to quality assessment and process improvement are increasingly being defined as the responsibility of everyone within the organization rather than being relegated to a single committee with no status within the organization. As a consequence, the value accorded quality management has increased within MCOs and provider groups and the infrastructure (including technology) is more likely to be appropriately resourced.

As a consequence of the operational shift of quality management from the margin to the center of services planning, provision, and monitoring, quality management has begun to make the transition from being viewed as something done to providers, to being regarded as a tool that health care professionals (and the service organizations of which they are increasingly a part) can routinely use to assess and improve the quality of services they deliver. Ultimately, this change in operational focus will be complete when practitioners assume direct ownership of quality management and come to regard it as a necessary and integral component of service delivery and a useful tool. When this occurs, it is most often the case in the growing number of integrated provider groups, particularly those that are able to accept risk.

Table 1 summarizes the major attributes of quality management as traditionally operating within health services organizations on one hand and those characteristics of quality management within mature, accountable systems of care on the other. The attributes labeled "traditional," then, describe aspects of quality management structure and process as they were typically encountered in health services environments; those labeled as "emerging" reflect the new, more central role of quality management.

TABLE 1. Transformation of the Attributes of Quality Management Technology in Behavioral Health

Traditional attributes of technology	Emerging attributes of technology
Eternal	Internal, participatory
Regulatory	Proactive, "owned" from within
Ancillary, isolated from service delivery	Integrated within service delivery
Sole "expert"	Integrated team performance
Single stakeholder	Multiple stakeholders
Focus on finding and "fixing" problems	Focus on improvement
Compliance oriented	Process "owned" by service system
Episodic	Continuous, ongoing
Retrospective	Concurrent
Ad hoc, atheoretical	Systematic, possessing a technology
Focus on "assuring" quality	Focus on the management of quality

There were traditionally two common manifestations of quality management within any service system: (1) the internal quality assurance committee, discussed above, maintained by the organization itself, and (2) the accrediting agency* that periodically performed site visits to service organizations to determine whether their structures and processes warranted public recognition in the form of accreditation. While only the latter manifestation was truly external to the organization and the process of service delivery, both in fact were regarded by the organization as external, reflecting, as we have discussed, the traditional marginalization of quality management. Just as accreditation was seen by the agency as something to "get through," so too was scrutiny by the quality assurance committee regarded as something to be endured. Both were seen as something imposed on service providers by people who not only were outside of the service delivery process, but also had little understanding of it. The roles of both entities were viewed, in essence, as wholly antagonistic to the truly valued role of the mental health professional: autonomously to provide psychotherapy.

Using Information to Manage Quality

More effective quality management programs succeed because of their ability truly to integrate quality assessment and improvement activities into service delivery. This might include, for example, routinely collecting clinical information that is used in an ongoing fashion to monitor certain aspects of service delivery (e.g., progress toward goals; number of days before first available appointment; access to specialty services) and implement quality improvement activities (rather than corrective actions) immediately. The focus is more often on aggregate data and less on individual episodes. The data are regarded as management indicators that may be used by those

*These agencies include independent accrediting organizations such as the National Committee on Quality Assurance (NCQA) and the Joint Commission for the Accreditation of Healthcare Organizations (JCAHO), which may serve a quasi-governmental function, and state or federal agencies such as state departments of insurance or the federal Health Care Financing Administration (HCFA).

involved in the relevant aspect of service delivery to monitor and implement their own quality improvement activities.

Current multifaceted quality management programs, commonly supported by sophisticated management information systems, employ a wide range of analytic techniques to assess aspects of quality and track efforts to improve. These information systems generate concurrent data reflecting many aspects of the service delivery system from, for example, timeliness of referral, to goal achievement, to appropriate use of specific interventions. These management information systems provide the information necessary for day-to-day or week-to-week management of critical aspects of the system. Hence, rather than attempt to "assure" quality, modern accountable systems attempt to manage quality and manage it continuously as a nonnegotiable component of service planning and delivery.

Easy access to a range of system management data gives the MCO or provider organization the capacity to implement two types of activities that appear to have significant potential for improving quality. The first is provider profiling, typically a multivariate analytic process for evaluating providers on a range of quality and performance indicators and giving those providers feedback on their performance that may be used as a basis for behavior change or skills enhancement. The second is the implementation of empirically derived practice guidelines that constitute "benchmarks" for practitioner behaviors. Given the availability of the relevant data on practice patterns for specific diagnoses, the MCO can monitor its providers' performance against the benchmarks defined by the guidelines.

WHAT FOLLOWS IN THIS VOLUME

Throughout the chapters that follow, the reader is presented with discussions of philosophical issues related to the new methods of services organization, financing, and delivery. Just as these systems have shown promise for increasing accountability to stakeholders and improving quality, so too have they demonstrated a potential for sacrificing quality in the interest of cost. In Chapter 2, Sharfstein and Stoline offer a particularly compelling discussion of the competing stakeholder interests that create tension among behavioral health providers, consumers, and purchasers in the context of managed care. By their nature, farreaching innovations such as those reshaping health services in the United States require careful evaluation and modification. It is over the coming 5–10 years that the systems that have grown so rapidly will truly be tested and the delicate balance between cost and quality will, it is hoped, be achieved.

Selections in Parts II and III describe some of the new technologies, or tools, being applied to the management of service delivery systems. Particular emphasis is given to two topics: (1) outcomes as indicators of quality, and (2) the use of practice guidelines, both to educate providers about appropriate services and to raise the overall quality of services by reducing variation in practice patterns. Both types of activities challenge two basic assumptions about the delivery of behavioral health services: That the process of care as well as its outcomes cannot be quantified or systematized, and that the therapeutic process is somehow diminished by the act of measurement or other scrutiny.

The chapters found in Part IV provide different perspectives on stakeholder involvement in defining professional practice and shaping systems of care. A critical aspect of the process through which systems will change and improve is informed and reasoned discussion aimed at balancing the values and needs of all relevant stakeholder groups. Many of the changes still to occur in health care will be the result of pressures from stakeholders, including consumers and organizations representing consumerist views (e.g., NCQA); federal and state authorities that (often responding to stakeholder lobbying) promulgate regulations affecting the structure and activities of MCOs and provider organizations as well as the scope and parameters of professional practice; and professional associations and related credentialing organizations that in their own ways shape professional behaviors and attitudes. It is these entities as much as the "marketplace" that will create service systems that themselves are accountable for outcomes of the services they provide.

The contents of this volume, taken as a whole, bear witness to the chaotic environment that is the health care system in the United States. Unresolved issues ranging from the large and complex (i.e., the appropriate role of regulation in health care and the interrelationships among regulatory, credentialing, and certifying entities) to the more specific but not necessarily less vexing (i.e., the appropriate role of practice guidelines in service delivery). This chaos is reflected in the starkly contrasting points of view offered even among the relatively small group of professionals constituting the authors' pool of this volume. It is not unusual for professionals involved in health services to express frustration or even despair about the changes that are occurring and the stresses that these changes bring to consumers, providers, and payers alike. A different perspective suggests that these same stakeholders now have an opportunity to actually shape a health system that will replace the one that evolved in such a haphazard fashion over the prior decades. If there is one dynamic that most characterizes views of health care in the 1990s, it is the stark contrast between those who view the current environment as disastrous and those who view it as providing an opportunity to develop a health system that effectively balances the need to make efficient use of resources with the imperative to improve quality of services.

REFERENCES

Brook, R. H., McGlynn, E. A., & Cleary, P. D. (1996). Quality of health care. Part 2: Measuring quality of care. *New England Journal of Medicine, 335*(13), 966–970.

Shueman, S. A., Troy, W. G., & Mayhugh, S. L. (1994). *Managed behavioral health care: An industry perspective.* Springfield, IL: Charles C. Thomas.

Wells, K., & Brook, R. (1988). Historical trends in quality assurance for mental health services. In G. Stricker & A. Rodriguez (Eds.), *Quality assurance in mental health* (pp. 39–63). New York: Plenum Press.

2

Challenges to the Preservation of Quality in Cost-Contained Behavioral Health Systems

STEVEN S. SHARFSTEIN AND ANNE M. STOLINE

INTRODUCTION

After three decades during which health care costs rose faster than the rate of general inflation, employers and insurance companies implemented dramatic, sometimes seemingly draconian, measures to bring health care costs under control. As a result of these interventions by payers, many clinical changes have swept through medicine (including behavioral health services), catalyzed by a reorganization of the financial and administrative underpinnings of the entire health care industry. As a result of these fundamental changes, health care professionals today face unprecedented challenges to the provision of high-quality care. These challenges are explored in this chapter.

Although a focus on quality of care is not new, what is unprecedented today is the aggressiveness of market-based, managed-care-directed efforts to reduce the use of hospital beds (i.e., inpatient acute care) and medical specialists. Cost is now the number one priority in the delivery of health care. Those systems or services that limit utilization and cost and provide acceptable quality will survive and prosper. Some of the cost-driven changes are subtle, with an impact on clinicians and patients that may be steadily eroding expectations of quality. The numbers of independent hospitals, group practices, and solo practitioners shrink as more health care providers join networks of care or are purchased by larger organizations. The independence of decision making that traditionally accompanied independent ownership and management has been replaced or significantly influenced by corporate policy making, not only administrative, but also clinical. Patients, formerly able to move freely among practitioners, now frequently are locked in by contract to particular care providers who are members of a health maintenance organization (HMO), a network, or other limited group.

Yet not all the challenges to provider quality of care are new. In fact, any health care delivery system contains one or another of the inherent challenges to the provi-

---

STEVEN S. SHARFSTEIN • Sheppard Pratt Health System, Baltimore, Maryland 21204, and Department of Psychiatry, University of Maryland, Baltimore, Maryland 21201. ANNE M. STOLINE • Women's Psychiatry Unit, Mercy Medical Center, Baltimore, Maryland 21202.

Handbook of Quality Management in Behavioral Health, edited by Stricker *et al.* Kluwer Academic / Plenum Publishers, New York, 2000.

sion of high-quality care. This chapter also surveys those "old" challenges to the provision of quality in services in order to provide a balanced presentation of a topic that is often the subject of heated discussion among those who look with nostalgia on the "good old days."

Until recently, little attention had been paid by health care professionals to measuring the quality of care. Thus, the current era, for all its challenges, also brings with it an opportunity for medical and other behavioral health practitioners to assess and subsequently improve their standards of care. This chapter provides an overview of questions to be asked as we begin to consider the quality of outcomes in behavioral health care.

THE "GOOD OLD DAYS"

Before exploring recent threats to quality in medical care, it is important to establish the fact that the focus on quality is itself a fairly recent phenomenon in health care. This could lead to the conclusion that quality was never studied because quality was never an issue; an incorrect conclusion indeed. In fact, the recent focus on quality highlights the historical neglect of the outcomes of medical care.

In the good old days before the health care cost crisis and development of modern cost containment interventions, physicians practiced with essentially complete autonomy. Once a new test or technology was developed and determined to be "safe," clinicians tended to incorporate it into practice indiscriminately, with few concerns about evaluating its effectiveness or efficiency.

Physicians were rewarded financially for their incremental use of tests and procedures through the fee-for-service insurance system, which reimbursed them unquestioningly for care provided. These "more-is-better" incentives prevailed in the health care system from the earliest days of medical insurance until the era of managed care.

The fee-for-service financial incentives conformed to the physician's own need for certainty. Facing diagnostic or management uncertainty, the clinician was free to order more tests or additional treatments to minimize that uncertainty. There was little need for patient or clinician to tolerate lack of certainty, and this fact fueled the expectation in the mind of the typical patient that the "best" care was owed to him or her, regardless of cost. With few data as to efficacy of many tests and treatments, patients also tended to expect good outcomes as the result of almost any intervention. (This also lowered their threshold for litigation when treatment failures inevitably occurred.) Thus, in addition to receiving financial gain, physicians were supported in this practice of providing as many diagnostic and treatment opportunities as possible by patients' expectations as well as by a reduced risk of malpractice litigation.

This approach to medical care, occurring within an open-ended financing system, no doubt contributed significantly to cost inflation. It is misleading, however, to conclude that health cost inflation was the only negative consequence of this approach to services financing. For example, it cannot be assumed that more is better with regard to quality of care. Many tests and treatments are associated with significant morbidity or mortality. Consequently, their addition to the treatment regimen worsens the potential outcome for the patient. Thus, a closer look at the good old days suggests that they were not, in fact, so good at all. Clinicians had autonomy and unlimited decision-making authority, but not all patients benefitted as much as they might have from the health care system.

Therefore, while we mourn the loss of autonomy and Aesclapion authority possessed by the medical profession in the good old days, we also should look with open minds at the current situation in health services management and financing. It may contain important kernels of truth about potentially *better* ways of practicing medicine.*

A NEW VOCABULARY OF HEALTH CARE

How do we talk about the recent changes in the health care system? Buyer and seller, producer and consumer are terms from economics that have become integral to the vocabulary of the health care industry today. They do not begin to describe the experience of clinical medicine for either patient or physician. Do we need to translate the unique, intimate, caring, and at times life-saving service known as medical care into market economic terms, and if so, how do we do it?

Of course, provision of medical care is more than an exchange of goods and services. Yet we rely on economic terms and concepts to capture most clearly the effects of cost control and services management so as to explore fully the impact of these strategies on the quality of care. Paradoxically, in order to design health care delivery systems that are most proficient at providing high-quality and caring services, we must consider those systems using stark market-based terms.

Resistance by health professionals to even a temporary shift in their assumptions about health care, possibly reflecting an unwillingness to consider the need for change, for many years has hindered rational discussion of these crucial issues. In today's rapidly changing health care marketplace, however, this failure to participate on the part of a significant proportion of clinicians itself becomes a threat to service quality. If health professionals themselves do not work for change and thereby help shape future systems, those systems that do get created may be insufficiently sensitive to the legitimate needs of patients and professionals.

COST CONTAINMENT STRATEGIES IN MANAGED CARE

Cost-contained behavioral health systems use what have come to be known as "managed care" techniques to control utilization and cost. But what is managed care? It is defined by the American Medical Association (AMA) as "systems or techniques that are used to affect access to and control payment for health care services" (1994, p. 1). In fact, a wide range of review methods and service delivery and financing models designed to control health care costs by controlling utilization of health care resources fall under the rubric of managed care. Most broadly defined, any intervention intended to control health care costs could be a component of managed care.

Another phrase commonly used is managed care organization (MCO). This could refer to an insurance company that uses managed care techniques, to an independent

*For an expanded discussion of this issue, see Stoline et al. (1993), pp. 137–198.

organization contracted by an employer or insurance company to managed the health services resource use, to an HMO, or to other entities involved in managing the delivery or financing of health services. Clearly, it is difficult to construct a precise definition of managed care, and as a consequence such entities are difficult to regulate. This imprecision then is itself a threat to quality.

This chapter narrows the scope of consideration, classifying managed care interventions by their targeted population or their outcome. The chapter focuses first on two general categories of managed care interventions: (1) those that target patients, and (2) those that target clinicians or clinical decision making. The subsequent section focuses specifically on the kinds of effects that managed care interventions have on health care delivery systems. The interventions discussed are employed very commonly in the current health care environment, although clearly their threats to quality vary in scope and severity. These distinctions are made where appropriate.

Managed Care Interventions Intended to Influence the Patient

Each of us on occasion has developed physical and psychological symptoms that cause us to consider seeking medical care. If we are covered by a health insurance plan, the insurer (or payer, in the case of a self-insured company benefit plan) saves money to the extent that we do not use our benefits to pay for our health care. Insurers, therefore, attempt to raise the threshold at which enrollees seek to become "patients" by using their health care benefits.* Strategies aimed at doing this constituted some of the earliest attempts to control costs, in some cases dating back to the 1970s. Most are still in use today.

Defining Limited Benefits

Defining a limited benefit is one of the simplest cost control methods aimed at patients. If the insurer does not offer coverage for a particular service, then of course it does not have to pay for that service. Psychiatric benefits have been particularly vulnerable to this strategy, given the stigma associated with seeking mental health care and the ambiguity surrounding both the definition of psychiatric problems and their appropriate treatments (Sharfstein, Muszynski, & Myers, 1984).

Long-term psychotherapy is one of the most obvious casualties of this strategy, as the number of annual therapy sessions allowed in the typical benefit plan is 20 or fewer sessions (Scheidemandel, 1993). Enrollees who intend to use more visits may shop for another policy or pay for additional treatment out of pocket. Enrollees who develop a need for care likely enter treatment with a short-term mind set, that is, "I'm covered for 20 sessions so that must be enough," and this may or may not be an appropriate expectation given the particular problem requiring treatment.

For those who could benefit from additional care, affordability becomes the deciding factor, and many patients will do without care or consider themselves treated if the alternative is to pay for their own care. Typically, it becomes the clinician's responsibility to complete care within the benefit limits. As a consequence, a patient who remains in distress at the end of treatment may be more likely to perceive fail-

*Systems that care for the uninsured indigent tend to establish a high threshold for seeking care through different methods, for example, long waiting times to receive care.

ure as the fault of the clinician than to blame the insurer or to attribute it to an inadequate benefit plan.

Higher Patient Costs

Higher copayments or deductibles are a second, straightforward cost control measure. Greater cost-sharing responsibility is intended to deter the enrollee from seeking care. For some, the discretionary decision not to seek care does not threaten health or functioning, while for others it poses a clear threat to their ability to function effectively in their everyday lives. For symptoms that to the enrollee clearly indicate necessity for care, he or she will contribute a higher percentage of the payment for services to treat those symptoms. Studies have shown that increasing patient cost sharing does reduce the amount of care that enrollees seek (Wells et al., 1982).

As a result of higher copayments, patients will tend to present for care with more serious complaints. The quality of care (in this case, outcome) may be compromised to the extent that irreparable damage has already occurred at the time of presentation (e.g., a stroke in the case of untreated hypertension or an acetaminophen overdose with hepatic impairment in the case of untreated depression). Ironically, under such circumstances a treatment course may be more costly, because the patient is sicker when care is initiated.

Reducing Patient Choice of Clinician

A more recent managed care strategy that targets enrollee choice about care is reduced choice of clinician. Through mental health carve-out organizations and other systems that use designated provider networks, enrollees are increasingly limited in their choice of clinician. Such policies may disrupt long-standing patient–clinician relationships or they may prevent enrollees from seeking appropriate specialty care as a result of requirements to obtain referral to specialists through primary care physicians or MCO staff (sometimes nonclinicians providing standardized telephone "triage"). The threats to quality here are obvious.

Many enrollees have opposed these policies. In response, some insurers recently have initiated "opt-out" or "point-of-service" plans, through which the enrollee may seek care from an out-of-network clinician at the time of service. Under such a model the enrollee pays a higher premium and copayment.

These cost control interventions generally are transparent to an enrollee, as such policies are spelled out in handbooks (variously referred to as evidence of coverage, explanation of benefit, etc.) provided to all beneficiaries. Providing such explanations does not necessarily preclude threats to quality of care, however, since an enrollee may not understand a particular policy or may not anticipate the implications of a particular policy for his or her own health care needs. Threats to quality of care include an inadequate benefit, deterrence from seeking care for specific impairments, disruption of long-standing relationships with trusted clinicians, and exclusion of appropriate clinicians from caring for enrollees.

As stated, these are some of the oldest cost control interventions and they have tended to grow sharper teeth over time. Yet, they are not very effective cost control methods. Policymakers have realized that once the enrollee makes the first decision to seek care, it is the clinician rather than the patient who makes most of the decisions about health care resource use. While these policies remain in place, insurers have learned that to be maximally effective in ratcheting down costs, they must use their strongest interventions in system design: those aimed at influencing and controlling clinician behavior. Such measures are described below.

Interventions that Influence Clinicians

Once a person decides to seek medical care for a particular problem, and thus assumes the role of patient, he or she relies heavily on a clinician's advice. Additional tests or treatments are ordered by clinicians as a result of the knowledge differential between the patient and the professional. Thus, apart from the costs of initial visits (which are generated by enrollees' decisions), clinicians generate virtually all additional health care costs.* Measures that influence clinical decision making, therefore, have tremendous cost saving potential.

The degree of reliance on the "supplier," combined with the importance of the "product" of medical care, distinguish medicine from other economies.† Patient trust is crucial to successful provision of medical care. The physician's responsibility to attend to and work in the best interest of the patient is the essence of this special relationship. Indeed, noted ethicist and physician Edmund Pellegrino stated that medicine, at heart, is a moral enterprise. Yet this ethical core, the moral heart of medicine, has not been spared in the era of managed cost control.

When a payer's focus is cost-based rather than care-based, a fundamental tension is created between the goals of payers and the goals of clinicians, and managed care might be more accurately termed "managed costs." Yet the struggle usually is not framed so openly. Instead, managed care entities have evolved strategies to influence clinical decision making, some of which have theoretical medical justification, but which are fundamentally aimed at reducing costs.

As a result of managed care measures, the extent of payers' control over clinical decisions is unprecedented. From an insurance system in which clinicians had essentially complete autonomy "at the bedside" (with retrospective reimbursement), a system has evolved in which clinical autonomy may be dissected from clinical responsibility. Cost control interventions that target clinicians in their role as decision makers about resource use pose some of the most serious threats to quality of care and the ethical practice of medicine. Several examples from the mental health sector demonstrate these strategies and their possible consequences.

Behavioral health care is often "carved-out" for management separate from physical medicine. These carve-outs tend to manage behavioral health services more tightly than they would be managed within a comprehensive medical benefit program, and they usually have stricter criteria for defining necessity and appropriateness of services. This tighter management is made possible by the more subjective nature of many psychiatric complaints (as compared to physical problems) and the consequent greater uncertainty about their appropriate treatment. Without availability of diagnostic tools other than observation and interview, the psychiatrist may often

*This is a simplification, of course. Common exceptions include emergency room visits initiated by ambulance drivers and patients who solicit tests and treatments for which they pay out of pocket (which need physician approval but are not physician initiated).

†Note that the patient is not referred to as the buyer, since insurance coverage complicates the patient's financial incentives in a medical "transaction."

find it difficult to demonstrate, in an objective manner, the presence of a specific diagnosable mental illness. Further, the stigma associated with psychiatric care often prevents patients and their families from engaging in lobbying to affect health policy; it also causes behavioral health services to be vulnerable to stringent cost containment measures.

Preauthorization

Preauthorization, a process whereby a determination of "medical necessity" is made, is the rule in virtually all managed plans. Most insurance and managed care organizations have developed their own unique set of requirements for defining the types of problems and levels of severity necessary to justify use of the benefit. Clinicians are asked to justify their use of financial resources through adherence to these rules. Unfortunately, clinicians are often not privy to the rules, which may differ significantly from company to company.

Most companies use practice guidelines or other criteria to determine necessity for treatment and appropriateness of the treatment type being recommended by the provider. But without generally agreed-upon standards of "quality," some of these protocols may provide for an inferior level of care. Furthermore, if patients are outliers, either in terms of severity of symptoms or dysfunction, comorbidity, or some other complication, the protocols or guidelines may be inadequate to account for such contingencies. Behavioral health care needs to be tailored to patient characteristics and conditions to a much greater extent that much of general medical care (consider, for example, criteria for appendectomy or treatment of pneumonia). Psychiatric patients may not fit narrowly defined criteria or protocols. For example, one managed care company denied inpatient admission to a suicidal patient because he owned a gun but had not made a specific threat to commit suicide. While the clinician's "intuition" (developed over many years of experience) may signal to that clinician a clear danger, the only choice under a managed care system may be to provide care without reimbursement. This type of situation is too common under managed care, where rigid policy may override clinical opinion.

Suicide is the most adverse event that can happen in psychiatry. Psychiatric patients commit suicide at a rate between five and ten times that of the general population. Yet suicide remains a rare event. Of 100 suicidal patients, that is, patients with suicidal ideation, perhaps only five to ten will actually attempt to kill themselves, and of those, one in eight may succeed. Clinicians who are responsible for the care of patients will err on the side of safety and will most likely want to hospitalize or keep hospitalized any patient with suicidal ideation. MCOs, however, noting the rarity of the event, may attempt to cut costs by relying on the low probability of a patient actually attempting suicide, noting that most patients will not act on their suicidal ideation. Since it is difficult if not impossible to predict a successful suicide, the clinical uncertainty gives the MCO the discretion of intervening to contain costs by denying high-cost hospitalizations to these patients.

Requests to Share Confidential Information

Managed care organizations challenge clinicians for ever more detailed descriptions of patients' distress, sometimes requiring very personal disclosures to demonstrate clinical need. The consequent erosion of confidentiality undermines the trust so necessary in a therapeutic relationship, and the quality of care must suffer in the process.

Pressure to Use Lower Levels of Care

The acute psychiatric hospital is the most expensive treatment setting, and its use has dropped precipitously in recent years as a result of tight management of this level of care. In general, a patient must be actively suicidal or homicidal to qualify for use of the inpatient benefit, and payment for additional services in such a setting is denied once these feelings have subsided. As a consequence, a patient may experience "revolving door" hospitalizations as he or she undergoes a series of inpatient crisis stabilization stays, followed by rapid decompensation in a lower level of care and readmission to acute care. Many clinicians, while agreeing that hospitalization was overused in the past, believe also that managed care companies, to too great an extent, make decisions about hospitalization on the basis of cost rather than clinical necessity. This poses a serious threat to quality of care.

Insurers have instituted "flexible" benefit plans that use formulae allowing substitution of services, for example, 2 days of partial hospitalization for 1 day of inpatient care. Often the enrollee is unaware that clinical decisions are restricted by this "Chinese menu" approach to treatment planning. Under such a plan, the responsibility falls to the clinician to structure treatment within limits imposed by the benefit. If suboptimal, this poses a threat to quality.

Bias against Longer-Term Psychotherapy

Psychotherapy, one of the main behavioral health services, has been significantly affected by managed care. As rather cynically described by one discouraged therapist,

> In the short run the cheapest way to provide psychotherapy is not to provide it. This solution is appealing to executives of insurance companies and HMOs.... But openly admitting that you do not provide psychotherapy interferes with sales and enrollments in HMOs, and the salesmen do not like it. Managed care is the next best fiscal alternative. The aim is to provide as little care as possible, without admitting that you are not providing adequate mental health care. (Karon, 1992, p. 55)

Inordinate skepticism by managed care companies has been used as justification to curtail the use of "long-term" psychotherapy (e.g., more than 20 sessions). By asserting that this type of treatment is ineffective or that it is the province of the "worried well," payers have justified denial of extended therapy benefits even if ostensibly included in enrollees' benefit plan. Furthermore, psychiatrists frequently find that they are not authorized to provide any psychotherapy. They are told, rather, that such services can be provided more economically by psychologists, social workers, and other masters-prepared therapists. Yet even the nonpsychiatrist increasingly finds that the type of psychotherapy approved for reimbursement by managed care entities is limited to short-term crisis intervention.

Bias toward Use of Medications

MCOs may reward clinicians who favor medication prescription over psychotherapy by giving them preference in patient referrals. As Pollock (1995) notes, patients and clinicians alike are dismayed by insurers' new emphasis on medications over therapy. Psychopharmacological treatment can be provided in fewer visits over a shorter period of time than verbal therapy. This treatment is less expensive and more efficient, and certainly is helpful for many patients. Often, however, psychotherapy is also indicated for a particular patient or a particular problem, either alone or in combination with medications. Quality care cannot be provided under a system that by policy precludes a determination of appropriateness based on clinical need of the individual patient. Each case is unique and requires a clinician who coordinates and provides care and has as his or her primary concern the best interest of the patient.

By providing invitations to corporate "educational" offerings or administrative meetings, MCOs suggest to providers that they are integral to the organization's success. Over time, many clinicians learn that changes to their typical clinical or administrative practices as requested by the MCO are necessary in order to maintain their place on networks and panels. Often there is no direct pressure for this type of conformity. Rather, subtle suggestion is sufficient to effect change. The clinician knows the consequences of declining such participation, including loss of patient referral volume, potential loss of established relationships with patients whose health benefits have become managed, and replacement on the network by more "managed-care-friendly" providers. The conflict inherent in adapting to MCO systems, including being asked to practice in ways that differ significantly from those learned in training, may cause substantial demoralization and a fear of hypocrisy, the "selling out" of one's personal and professional values.

This trend affects specialties other than behavioral health. For example, physicians have been alarmed by the corporate shift to relatively low-cost providers, for example, those with less education or less experience. Recognizing the potential cost savings, payers have embraced a move toward primary care medicine, reflected in a recent increase in medical school graduates seeking training in primary care and family medicine. Under a model where primary care physicians act as gatekeepers to specialist care, appropriate care may be withheld from patients. This trend has had a particularly significant impact on the practices of clinicians affiliated with academic medical centers.

A crisis intervention philosophy dominates the managed mental health sector. HMOs and other cost-contained systems have tended to take a short-term approach to service; the philosophy promised by the "health maintenance" moniker has not been translated into care provision (Wright, 1992).* Although refusing to cover long-term therapy may be considered analogous to treating a stroke rather than the hypertension that caused it, companies have found it cheaper not to cover services such as longer-term treatment. This short-term perspective is evident not only with HMOs, but also with insurance companies and payers such as government agencies and employers. The short-term profits have made such strategies attractive. The costs in terms of negative health effects are unknown and such effects would be tremendously difficult to identify or track. But while it has not to date been possible to identify adverse health consequences in enrollee pools whose benefit coverage has a short-term orientation, the threats to quality posed by withholding care to benefit the bottom line seem obvious.

A variety of other strategies are used to influence clinical decisions (i.e., effect

*Wright (1992) provides a number of specific examples of HMO administrative policies that create disincentives for clinicians to provide therapy and for patients to receive it.

denial of reimbursement for services). Therapists may receive approval for additional sessions in increments such as three or five sessions, effectively curtailing any long-term planning in their work with patients. They may be told that a patient's condition is chronic (e.g., a borderline personality disorder), and hence, that treatment is not covered under the benefit plan. Treatment denials may be made by clinicians employed by the MCO who have less education or experience than the professional providing the services. Appeals of denials are costly in terms of time and money lost.

Managed care organizations may not need to deny payment for care directly. Clinicians know that companies are monitoring their practice patterns, and that ongoing enrollment in managed care panels or even hospital privileges depends on cost-efficiency. Therapists who routinely proffer treatment plans for long-term psychotherapy may find themselves removed from provider panels or networks. Disincentives may be created to treat patients with complicated psychopathology or comorbid conditions, as a significant number of such patients may result in "bad" statistics in the clinician's profile (Lazarus, 1994) if the managed care company does not use risk adjustment in its profiling. The incentive may be to transfer such outlier patients quickly; treating difficult patients like "hot potatoes" is a threat to quality care.

Use of Networks

In the private sector, creation of a network or panel of hospitals, group practices, or individual clinicians was a relatively early managed care intervention. Such a use of networks can enhance quality of care through creation of a care-driven system of service delivery. In theory, a well-organized network could provide for coordination of care for the enrollee population through designation of particular facilities as specialty providers of a range of services. It could increase coherence in the nonsystem of primary through tertiary services that today are used by patients in a fairly random fashion. Neither network nor panel use, however, has reached this level of sophistication. Achievement of this level is potentially expensive in terms of both development and maintenance of the network. Instead, MCOs usually use networks in a fairly simplistic manner, to control referral to particular clinicians and facilities to save costs.

Managed care organizations may use financial incentives to influence clinical decisions. Through network contracts, today's providers agree to contractual arrangements specified by the payer. Such contracts contain financial and clinical parameters consistent with the corporate philosophy and objectives. Providers may be asked to agree to "gag rules," that is, contract provisions forbidding them to communicate differences in opinion on corporate policies that "could undermine the confidence of enrollees, potential enrollees, their employers, their unions, or the public" (Woolhandler & Himmelstein, 1995, p. 1707). "Efficient" clinicians whose average inpatient lengths of stay are short or who demonstrate a small mean number of outpatient psychotherapy visits may be considered desirable for membership on networks or panels. Some clinicians, however, are hospital employees who find that agreements about issues such as target lengths of stay are made for them by financial administrators. As a result, they may be pressured to make treatment decisions based more on financial considerations over which they have no control than on clinical considerations.

Clinicians experienced in providing long-term therapy find their patient pools shrinking as managed care organizations divert patients to more "efficient" providers or refuse to authorize extended treatment plans. When applying for membership on panels or networks such clinicians may be told that they are closed.*

Financing Arrangements

To maintain patient volume, many clinicians accept reduced fee-for-service payments. More controversial payment arrangements create "less-is-more" provider incentives in which providers may agree to limit their use of diagnostic or treatment services or may receive bonuses for such practice. Clinicians may be paid by capitation, through financial withholds until year's end (to be paid out if the clinician's or group's ordering profile permits profit), or through other arrangements.

Certain reimbursement practices used for hospital care may also provide less-is-more incentives. Although an oversimplified description, the Medicare prospective payment or diagnosis-related grouping (DRG) system essentially pays hospitals a fixed fee to treat a patient with a given diagnosis. The hospital benefits to the extent that fewer resources are used in the patient's care. For such a system to be feasible, hospitals must create incentives for their clinicians to practice in ways that are consistent with this financial arrangement.

Is the more-is-better incentive created by fee-for-service insurance reimbursement as potentially harmful to patients as the less-is-better incentive? In recent years, some of the most egregious financing arrangements have been affected by regulation or prohibited by law. At the same time, however, whatever the financial arrangements, patients rely on physicians to look out for their best interests. While assuming that clinicians continue to hold their moral responsibility above the profit motive, regulators must remain vigilant in identifying those clinicians straying from these principles.

A final risk of the growing influence of managed care on direct clinical decision making is that it is largely opaque to patients, again due to the knowledge differential between the patient and the clinician. As a result, patients may believe that they have purchased health coverage that entitles them to a specified set of benefits, but if the benefit plan is managed, there is no guarantee that services will be received even if a clinician believes them to be necessary. Patients are at risk for becoming pawns in a system in which they have always been passive but have trusted clinicians to do what is in their best interest. Some cost control interventions place this relationship at risk, and their hidden nature poses an additional threat to the quality of care.†

This brief overview of managed care interventions that target clinical decision making highlights the most serious threats that behavioral health providers perceive from managed care. Clinicians feel that their judgment has been inappropriately challenged in the name of cost containment and corporate profit and that their relationships with their patients have been threatened. Apart from the "hassle factor," which has essentially become part of the time and emotional cost of doing business, clinicians fear that quality medicine is in a downward slide and do not know what will stop it. Many feel powerless to reverse the tide. What needs to be said about the threats to quality associated with managed care's intrusion into the consulting room?

*Complaints about this type of restraint on practice has led to national calls for "any willing provider" legislation.

†There are many potential reasons for patient ignorance of this type of cost control, including a paternalistic or maternalistic clinician style, clinician discomfort with disclosing the impact of the patient's particular payer on clinical decisions, and outright administrative fiat against such disclosure.

EFFECTS ON HEALTH CARE DELIVERY SYSTEMS

This final broad category includes modifications to health care delivery systems resulting from managed care that both directly and indirectly affect clinical practice.

Until the "cost crisis" and cost control efforts began in the 1970s, the US health care system embodied an effort to enrich, expand, and improve the health care resources available and offered to patients. In sharp contrast, most of the changes described below represent attempts to eliminate "fat" from the health care system by reducing resources perceived as expendable in the delivery of care. The primary objective of many of these changes is to reduce the number of hospital beds and specialists that are perceived as excessive and therefore related to unnecessary higher costs. The changes vary in the severity of their threats to quality of care, particularly since some of the changes are easily visible to clinicians, enrollees, and patients, while others are quite subtle, such that participants may not realize their impact on access to care and utilization. The evolution in health care delivery tends to affect all enrollees equally, although, of course, some are able to use their own funds to afford additional services or to circumvent the benefit system altogether (e.g., wealthy psychotherapy patients paying for care entirely out of pocket). In the view of many clinicians, however, the most destructive aspect of this type of evolution is its gradual eroding nature, which over time lowers everyone's expectations regarding medical care (similar to the acceptance of unsafe streets and inferior education). These resource-reducing decisions are often made by payers over strong objections of clinicians, and they are a significant source of demoralization among clinicians.

It is argued that the costs of administrative overhead and profit margins of managed care companies are excessive and that such costs are covered by limiting patient care. While such arguments are well publicized in the media, most enrollees probably do not appreciate the connection between high corporate salaries and the strict rules affecting their access to and use of medical resources. High profits and a strong stock market showing may be good business, but it is obvious that these factors are not necessarily associated with good quality medicine.

In public sector programs budget appropriations have been used to control costs. Inflation in the health care sector has for years exceeded inflation in the general economy. Therefore, if budgets increase each year by less than the rate of inflation, their purchasing power is reduced (i.e., fewer services can be provided to patients). This is particularly worrisome in those states that have implemented cost-contained public health care systems. With a conservative Republican Congress and a nationwide trend in the direction of increased services management, this phenomenon becomes an increasing threat to quality of care in the public sector.

System Change Resulting from Implementation of Managed Care

Reductions in inpatient volume through diversion to outpatient programs, reduced lengths of stay, and lower reimbursement have led to compensatory measures by hospitals. One of the most notable is a reduction in the inpatient workforce. This shrinking of inpatient staffs (sometimes via "benchmarking") has reduced the therapeutic richness of the inpatient milieu. It has also intensified the stress experienced by the remaining inpatient staff, thereby heightening exposure to risk from a more severely ill and potentially dangerous patient population.

Disruptions in Continuity of Care

A second system effect is disruption in continuity of care. Through a variety of phenomena, including limited provider networks and panels, continually mutating managed care regulations and policies, and some corporate philosophies in which clinicians are interchangeable, today's patient has a much more difficult time establishing a consistent relationship with clinicians. To the extent that these disruptions discourage visits, they save corporate dollars. These disruptions, however, also impair trust, discourage aftercare compliance, and threaten treatment adequacy, particularly for psychiatric populations. In addition to these threats to quality of care, lack of continuity makes it less likely that a patient's history will be well-known to his or her provider.

Loss of Confidentiality

Managed care has severely undermined the traditional pattern of patient–clinician confidentiality. From telephonic reviews to written treatment plans, the breadth and depth of information requested about patients has steadily increased. As with other compromises required of providers to survive in today's systems, over time many clinicians have become inured to this aspect of care, resigned to the fact that without it authorization for care or its reimbursement may be jeopardized. Trade-offs are evident, however, including a reduction in patient's comfort with sharing personal information. Particularly within the psychotherapeutic process, the potential shallowness of communication between patient and provider reduces the potential for healing and consequently reduces the quality of care.

These are issues and questions of values. Has "fat" or "meat" been removed from the system? Is continuity important? What about an ongoing and consistent relationship with a clinician? How important is confidentiality? Have the concerns discussed here become old-fashioned in the context of today's health services marketplace? Today, the pendulum has swung from a focus on traditional clinical values to an emphasis on cost control. How far will the pendulum swing?

THREATS TO PROFESSIONAL EDUCATION

Medical education as well as the education of other allied health professionals is suffering as a result of managed care and other changes in health services financing. Academic medicine is at a disadvantage in today's cost-conscious marketplace. Many managed care companies do not reimburse for services provided by resident physicians. As a result, attending physicians must evaluate and treat patients early, often before residents have had a chance to do so. Short lengths of stay diminish opportunities to observe the course of treatment and recovery. Many companies also refuse to authorize resident physicians to provide outpatient treatment, and some even require 3 years of independent practice before a clinician is qualified for membership on their networks. These changes will more severely affect the quality of care as time goes on. The hands-on learning necessary in medicine as well as allied health services is different from classroom learning. Apprenticeship balanced with independent clinical experience is crucial to the quality of the education and therefore to the quality of care physicians provide. As a result of today's managed care regulations, physicians entering practice are likely to have less experience than their colleagues who received their degrees in the past. To the extent that their education is inadequate, quality of medical care is diminished now and in the future. Similar dynamics are effecting training of other behavioral health professionals.

Due to their higher costs related to training of health professionals, many academic medical centers find themselves unable to compete for entry into networks. While everyone would like access to a tertiary care specialist if necessary, the market seems unable to bear their higher cost. Over time, this is likely to result in a homogenization of medical care across facilities. To the extent that the best no longer reach their full potential, the quality of medical care is diminished now and in the future.

CHALLENGES FOR TODAY'S HEALTH CARE INDUSTRY

Outcomes are the products of medical care. In the absence of empirical evidence regarding efficacy, it is imperative that clinicians, academic medical centers, and the managed care industry join together to develop rigorous outcome studies so that decisions about reimbursement are not made solely on the basis of cost.

One of the best outcome studies ever conducted was the Rand Medical Outcomes Study, a large-scale effort to examine outcomes and the effect of health services financing (fee-for-service compared to prepaid) on outcomes (Wells, 1995; Rogers, Wells, Meredith, Sturm, & Burnam, 1993; Sturm & Wells, 1995). One finding of this study was that quality improvement measures that roughly follow practice guidelines for depression can improve outcomes, but only at increased treatment costs. Shifting patients away from mental health specialists decreases costs but worsens functional outcomes. The Rand study suggests that a combination of strategies can improve outcomes, lower treatment costs, and increase value in medical care, as long as substantial quality improvement activities are implemented in general medical practice.

A number of other studies suggest effective strategies for measuring outcome. For example, Thompson, Burns, Goldman, and Smith (1992) recommend several approaches to studying outcome, including: (1) collection of case-level in addition to system-level data; (2) use of standardized and validated instruments and rating systems; (3) implementation of procedures to ensure collection of clinically valid ratings and periodic assessment of interrater reliability; (4) monitoring of data collection by a clinician not directly involved in the study; and (5) use of multiple treatment outcome measures, including patients' clinical status, follow-up after discharge, and readmission rates.

Allgulander (1994) suggests evaluating care on the basis of appropriateness, equity, accessibility, effectiveness, acceptability, and efficiency. Examples of indicators of the effectiveness of psychiatric treatment include rates of noncompliance with treatment recommendations, adverse drug events, incidence of violent assaults, and use of restraints in treatment. Allgulander suggests patient and family education and satisfaction as other key outcome indicators.

A key challenge to the health delivery system therefore is to develop an outcome-driven approach with input and consensus from all critical stakeholders. For clinicians, the challenge is to keep the patient's best interest as the primary value, while accepting the principles that more is not always better and that cooperating with managed care organizations while providing high-quality care to patients is both possible and necessary. It is up to the clinician to maximize the benefit from available resources for the individual patient as well as for the community. The ultimate guardians of quality are clinicians who, by oath and ethics, must put their patients' needs first and their own economic interest second.

Until all stakeholders can agree on definitions of quality and work together to develop meaningful outcome studies, governmental oversight and regulation of the managed care industry will be required to ensure that cost containment does not compromise quality of care. The challenge to legislators is to write effective law and regulation that will adhere to the amorphous, ever-mutating conglomeration of systems and organizations that form the current health care environment. A reorganization of the health care industry into a universal system of care may be necessary in order to effect this change.

REFERENCES

Allgulander, C. (1994). Can quality care in psychiatry be purchased? *Nordisk Journal of Clinical Psychiatry, 48,* 167–172.

American Medical Association. Department of Medical Review. (1994). *Principles of managed care.* Chicago: Author.

Garnick, D. W., Hendricks, A. M., Dulski, J. D., Thorpe, K. E., & Horgan, C. (1994). Characteristics of private-sector managed care for mental health and substance abuse treatment. *Hospital and Community Psychiatry, 45*(12), 1201–1205.

Karon, B. P. (1992). Problems of psychotherapy under managed health care. *Psychotherapy in Private Practice, 11*(2), 55–63.

Lazarus, A. (1994). Dumping psychiatric patients in the managed care sector. *Hospital and Community Psychiatry, 45*(6), 529–530.

Mone, L. C. (1994). Managed care cost effectiveness: Fantasy or reality? *International Journal of Group Psychotherapy, 44*(4), 437–448.

Pollock, E. J. (1995). Managed care's focus on psychiatric drugs alarms many doctors. *The Wall Street Journal,* December 1, 1, A11.

Rogers, W. H., Wells, K. B., Meredith, L. S., Sturm, R., & Burnam, M. A. (1993). Outcomes for adult outpatients with depression under prepaid or fee-for-service financing. *Archives of General Psychiatry, 50,* 517–525.

Scheidemandel, P. (1993). *The coverage catalog* (3rd ed.). Washington, DC: American Psychiatric Press.

Sharfstein, S. S., Muszynski, S., & Myers, E. (1984). *Health insurance and psychiatric care: Update and appraisal.* Washington, DC: American Psychiatric Press.

Sturm, R., & Wells, K. B. (1995). How can care for depression become more cost-effective? *Journal of the American Medical Association, 273*(1), 51–58.

Stoline, A. M., Weiner, J. P., (1993). *The new medical marketplace: A physician's guide to the health care system* (2nd ed.). Baltimore: Johns Hopkins University Press.

Thompson, J. W., Burns, B. J., Goldman, H. H., & Smith, J. (1992). Initial level of care and clinical status in a managed mental health program. *Hospital and Community Psychiatry, 43*(6), 599–603.

Wells, K. B. (1982). *Cost sharing and the demand for ambulatory mental health services.* Santa Monica, CA: Rand Corporation.

Wells, K. B. (1995). Cost containment and mental health outcomes: Experiences from US studies. *British Journal of Psychiatry, 166*(Suppl. 27), 43–51.

Woolhandler, S., & Himmelstein, D. U. (1995). Extreme risk—The new corporate proposition for physicians. *New England Journal of Medicine, 333,* 1706–1708.

Wright, R. H. (1992). The cons of psychotherapy in managed health care. *Psychotherapy in Private Practice, 11*(2), 71–77.

II

TOOLS FOR QUALITY MANAGEMENT

3

Protecting the Consumer

Issues in the Development and Implementation of Practice Guidelines

JUDITH EMERSON AND GEORGE STRICKER

Quality assurance for mental health services has been around for many years primarily as a function of oversight agencies such as the Joint Commission on Accreditation of Healthcare Organizations (JCAHO). Quality assurance has been housed in semi-obscure offices within hospitals and clinics given the task of making sure their particular organization complies with various regulations. More recently, as managed health care has grown, there has been increasing interest in quality among purchasers, health care plan administrators, practitioners, and consumers. Purchasers want to know the value of what they are buying, plan administrators want to demonstrate quality services as well as cost containment, practitioners want to know that cost management does not interfere with the provision of appropriate and necessary treatment, and consumers are concerned about access to good quality care. New models of quality measurement and management are emerging in response to these varied interests.

One quality management tool endorsed by JCAHO and the National Committee for Quality Assurance (NCQA) consists of monitoring adherence to clinical practice guidelines (JCAHO, 1994; NCQA, 1994). Interest in practice guidelines was intensified by discovery of substantial geographic variation in medical care utilization related to differences in resource availability rather than severity of illness or clinical need (Wennberg, Freeman, & Culp, 1987). While similar studies have not been done for mental health, subjectivity in establishing medical necessity and an assortment of theoretical approaches to treatment suggest that mental health care may vary as much as medical care. Clinical practice guidelines are a mechanism for standardizing mental health services and understanding practice variability, a key concept in continuous quality improvement (Berwick, 1991). Practice guidelines are not intended to eliminate clinician autonomy or reduce the need for clinical judgment but to facilitate consistency of care. Application of practice guidelines to stabilize and standardize mental health care delivery is only possible, however, to the degree that well-accepted,

---

JUDITH EMERSON • Portland Veterans Administration Medical Center, Portland, Oregon 97207.
GEORGE STRICKER • The Derner Institute, Adelphi University, Garden City, New York 11530.

Handbook of Quality Management in Behavioral Health, edited by Stricker *et al.* Kluwer Academic / Plenum Publishers, New York, 2000.

empirically grounded guidelines are available. This chapter contains a review of practice guidelines for the evaluation and treatment of mental, emotional, and behavioral disorders and a discussion of related considerations.

IDENTIFYING PRACTICE GUIDELINES FOR MENTAL HEALTH

In 1994, the Office of the Assistant Secretary of Defense for Health Affairs requested that Science Applications International Corporation (SAIC) conduct a side-by-side comparison of existing practice guidelines for mental health.* The charge was to collect, review, and evaluate published guidelines from all sectors of the mental health care industry, including the published literature, professional organizations, federal and state agencies, and managed care companies.

Compiling a list of practice guidelines is not as straightforward a task as it might seem. Self-proclaimed guidelines for clinical practice range from small empirical studies and opinion papers to large, government-sponsored task force efforts. Hence, simply looking for "practice guideline" in the title is insufficient. Depending on the sponsoring organization, titles for guidelines may include any one or more of several adjectives (clinical, practice, therapeutic, treatment, best, improvement) combined with any one of several nouns (guidelines, parameters, protocols, pathways, standards, options, policies) (Browne, 1995). For example, the American Medical Association (AMA) has collected and disseminated information on what they call "practice parameters" (AMA, 1994a,b), whereas the American Psychiatric Association (APA) has released a series of "practice guidelines" (Migdail, Youngs, & Bengen-Seltzer, 1995), and the Substance Abuse and Mental Health Services Administration (SAMHSA) has issued "treatment improvement protocols."

Searching literature databases by keywords is another common approach to document identification. MEDLINE has a "practice guideline" document-type specification that appears useful at first glance. However, one listing of references with this specification yielded close to 1000 papers (Migdail et al., 1995). Some of these were simply prescriptions for treatment based on one or two authors' clinical opinions. Many others were research studies or secondary review papers that may have included brief treatment recommendations along with the primary research findings. The MEDLINE category appears to be overly inclusive.

Many documents have shaped clinical practice but are not generally thought of as practice guidelines. For years, textbooks have provided training for new clinicians with recommendations grounded in empirical studies. These books are the de facto practice guidelines for beginning practitioners but are not usually labeled as such. Professional organizations have historically published consensus papers to inform members of current practices, but not all of these documents are considered practice guidelines even though they influence practice patterns.

For the SAIC review it was decided that to qualify as a practice guideline a document had to describe assessment or treatment approaches for mental, emotional, or behavioral problems or conditions and it had to be endorsed by a recognizable organization; individually authored empirical studies, position papers, or review articles were not included. Guidelines were identified through a combination of

*This work was funded by the Office of the Assistant Secretary of Defense for Health Affairs, contract number MDA906-93-D-0003.

(1) literature database searches (MEDLINE, PsychINFO, CINAHL, and HEALTH), (2) telephone surveys of state mental health departments, and (3) surveys of the largest managed behavioral health care organizations (enrollments of 1,000,000 or more). Sixty-five documents were identified, reviewed, and compared in a report submitted to the government on November 30, 1994. The list of guidelines was updated between December 1994 and June 1995, as part of a subsequent task, resulting in 71 documents (references are listed at the end of the chapter). The following descriptions are drawn from review of the 71 practice guidelines for mental health. It should be noted that practice guidelines are continually being developed and revised to address emerging treatment innovations and research findings. The list of documents used in the SAIC review and the data reported in this chapter are only a snapshot of one point in time.

Guideline Sponsors

Guidelines produced by professional organizations have primarily been published in peer-reviewed journals and are easily identifiable and accessible. Federal documents generally come from the government printing office and are also fairly easy to find. Documents developed by state mental health departments and managed care companies are harder to access. Individuals contacted in the SAIC survey of state agencies and managed care companies were not always sure what practice guidelines were, even after an explanation was given. However, 28 states indicated having some type of guidelines, and 17 sent their materials. Of these, only three fit the working definition of practice guidelines. The remaining papers were either state statutes and regulations or department procedural manuals. Telephone requests made to managed care companies were also met with confusion and sometimes with guarded responses. Not everyone understood exactly what was being requested, and some stated that their information was proprietary. Twelve companies indicated that they had guidelines and eight agreed to send their materials. Five of the documents turned out to be utilization review criteria. Three responses yielded four documents that met the definition of practice guidelines.

The majority of practice guidelines were developed by professional organizations (72%). A smaller number (18%) were sponsored by federal agencies, and even fewer still were endorsed by either state mental health departments (4%) or managed care organizations (6%) (see Table 1).

Target Audiences

The intended guideline audience revealed something about the scope of the practice guideline documents (see Table 2). Most of the guidelines were written for psychiatrists by psychiatric professional organizations (41%). Additional guidelines were written for other physicians, such as pediatricians and primary care physicians (21%). Other professional groups also wrote guidelines directly to their memberships but in much smaller numbers, such as the APA (4%), the American Nurses Association (3%), and the National Association for Social Work (1%). Professional organizations understand the limits of their authority, and therefore produce documents tailored to the special skills and interests of their own memberships. Unfortunately, these documents do not always translate across professions. Federal agencies, state mental health departments, managed care organizations, and a few professional groups addressed their protocols to all mental health providers (30%). These documents assume that any

TABLE 1. Organizations Sponsoring Practice Guidelines for Mental Health

	Number of guidelines
Professional organizations	
American Psychiatric Association	20
Royal Australian and New Zealand College of Psychiatrists	10
American Academy of Child and Adolescent Psychiatry	4
American Academy of Pediatrics	3
American College of Physicians	3
American Psychological Association	3
American Nurses Association	2
American Association for Partial Hospitalization	1
American College of Obstetricians and Gynecologists	1
American Society of Addiction Medicine	1
International Society for the Study of Dissociation	1
Mental Health Foundation	1
National Association of Social Workers	1
Federal agencies	
Substance Abuse and Mental Health Services Administration	7
National Institutes of Health	4
Agency for Health Care Policy and Research	2
State mental health departments	
Arizona Department of Health Services	1
California Department of Mental Health	1
State of Oregon Health Division	1
Managed care organizations	
CIGNA Corporation	1
CMG HEALTH, Inc.	1
MCC Managed Behavioral Care, Inc.	1
United Healthcare Behavioral Services	1

clinician licensed for independent practice in mental health care could implement such guidelines similarly; an ambitious assumption.

GUIDELINE TOPICS

The practice guidelines reviewed were written to address specific topics that fall into three domains: (1) *Diagnostic and Statistical Manual of Mental Disorders,* 4th edition

TABLE 2. Intended Audiences for Practice Guidelines by Type of Sponsoring Organizations

	Professional organizations (n = 51)	Federal agencies (n = 13)	State mental health (n = 3)	Managed care (n = 4)	Total (N = 71)
Psychiatrists	28	1	0	0	29
All MH professionals	5	9	3	4	21
Physicians	12	3	0	0	15
Psychologists	3	0	0	0	3
Nurses	2	0	0	0	2
Social workers	1	0	0	0	1

TABLE 3. Topics Addressed in Practice Guidelines by Type of Sponsoring Organizations

	Professional organizations (n = 51)	Federal agencies (n = 13)	State mental health (n = 3)	Managed care (n = 4)	Total (N = 71)
Diagnoses					
Alcohol/drug abuse	7	7	0	0	14
Mood disorders	7	3	0	0	10
Anxiety disorders	4	1	0	0	5
Multiple disorders	1	0	1	3	5
Personality disorders	4	0	0	0	4
Disruptive behavior disorders	3	0	0	0	3
Eating disorders	3	0	0	0	3
Psychotic disorders	2	0	0	0	2
Dissociative disorder	1	0	0	0	1
Organic mental disorders	0	1	0	0	1
Somatoform disorders	1	0	0	0	1
Clinical methods					
Level of care placement	2	0	1	1	4
Psychopharmacology	3	0	1	0	4
Electroconvulsive therapy	2	1	0	0	3
HIV/AIDS	2	0	0	0	2
Ethnic/cultural issues	1	0	0	0	1
Psychological testing	1	0	0	0	1
Qualitative EEG	1	0	0	0	1
Seclusion and restraint	1	0	0	0	1
Tardive dyskinesia	1	0	0	0	1
Professional activities					
Nursing practice	2	0	0	0	2
Psychology practice	1	0	0	0	1
Social work practice	1	0	0	0	1

(DSM-IV) (APA, 1994a) diagnostic disorders (69%), (2) clinical methods (25%), and (3) professional activities (6%) (see Table 3). Substance-related disorders have been a primary interest of both professional organizations and the federal government. Mood disorders also have been the subject of a number of guidelines. Other diagnostic groups have received much less attention. The absence of practice guidelines for the treatment of schizophrenia in adults at the time the SAIC review was conducted was surprising, considering the amount of research available and the amount of public funding allocated to serve individuals with this disorder. The APA has since released a schizophrenia guideline. Australian psychiatrists devoted a significant amount of effort to personality disorders, primarily from a psychodynamic point of view, whereas none of the American organizations described treatment for these conditions. Other diagnoses, such as posttraumatic stress disorder (PTSD), did not appear at all. The Veterans Health Administration has since developed a PTSD guideline. One guideline, produced by the Center for Substance Abuse Treatment, targeted traditional dual diagnoses of substance abuse and mental disorders, but no other guidelines addressed combined diagnostic presentations, such as comorbid anxiety and depressive disorders or mood disorders in the presence of personality disorders.

The managed care guidelines attempted to cover multiple topics and provided mostly diagnostic-specific and level-of-care recommendations. Closer examination of these documents indicated that sections were actually "borrowed" from published guidelines written by professional organizations, sometimes without citation. These attempts to cover many diagnoses and to disseminate information from a number of practice guidelines to busy practitioners were admirable, but sometimes resulted in oversimplification.

Guidelines for specific clinical methods were primarily addressed by the American professional groups. This may reflect apprehension about high-risk interventions, such as electroconvulsive therapy (ECT) and the use of neuroleptics, in a litigious society. More likely they express unique concerns of each discipline, such as psychologists' interest in testing integrity and psychiatrists' attempts to reduce harm to patients. The four documents describing professional practice were the most general documents of those reviewed and focused primarily on definitions of particular professional roles. Many clinical concerns were not included in guidelines, such as appropriate documentation, treatment termination considerations, or how therapeutic change can be measured. The SAIC review revealed gaps in the overall map of practice guideline content. While the most frequent or risky conditions and interventions have been written about, many other practice elements with lower profiles have not.

Purposes of Practice Guidelines

Most of the documents reviewed were endorsed by nationally recognized professional organizations or government agencies with the stated purpose of practitioner education. For example, the APA, via the Steering Committee on Practice Guidelines, has published a number of guidelines targeting specific DSM-IV disorders. Their stated purpose is to assist psychiatrists in clinical decision making. The following statement of intent prefaces the 1994 bipolar disorder document:

> This report is not intended to be construed or to serve as a standard of medical care. Standards of medical care are determined on the basis of all clinical data available for an individual case and are subject to change as scientific knowledge and technology advance and patterns evolve. These parameters of practice must be considered guidelines only. Adherence to them will not ensure a successful outcome in every case, nor should they be construed as including all proper methods of care or excluding other acceptable methods of care aimed at the same results. The ultimate judgment regarding a particular clinical procedure or treatment plan must be made by the psychiatrist on the basis of the clinical data presented by the patient and the diagnostic and treatment options available in the particular clinical setting. (APA, 1994b, p. iv)

AMA and AHCPR offer similar introductions to their respective guideline documents. Each describes their unique strategies, based on thorough evaluation of scientific literature and expert clinical opinion, to assist practitioners in making decisions regarding diagnosis, prevention, and treatment. The Center for Substance Abuse Treatment (CSAT), a division of SAMHSA, also introduced its guideline series with their statement of purpose: To transfer knowledge from clinical, research, and administrative experts to alcohol and drug treatment providers across the United States in order to improve quality.

The themes that emerge from these various descriptions of intention are (1) that practice guidelines are recommendations offered to clinicians to direct practice, (2) that they are based on the best available scientific information and clinical judgment, and (3) that their primary purpose is education. None of the guideline sponsors suggest treatment or intervention mandates. They recommend that the information provided be used by clinicians in the context of the individual patient. This philosophical stance supports the autonomy of providers in making the final decision about treatment, even though guideline consultation is expected to be part of that decision-making process. AHCPR goes one step further and counsels that patients too become educated about best practices and participate in treatment decisions (AHCPR, 1993).

CHARACTERISTICS OF IDEAL PRACTICE GUIDELINES

SAIC was not only to identify practice guidelines but also to evaluate them. This required consideration of guideline characteristics and how they could be compared. Although endorsement by an authoritative organization often defines practice guidelines, such sponsorship does not necessarily ensure document veracity. The guidelines reviewed varied in scope and methodological development. Three guideline criteria sets were identified and utilized to evaluate the strengths and weaknesses of the practice guidelines.

A task force of the APA formed a template for developing and evaluating practice guidelines. The report states that "guidelines that will be developed according to this template should be based on careful, judicious, and systematic weighing of research *and* clinical expertise" (APA, Task Force on Psychological Intervention Guidelines, 1995, p. 1). In order to guide the reader who is considering research evidence, two axes (dimensions) were constructed. The first dimension was concerned with efficacy, or the demonstration through sound evidence gathered in scientifically controlled settings, of the effects of treatment. The second dimension was concerned with generalizability (effectiveness), or the ability of the evidence to be transportable to a clinical setting. The following criteria are offered as defining model practice guidelines, including efficacy (1), clinical utility (3, 4, 5) and methods of guideline construction (2, 6–11):

1. Empirical confirmation of interventions is necessary. The strength of empirical evidence is rated based on the following hierarchy and takes into consideration the quality of the supporting studies and the number of replications. (The first is the most stringent and provides the most confidence in treatment efficacy. Confidence lessens with each successive criteria.)
    a. Randomized controlled trials demonstrating that the recommended treatment is superior to nonspecific treatment effects (placebo).
    b. Randomized controlled trials demonstrating that the recommended treatment is superior to no-treatment conditions.
    c. Quantified clinical observations.
    d. Strongly positive clinical consensus.
    e. Mixed clinical consensus.
    f. Strongly negative clinical consensus.
    g. Contradictory evidence.
2. Clinical consensus should be interdisciplinary. Guideline development panels should also be interdisciplinary with input from providers who have broad experience and are free from conflicts of interest. Input should also come from consumers.

3. The degree of generalizability across patient, provider, and setting characteristics should be considered and the robustness of the intervention included.
4. Assessment of guideline implementation feasibility is needed, including the likelihood of patient acceptance of the treatment and availability of providers.
5. Analysis of the costs and benefits of both providing and withholding the intervention should be reported.
6. Methods for evaluating guideline efficacy across providers need to be specified.
7. The development process includes dissemination of the recommendations to concerned parties for review.
8. The goal, processes, and methods of the guideline development are reported.
9. Desired guideline outcomes should be specified.
10. Methods for evaluating the reliability and validity of the guideline should be described.
11. Planned periodic review of guidelines is necessary.

The Institute of Medicine (IOM) also developed a list of the characteristics of exemplary practice guidelines. The following eight criteria are suggested (IOM, 1992):

1. *Validity*: Practice guidelines are considered valid if, when they are followed, they lead to the health and cost outcomes projected for them. Validity assessments should include the strength and quality of the evidence cited, the means used to evaluate this evidence, and the relationship between the evidence and the recommendations. Practice guidelines should be accompanied by a comparison of health and cost outcomes for the recommended interventions and for alternative interventions. Outcome assessments should consider patient perceptions and preferences.
2. *Reliability/reproducibility*: Given the same evidence and development methods, another group of experts should be able to produce essentially the same statements. Given the same clinical circumstances, practitioners should be able to apply the guidelines consistently.
3. *Clinical applicability*: Practice guidelines should define the targeted patient populations and recommendations should indicate to which population individual statements apply.
4. *Clinical flexibility*: Practice guidelines should identify exceptions to the recommendations and discuss how to identify and consider patient preferences.
5. *Clarity*: Practice guidelines must be presented in a logical and easy-to-follow way with unambiguous language and precisely defined terms.
6. *Multidisciplinary process*: The development process must include participation by "key affected groups," and may include these groups in development panels. Participation by these groups may include providing evidence and viewpoints and reviewing drafts of the guidelines.
7. *Scheduled review*: Practice guidelines must include statements about when they should be reviewed to determine whether revisions are needed. Revisions may be warranted by new clinical evidence or professional consensus, or by a lack of such evidence or consensus.

8. *Documentation*: Panels should meticulously document the procedures followed in development, the participants involved, the analytical evidence used, and the assumptions and rationales accepted.

The Clinical Efficacy Assessment Project of the American College of Physicians (ACP) also has put forth what they consider to be important attributes of practice guidelines. Their criteria include the following (Johnson-White, 1994):

1. Is the guideline topic relevant?
2. Could the recommendation change or reinforce practices?
3. Is there a description of the development process?
4. Is the guideline endorsed by a reputable organization?
5. Are practice options and outcomes clearly specified?
6. Was an explicit process used to select and combine evidence?
7. Was an explicit process used to assign values to potential outcomes of practice options?
8. Were evidence and judgments subjected to a credible external review process?
9. Is the guideline likely to account for important recent developments?
10. Are clear recommendations made?
11. Are important caveats identified?
12. Are the objectives of the guideline consistent with organizational objectives?
13. Are the recommendations applicable to the organization's patients?
14. Do the predicted benefits, harms, and costs merit the effort of guideline implementation?

As one would expect, there is significant overlap in these three practice guideline criteria sets. The overall areas of concern can be summarized into ten categories that include reliability, validity, development panel, methodology, scheduled review, clinical applicability, clinical flexibility, clarity, endorsement, and cost-benefit analysis (Table 4).

Reliability and Validity

All three criteria sets give some consideration to practice guideline reliability and validity. Reliability refers to the stability of the recommendations across time and sponsoring organizations. The question to be considered is whether another guideline

TABLE 4. Guideline Evaluation Criteria

Area of concern	APA	IOM	ACP
Reliability	×	×	
Validity	×	×	×
Development panel	×	×	
Methodology	×	×	×
Scheduled review	×	×	×
Clinical applicability	×	×	×
Clinical flexibility	×	×	×
Clarity		×	×
Endorsement			×
Cost-benefit analysis	×		×

panel given the same evidence would develop similar recommendations. It is unlikely that a sponsoring organization would commission two panels to generate identical guidelines in order to establish reliability, due to the cost of guideline development. A more realistic way to measure reliability might be to compare guidelines developed by different agencies that address the same conditions or clinical concern. Differences then could be explored and potential guideline limitations identified.

Validity of practice guidelines means that they fulfill their stated purposes. As indicated earlier, the purpose for guidelines is to improve quality of care, by educating providers. Testing how well this is accomplished may involve monitoring quality indicators while implementing guidelines. More specifically, construct validity measures the integrity of the ideas presented. One marker of this is how well grounded guidelines are in empirical evidence. Face validity, another type of validity, means that the users of the guidelines think they make sense and that they appear reasonable. This type of validity is necessary for faithful guideline implementation and can be established by disseminating guidelines to potential user groups for comment prior to finalization.

Development Methodology

The IOM and APA recommend that the guideline development panel be multidisciplinary and include representatives of affected groups including providers and consumers. Furthermore, the APA states that panel members should represent a broad range of expertise, that individual conflicts of interest should be avoided, and that panel members should be listed in the final guideline document. Multidisciplinary input is important for practices, such as psychotherapy, where providers from several disciplines are providing the service. Specialty guidelines have been developed, however, that address discipline-specific methods, such as ECT or psychological testing. In these cases, the appropriate expert panel may be more limited. The intent about panels is to include representative users of the guidelines along with members of other relevant groups, including consumers. This ensures that those who are impacted by the guidelines have a voice in their development.

All three organizations suggest that an explicit development process be documented and used to compile evidence and opinions and to design recommendations. Specific development concerns include literature search strategies, how empirical data from various sources are integrated, rating the strength of empirical evidence, how clinical consensus is arrived at, use of expert advisors, inclusion of professional groups or other concerned parties, and independent external review of the guidelines. Furthermore, the APA criteria recommend a hierarchy for evaluation of the evidence used.

Guideline recommendations are expected to change over time as new clinical methods are developed and tested. Hence, there is the need for scheduled review and updating of guideline recommendations. All three organizations support this practice. Guidelines that are several years old may need to be carefully scrutinized before they are implemented.

Ease of Guideline Use

Ease of use is related to how applicable guidelines are to various patient populations, how flexible the recommendations are, and how clearly they are written. Applicability, as used in the IOM document, is similar to guideline generalizability, as described by APA, and refers to how widely guideline recommendations can be applied to varying clinical populations without decreasing validity. One of the difficulties in generalizing from clinical trials is that treatment studies are usually conducted with relatively "pure" diagnostic samples defined by specified symptoms, behaviors, or test score cutoffs. Unfortunately, very few patients present with "pure" conditions. In fact, comorbidity or other confounding factors are the norm. In addition, clinical trials rely on treatment manuals, and adherence is strictly monitored. This rarely is the case in the field setting (Stricker, 1996). Guideline flexibility refers to the number of options that are built into the guidelines allowing for patient differences, patient preferences, or other mitigating circumstances. Flexibility is evident to the degree that the target populations are identified and modifications for varying circumstances are included.

Clarity of the practice guideline relates to the precision of the language used and the format of the document. Vague or awkward descriptions are likely to be misinterpreted. Busy clinicians require information that is quickly accessible and assimilated, easily understood, and readily applied. Long, overly detailed documents are less likely to be used.

Endorsement and Cost-Benefit Analysis

The ACP criteria for assessing practice guidelines include a question about the reputation of the endorsing organization. Part of the concern here is potential conflict of interest. Could members of the endorsing organization stand to profit from implementation of the recommendations? Have potential conflicts been described and accounted for? The APA criteria speak to similar conflict of interest concerns when describing the characteristics of the development panel. Another point is the experience of the sponsoring organization. Have they produced previous documents of acceptable merit? The reputation of the organization with providers and consumers also can contribute to face validity.

Cost-benefit analysis means consideration of the cost of treatment implementation relative to expected results. Direct costs (dollars) and indirect costs (time, effort, distress) should be estimated for providing and for withholding treatment along with anticipated outcomes. This information is necessary for clinicians and consumers to decide whether the recommendations of the guideline are "worth it" in their particular case. It is conceivable that a decision would be made not to implement recommended interventions.

The IOM, APA, and ACP practice guideline criteria described above are ideal. Available practice guidelines vary in how closely they match these characteristics. The ten areas of concern discussed are useful for individuals developing and modifying guidelines, for quality assurance policymakers selecting guidelines for implementation, and for mental health providers and consumers who are deciding about the merits of specific guideline recommendations.

METHODOLOGICAL STRENGTHS AND WEAKNESSES OF AVAILABLE GUIDELINES

The 71 practice guidelines identified by the SAIC in 1994 and 1995 were evaluated and compared using the combined criteria of the APA, IOM, and ACP. The purpose

TABLE 5. Methodology Reported by Type of Sponsoring Organization

	Professional organizations (n = 51)	Federal agencies (n = 13)	State mental health (n = 3)	Managed care (n = 4)	Total (N = 71)
Clinical consensus	37	13	0	3	53
Expert opinion	18	9	0	0	27
Literature search	22	2	0	3	27
Multidisciplinary panel	10	12	0	0	22
External review	12	9	0	0	21
Survey	11	0	0	1	12
Meta-analysis	4	1	0	0	5
Strength of the evidence	2	2	0	0	4
Guideline update planned	7	9	2	1	19

was to determine the overall quality of available practice guidelines and to discern which were the "best." In order to make these assessments, the methods used to develop each guideline were scrutinized (Table 5). Twenty-nine of the 51 documents from professional organizations, all 13 documents from federal agencies, none of the 3 from state mental health departments, and 3 of the 4 from managed care organizations reported their methodology. Twenty-six (37%) documents did not include a description of the development process, somewhat complicating the task. Methodology was inferred when references to literature or working groups were made. For some documents, particularly the state mental health materials, the methodology could not be discerned at all. These documents are not included in the findings that follow. Nine approaches to guideline development were reported, usually with more than one per guideline, including: clinical consensus building processes, expert opinion panel, literature searches, multidisciplinary working panel, external review by various groups or organizations, survey, and meta-analysis of empirical studies. Two additional observations were noted in the review: evaluation of the strength of the evidence used and planned guideline update.

A little less than one third of the guidelines (31%) reported a multidisciplinary development panel. To be coded as multidisciplinary, the panel had to include professionals from at least two disciplines. Some of the panels considered to be multidisciplinary were, in fact, dominated by a single profession. Federally sponsored guidelines had the highest frequency of input from various clinical and interest groups (12 out of 13) and the professional organizations had the lowest incidence of integrated panels (10 out of 51). The most frequently used method of guideline development was clinical consensus (75%). Various ways of gathering external opinions were reported, including opinions from recognized experts (38%), surveys of the organization's membership (17%), and external review of the protocol by various concerned organizations (30%). Surprisingly few documents (38%) described a systematic literature search and review. It is assumed that such a review would be necessary to identify and include relevant research findings. Very few guideline documents (6%) rated the strength of the evidence used to support the recommendations made. Five (7%) undertook the ambitious activity of combining published research findings via meta-analysis. Twenty-seven percent of the reports described a planned review and update of the protocol in the future.

In summary, a description of the methodology used in guideline development was missing from more than a third of the documents reviewed, making it difficult to evaluate their merits. Integrated reviews of empirical evidence with some rating of the strength of supporting research was the least reported methodology. Professional organizations, the largest group of guideline developers, were the least likely to include multidisciplinary input and reported clinical consensus and expert panels as the primary methodology. In spite of significant effort toward practice guideline development, the mental health field still has few guidelines that meet the standards put forth by the IOM, APA, and ACP.

There are several assumptions about practice guidelines that were contradicted by the findings of the SAIC study. First are the notions that guidelines exist for most known conditions and that treatment recommendations can be easily implemented by most mental health professionals. Diagnoses for children and adults, such as major depression or conduct disorder, have guidelines but are primarily written for single professional groups. These guidelines do not always translate across disciplines. Less frequent conditions do not yet have guidelines. Apart from traditional dual diagnoses in substance abuse treatment, there are no guidelines specifically written for treatment of complex conditions.

A second assumption is that practice guidelines are primarily based on scientific evidence and therefore represent the highest state of the art. Actually, more guideline recommendations are made on the basis of clinical consensus and opinions of expert panels than on randomized controlled treatment trials. Endorsement of and faith in the scientific method varies among authors and there are variations among guideline sponsors, in that some report the strength of the empirical evidence used and others do not. Treatment recommendations based on randomized trials have their own limitations, because generalizability from a "pure" experimental sample to the less clear-cut cases found in clinical practice is unknown. No guideline development panels have reported measuring the effectiveness of their recommendations in non-controlled conditions.

IMPLEMENTING PRACTICE GUIDELINES IN MENTAL HEALTH CARE

As stated earlier, practice guidelines are intended to educate practitioners and thereby improve the quality of care. Developing methodologically sound guidelines is only the first step. The larger task is inducing practitioners to study and consider guideline recommendations. In fact, attempts at implementation of practice guidelines by managed care and other provider organizations are still rudimentary. These organizations are interested in standardizing practice patterns because purchasers have expressed interest in "value," a concept that includes both cost and quality.

Informing and Guiding Clinical Decision Making

In order for guidelines to impact care, they need to be accepted by clinicians. One of the biggest problems health care organizations have described in aligning clinical care with accepted protocols is getting clinicians to read, understand, and regularly consult the practice guideline information. Busy practitioners do not appear to have the time or motivation to incorporate clinical protocols into practice without some additional tools and incentives. Efforts to bring mental health care practice patterns in line with guideline recommendations have to go beyond simple distribution of the documents; system interventions may be needed.

The review of practice guidelines conducted by SAIC revealed caveats included by the authors in anticipation of implementation barriers (Table 6). These considerations provide insight into some of the adjustments clinicians may need to make. Client developmental level was the most frequently cited implementation consideration (35%). Ethnic–cultural–linguistic diversity of individuals being treated and patient acceptance of treatment were both noted in 25% of the guidelines reviewed. Twenty-three percent addressed differing treatment needs across gender, 17% discussed possible cost barriers, 14% considered clinician characteristics, 14% talked about treatment setting concerns, and a few considered the availability of clinicians with appropriate training, clinician acceptance of the guidelines, or the effects of clinician reimbursement arrangements.

The AMA has made some suggestions for increasing clinician awareness and use of guidelines (AMA, 1994a). They state that the first step may be to modify or even rewrite a published guideline to meet local needs. Dissemination of the modified guideline then should be accompanied by endorsement from respected health care professionals in the organization or in the community. Random audits can be made to evaluate clinician behavior relative to the guidelines and to provide feedback on compliance. The auditing process should be explained to clinicians in advance as a continuous quality improvement tool to improve quality rather than as a way to control or punish diversity. Another mechanism suggested by the AMA is the use of computer flags and other reminders imbedded in electronic clinical databases at key decision points, such as treatment planning and review. The AMA further emphasizes that practice guidelines should not be absolute rules and that practice deviation must be allowed. Deviations and their rationales should be recorded, however, as this information can contribute to new insights and applications as well as to the detection of inappropriate care.

Two research projects funded by the AHCPR are currently underway to evaluate

TABLE 6. Implementation Impediments Addressed by Type of Sponsoring Organization

	Professional organizations (n = 51)	Federal agencies (n = 13)	State mental health (n = 3)	Managed care (n = 4)	Total (N = 71)
Ethnic/cultural/linguistic	10	6	1	1	18
Gender	7	7	2	0	16
Developmental level	16	5	2	2	25
Clinician characteristics	5	5	0	0	10
Treatment setting	6	3	1	0	10
Reimbursement pattern	2	1	0	0	3
Patient acceptance	11	6	1	0	18
Clinician acceptance	2	2	0	0	4
Availabilty of clinicians	3	2	0	0	5
Costs	5	7	0	0	12

methods for increasing guideline acceptance and use by clinicians. Kaiser Permanente Northwest Region and Group Health Cooperative of Puget Sound are studying implementation of the AHCPR guideline Treatment of Depression in Primary Care. They began by rewriting the guidelines for easier use by busy primary care physicians (44 pages instead of 327) and increased the focus on screening rather than diagnosis, emphasized lower-cost medications, and addressed access to care issues not covered in the original document. The studies consists of two interventions aimed at primary care physicians. The first intervention is "academic detailing," which involves one-to-one, face-to-face teaching by peers. The second intervention involves a combination of academic detailing and continuous quality improvement initiatives. Within each region, primary care physicians are randomly assigned to either one of the interventions or to a control condition. The effects of each intervention on patient psychiatric symptoms and general health will be measured (Migdail et al., 1995). Preliminary findings indicate that clinicians do not object to practice guideline implementation (Shye & Brown, 1995), and that initial practices were not in compliance with the AHCPR guidelines for depression. Specifically, fewer than half of the patients diagnosed and treated for depression made a return clinic visit within 2 months (Horowitz et al., 1996).

A second study examining implementation of the AHCPR Treatment of Depression in Primary Care guidelines is being conducted by Rand. Again, the intervention is to educate primary care physicians and the outcome is measured by patient depressive symptomatology. This study involves three independent service delivery sites, each with 12–19 general medical clinics. At each site, clinics are randomly assigned to one of three conditions: medication, psychotherapy, and control. Physicians in the medication condition are informed of the results of patient screening for depression, receive 3 hours of didactic training on antidepressant medication, participate in monthly case conferences, and have individual psychiatric consultation available. Physicians in the psychotherapy condition receive 3 hours of training in cognitive psychotherapy, including the goals of treatment and expected outcomes. They can refer patients to psychotherapy groups provided at each clinic and receive system support in the form of expert leadership teams and nurse follow-up with patients. The third condition consists of usual care, where exposure to the practice guidelines is standardized by simply providing copies to the clinics (Vibbert & Youngs, 1995).

Benchmarks for Quality Management

As stated at the beginning of this chapter, quality oversight agencies such as the JCAHO and NCQA are requiring health plans to identify, disseminate, and monitor practice guidelines as a condition of accreditation. The NCQA accreditation standards for managed behavioral health care organizations state that practice guidelines should be based on "scientific evidence and knowledge of best practices ... with input from practitioners, providers (and) members," and that the organization should "measure adherence to at least two of the guidelines ... (and) implement an explicit process for managing exceptions to guideline use" (NCQA, 1997, p. 61). How this is accomplished is left up to the managed care organization.

The NCQA's influence has developed from purchasers' desire for accountability. In response to purchasers' requests for information, the NCQA has headed a performance monitoring movement to measure and compare health plan functioning. Much attention in behavioral health care has been given to one aspect of performance monitoring, namely, outcomes (IOM, 1997; Coughlin, Simon, Soto, Youngs, & Vibbert, 1997). Managed care organizations and other provider groups are rushing to measure the outcomes of mental health treatment, specifically symptom and functional improvement, general health, and satisfaction. Less attention has been given to measuring the processes of care. Once outcome benchmarks have been established, the next question will be outcomes of what, and how can we make our outcomes better? An understanding of the processes of care will be needed to answer these questions, and it is conceivable that measures of practice guideline implementation will be one of the processes linked with treatment outcomes to identify ways of improving care.

CONCLUDING COMMENTS

Protecting the consumers of mental health care means attending to the issue of quality. Continuous quality improvement methodology informs us that quality of care improves as unintentional variation decreases. Hence, variance in clinical practice must be understood and managed to improve quality and protect consumers. This means that providers become consistent in their clinical decision making and digress from accepted practices only by conscious choice to accommodate individual client needs. Deviation would then represent innovation or thoughtful practice, rather than incompetence. Guideline authors recognize that clinical decisions ultimately rest with the practitioner who faces the unique circumstances of each individual case. It is unintentional variation that practice guidelines can help to reduce.

A review of existing guidelines indicated that practice guideline development is by no means a perfect or completed task. There are conditions and treatments that have yet to be addressed and improvements to be made in methodology. Implementation of practice guidelines is a challenge that has not yet been mastered. Simply providing clinicians with guideline documents appears to be insufficient. System interventions and support are needed to impact practice patterns.

Whatever the true value of practice guidelines, they come from a long history of concern with quality and are here to stay. More guidelines will be written and health care stakeholders will continue to be interested in the question of practice variation. Mental health providers need to understand the strengths and limitations of clinical guidelines in order to thoughtfully apply them. Further empirical investigation is needed, however, before anyone will truly understand the impact of practice guidelines on quality of care.

REFERENCES

Agency for Health Care Policy and Research (AHCPR). (1993). *Depression in primary care: Vol. 1. Detection and diagnosis*. Rockville, MD: Author.

American Medical Association (AMA). (1994a). *Implementing practice parameters on the local/state/regional level*. AMA Office of Quality Assurance and Medical Review. Chicago: Author.

American Medical Association (AMA). (1994b). *Directory of practice parameters: Titles, sources, and updates, 1994 edition*. Chicago: Author.

American Psychiatric Association (APA). (1994a). *Diagnostic and statistical manual of mental disorders* (4th ed.). Washington, DC: Author.

American Psychiatric Association (APA). (1994b). Practice guidelines for the treatment of patients with bipolar disorder. *American Journal of Psychiatry, 151*(12)(Suppl.), 1–36.

American Psychological Association (APA) Task Force on Psychological Intervention Guidelines. (1995). *Template for developing guidelines: Interventions for mental disorders and psychosocial aspects of physical disorders*. Approved by the American Psychological Association Council of Representatives, February 1995, Washington, DC.

Berwick, D. M. (1991). Controlling variation in health care: A consultation from Walter Shewhart. *Medical Care, 29*(12), 1212–1225.

Browne, R. A. (1995, June). *Practice guidelines: The challenges ahead*. Presentation made at the Behavioral Healthcare Outcomes, Guidelines and Report Card Summit, Institute for Behavioral Healthcare, Minneapolis, MN.

Center for Substance Abuse Treatment. (1994). *Intensive outpatient treatment for alcohol and other drug abuse* (DHHS Publication No. SMA 94-2077). Washington, DC: US Government Printing Office.

Coughlin, K. M., Simon, K., Soto, L., Youngs, M. T., & Vibbert, S. (Eds.). (1997). *The 1997 behavioral outcomes and guidelines sourcebook*. New York: Faulkner & Gray.

Horowitz, C. R., Goldberg, H. I., Martin, D. P., Wagner, E. H., Fihn, S. D., Christensen, D. B., & Cheadle, A. D. (1996). Conducting a randomized controlled trial of CQI and academic detailing to implement clinical guidelines. *Journal on Quality Improvement, 22*(11), 734–750.

Institute of Medicine (IOM). (1992). *Guidelines for clinical practice: From development to use*. Washington, DC: National Academy Press.

Institute of Medicine (IOM). (1997). *Managing managed care*. Washington, DC: National Academy Press.

Johnson-White, L. (1994, May). *Clinical efficacy assessment project*. Presentation at the Faulkner and Gray Medical Outcomes Conference IV, Washington, DC.

Joint Commission on Accreditation of Healthcare Organizations (JCOHA). (1994). *1994 accreditation manual for health care networks* (vol. I). Oakbrook Terrace, IL: Author.

Migdail, K. J., Youngs, M. T., & Bengen-Seltzer, B. (1995). *The 1995 behavioral outcomes and guidelines sourcebook*. Washington, DC: Faulkner & Gray's Healthcare Information Center.

National Committee for Quality Assurance (NCQA). (1994). *Standards for the accreditation of managed care organizations*. Washington, DC: Author.

National Committee for Quality Assurance (NCQA). (1997). *Surveyor guidelines for the accreditation of managed behavioral healthcare organizations*. Washington, DC: Author.

Shye, D., & Brown, J. B. (1995). Primary care HMO clinicians' opinions about clinical practice guidelines. *HMO Practice, 9*(3), 111–115.

Stricker, G. (1996). Empirically validated treatment, psychotherapy manuals, and psychotherapy integration. *Journal of Psychotherapy Integration, 6*, 217–226.

Vibbert, S., & Youngs, M. T. (Eds.). (1995). *The 1996 behavioral outcomes and guidelines sourcebook*. New York: Faulkner & Gray.

Wennberg, J. E., Freeman, J. I., & Culp, W. J. (1987). Are hospital services rationed in New Haven or over-utilized in Boston? *Lancet, 1*, 1185–1188.

PRACTICE GUIDELINES REVIEWED BY SAIC

Major American Journals and Professional Organizations

American Academy of Child and Adolescent Psychiatry. (1991). Practice parameters for the assessment and treatment of attention-deficit hyperactivity disorder. *Journal of the American Academy of Child and Adolescent Psychiatry, 30*(3), I–II.

American Academy of Child and Adolescent Psychiatry. (1992). Practice parameters for the assessment and treatment of conduct disorders. *Journal of the American Academy of Child and Adolescent Psychiatry, 31*(2), IV–VII.

American Academy of Pediatrics. (1987). Medication for children with an attention deficit disorder. *Pediatrics, 80*(5), 758–760.

American Academy of Pediatrics. (1989). Screening for drugs of abuse in children and adolescents. *Pediatrics, 84*(2), 396–398.

American Academy of Pediatrics. (1990). Selection of substance abuse treatment programs. *Pediatrics, 86*(1), 139–140.

American College of Obstetricians and Gynecologists. (1993). Depression in women. ACOG technical bulletin number 182—July 1993. *International Journal of Gynaecology and Obstetrics, 43*(2), 203–211.
American College of Physicians. (1984). The dexamethasone suppression test for the detection, diagnosis, and management of depression. *Annals of Internal Medicine, 100*, 307–308.
American College of Physicians. (1986). Eating disorders: Anorexia nervosa and bulimia. *Annals of Internal Medicine, 105*, 790–794.
American College of Physicians. (1989). Disulfiram treatment of alcoholism. *Annals of Internal Medicine, 111*(11), 943–945.
American Nurses Association. (1988). *Standards of addictions nursing practice with selected diagnoses and criteria* (American Nurses Association Publications; i–iv, 1–58; Jan.). Kansas City, MO: Author.
American Nurses Association. (1994). *Statement on psychiatric-mental health clinical nursing practice and standards of psychiatric-mental health clinical nursing practice* (American Nurses Association Publications; i–iv, 1–47; Jan.). Washington, DC: Author.
American Psychiatric Association. (1985a). *Seclusion and restraint: The psychiatric uses*. Washington, DC: American Psychiatric Press.
American Psychiatric Association. (1985b). Tricyclic antidepressants—Blood level measurements and clinical outcome: An APA task force report. *American Journal of Psychiatry, 142*(2), 155–162.
American Psychiatric Association. (1987). The dexamethasone suppression test: An overview of its current status in psychiatry. *American Journal of Psychiatry, 144*(10), 1253–1262.
American Psychiatric Association. (1989). *Treatments of psychiatric disorders: A task force report of the American Psychiatric Association*. Washington, DC: American Psychiatric Press.
American Psychiatric Association. (1990a). *Benzodiazepine: Dependence, toxicity, and abuse*. Washington, DC: American Psychiatric Press.
American Psychiatric Association. (1990b). *The practice of electroconvulsive therapy: Recommendations for treatment, training and privileging*. Washington, DC: American Psychiatric Press.
American Psychiatric Association. (1991). Quantitative electroencephalography: A report on the present state of computerized EEG techniques. *American Journal of Psychiatry, 148*(7), 961–964.
American Psychiatric Association. (1992a). AIDS policy: Guidelines for inpatient psychiatric units. *American Journal of Psychiatry, 149*(5), 722.
American Psychiatric Association. (1992b). AIDS policy: Guidelines for outpatient psychiatric services. *American Journal of Psychiatry, 149*(5), 721.
American Psychiatric Association. (1992c). *Tardive dyskinesia: A task force report of the American Psychiatric Association*. Washington, DC: American Psychiatric Press.
American Psychiatric Association. (1993a). Practice guideline for eating disorders. *American Journal of Psychiatry, 150*(2), 212–228.
American Psychiatric Association. (1993b). Practice guideline for major depressive disorder in adults. *American Journal of Psychiatry, 150*(4)(Suppl.), 1–26.
American Psychiatric Association. (1994a). Position statement on methadone maintenance treatment. *American Journal of Psychiatry, 151*(5), 792–794.
American Psychiatric Association. (1994b). Practice guideline for the treatment of patients with bipolar disorder. *American Journal of Psychiatry, 151*(12)(Suppl.), 1–36.
American Psychiatric Association. (1994c). *American psychiatric association practice guideline for the treatment of patients with substance use disorders: Alcohol, cocaine, opioids*. Draft document. Washington, DC: Author.
American Psychological Association. (1985). *Standards for educational and psychological testing*. Washington, DC: Author.
American Psychological Association. (1987). General guidelines for providers of psychological services. *American Psychologist, 42*, 712–723.
American Psychological Association. (1993). Guidelines for providers of psychological services to ethnic, linguistic, and culturally diverse populations. *American Psychologist, 48*(1), 45–48.
American Society of Addiction Medicine. (1991). *Patient placement criteria for the treatment of psychoactive substance use disorders*. Washington, DC: Author.
Bernstein, G. A., & Shaw, K. (1993). Practice parameters for the assessment and treatment of anxiety disorders. *Journal of the American Academy of Child and Adolescent Psychiatry, 32*(5), 1089–1098.
Block, B. M., & Lefkovitz, P. M. (1991). *Standards and guidelines for partial hospitalization*. Alexandria, VA: American Association for Partial Hospitalization.
International Society for the Study of Dissociation. (1994). *Guidelines for treating dissociative identity disorder (multiple personality disorder) in adults*. Skokie, IL: Author.

Kane, J. M., Evans, D. L., Fiester, S. J., Mirin, S. M., Pincus, H. A., Schatzberg, A. F., Cole, J. O., & Popper, C. W. (1992d). Psychopharmacological screening criteria. *Journal of Clinical Psychiatry, 53*(6), 184–196.

Lader, M., & Russell, J. (1993). Guidelines for the prevention and treatment of benzodiazepine dependence: Summary of a report from the Mental Health Foundation. *Addiction, 88*(12), 1707–1708.

McClellan, J., & Werry, J. (1994). Practice parameters for the assessment and treatment of children and adolescents with schizophrenia. *Journal of the American Academy of Child and Adolescent Psychiatry, 33*(5), 616–635.

Miller, S. I., & Phillips, K. L. (1992e). Chemical dependency disorders: Guidelines for review of inpatient therapy and rehabilitation. In M. R. Mattson (Ed.), *Manual of psychiatric quality assurance* (pp. 161–166). Washington, DC: American Psychiatric Association.

National Association of Social Workers. (1984). *NASW standards for the practice of clinical social work.* Silver Spring, MD: Author.

Weiner, R. D., Fink, M., Hammersley, D. W., Moench, L., Sackeim, H., & Small, I. F. (1992). Electroconvulsive therapy guidelines and criteria. In R. M. Mattson (Ed.), *Manual of psychiatric quality assurance* (pp. 181–187). Washington, DC: American Psychiatric Association.

Wilson, G. F., & Phillips, K. L. (1992a). Eating disorders: Quality assurance and utilization review guidelines. In M. R. Mattson (Ed.), *Manual of psychiatric quality assurance* (pp. 167–172). Washington, DC: American Psychiatric Association.

Wilson, G. F., & Phillips, K. L. (1992b). Residential treatment centers: Quality assurance and utilization review guidelines. In M. R. Mattson (Ed.), *Manual of psychiatric quality assurance* (pp. 173–180). Washington, DC: American Psychiatric Association.

Federal Agency Documents

Agency for Health Care Policy and Research. (1993a). *Depression in primary care: Volume 1. Detection and diagnosis.* Washington, DC: US Government Printing Office.

Agency for Health Care Policy and Research. (1993b). *Depression in primary care: Volume 2. Treatment of major depression.* Washington, DC: US Government Printing Office.

Center for Substance Abuse Treatment. (1993a). *State methadone treatment guidelines* (DHHS Publication No. SMA-93-1991). Washington, DC: US Government Printing Office.

Center for Substance Abuse Treatment. (1993b). *Pregnant, substance-using women* (DHHS Publication No. SMA-93-1998). Washington, DC: US Government Printing Office.

Center for Substance Abuse Treatment. (1993c). *Screening and assessment of alcohol- and other drug-abusing adolescents* (DHHS Publication No. SMA-93-2009). Washington, DC: US Government Printing Office.

Center for Substance Abuse Treatment. (1993d). *Guidelines for the treatment of alcohol- and other drug-abusing adolescents* (DHHS Publication No. SMA-93-2010). Washington, DC: US Government Printing Office.

Center for Substance Abuse Treatment. (1993e). *Screening and assessment for alcohol and other drug abuse among adults in the criminal justice system* (DHHS Publication No. SMA-94-2076). Washington, DC: US Government Printing Office.

Center for Substance Abuse Treatment. (1993f). *Intensive outpatient treatment for alcohol and other drug abuse* (DHHS Publication No. SMA-94-2077). Washington, DC: US Government Printing Office.

Center for Substance Abuse Treatment. (1993g). *Assessment and treatment of patients with coexisting mental illness and alcohol and other drug abuse* (DHHS Publication No. SMA-94-2078). Washington, DC: US Government Printing Office.

National Institutes of Health. (1984). Mood disorders: Pharmacologic prevention of recurrences. *National Institutes of Health Consensus Statement, 5*(4), 1–23.

National Institutes of Health. (1985). Electroconvulsive therapy. *National Institutes of Health Consensus Statement, 5*(11), 1–8.

National Institutes of Health. (1987). Differential diagnosis of dementing disease. *National Institutes of Health Consensus Statement, 6*(11), 1–27.

National Institutes of Health. (1991). Treatment of panic disorder. *National Institutes of Health Consensus Statement, 9*(2), 1–24.

Substantial Foreign Papers

The Quality Assurance Project. (1982). A treatment outline for agoraphobia. *Australian and New Zealand Journal of Psychiatry, 16*(1), 25–33.

The Quality Assurance Project. (1983). A treatment outline for depressive disorders. *Australian and New Zealand Journal of Psychiatry, 17*(2), 129–146.
The Quality Assurance Project. (1984). Treatment outlines for the management of schizophrenia. *Australian and New Zealand Journal of Psychiatry, 18*(1), 19–38.
The Quality Assurance Project. (1985a). Treatment outlines for the management of anxiety states. *Australian and New Zealand Journal of Psychiatry, 19*(2), 138–151.
The Quality Assurance Project. (1985b). Treatment outlines for the management of obsessive–compulsive disorders. *Australian and New Zealand Journal of Psychiatry, 19*(3), 240–253.
The Quality Assurance Project. (1985c). Treatment outlines for the management of the somatoform disorders. *Australian and New Zealand Journal of Psychiatry, 19*(4), 397–407.
The Quality Assurance Project. (1990). Treatment outlines for paranoid, schizotypal and schizoid personality disorders. *Australian and New Zealand Journal of Psychiatry, 24*(3), 339–350.
The Quality Assurance Project. (1991a). Treatment outlines for antisocial personality disorder. *Australian and New Zealand Journal of Psychiatry, 25*(4), 541–547.
The Quality Assurance Project. (1991b). Treatment outlines for avoidant, dependent and passive–aggressive personality disorders. *Australian and New Zealand Journal of Psychiatry, 25*(3), 404–411.
The Quality Assurance Project. (1991c). Treatment outlines for borderline, narcissistic and histrionic personality disorders. *Australian and New Zealand Journal of Psychiatry, 25*(3), 392–403.

Managed Care Organization Practice Guidelines

CIGNA Corporation. (1991). *CIGNA level of care guidelines for mental health and substance abuse.* Philadelphia: Author.
CMG Health Inc. (1994). *Clinical management guidelines.* Owings Mills, MD: Author.
MCC Managed Behavioral Care, Inc. (1991). *MCC preferred practices—Guide.* Eden Prairie, MN: Author.
United HealthCare Behavioral Services. (1994). *Manual of preferred clinical practices.* Minneapolis, MN: Author.

State Mental Health Department Guidelines

George, R. A., McFarland, B. H., Angell, R. H., & Pollack, D. A. (1994). *Guidelines and standards of care for mental health treatments in the Oregon health plan.* Salem, OR.
Arizona Department of Health Services. (1994). *Behavioral health services: Service level checklist, admission criteria for acute inpatient psychiatric hospitalization, clozapine therapy.* Phoenix, AZ: Author.
California Department of Mental Health. (1994). *Psychotropic medication guidelines.* Sacramento, CA: Author.

4

Information Management for Clinical Decision Making

RON L. MEREDITH, STEPHEN L. BAIR, AND G. R. FORD

THE USE OF COMPUTERS IN BEHAVIORAL HEALTH

The "information age" will result in revolutionary changes for the behavioral health care industry. The industry is witnessing an unprecedented capacity to quickly access and process enormous amounts of information. Collecting, storing, analyzing, interpreting, and reporting clinical data promise to dramatically affect the design, delivery and scope of behavioral health care services. Computer technology will not only facilitate the practice of behavioral health care, it will force changes in the delivery systems themselves.

Early applications of computer technology in clinical practice were characterized by attempts to simulate psychotherapy (DeMuth, 1984) and to use computers to score and interpret psychological assessment instruments (Fowler, 1985). While practitioners have been enmeshed in the various exigencies of the managed care movement during the last decade, an emerging technology has developed that will shift the "cottage industry" standards of most clinical practices into "high-tech" behavioral health care centers. Behavioral health care is on the verge of a rather remarkable revolution in how data are collected, processed, and analyzed. Clinical decision making will be both facilitated and shaped by the computer systems that will soon form the infrastructure of complex health care delivery systems. Clinical skill and sensitivity will be augmented by fingertip access to computerized information and products. Research suggests that most providers are not well prepared for these changes.

Surveys by Farrell (1989) and Rosen (1995) suggest that psychologists, while being fairly typical of behavioral health care providers, have not yet availed themselves of the emerging technology (see Table 1). According to Rosen (1995), about 72% of psychologists are currently using a computer in some capacity. This compares with a report of about 55% utilization 6 years ago (Farrell, 1989). Only about 50% use computers to process financial records and fewer than 25% have used computers to administer, score, or interpret psychological tests.

Cagney and Woods (1994) note that "To many providers, the term 'clinical

RON L. MEREDITH, STEPHEN L. BAIR, AND G. R. FORD • University of Alabama at Birmingham, Birmingham, Alabama 35294-0018.

Handbook of Quality Management in Behavioral Health, edited by Stricker *et al.* Kluwer Academic / Plenum Publishers, New York, 2000.

TABLE 1. Use of Computers by Psychologists[a]

	Percentage
Psychologists using computers in clinical practice	72
Hardware	
IBM compatibles	66
Laser printers	50
Modems	60
Connectivity	
Connectivity to on-line service	24
Clerical/adminstrative	
Word processing	69
Financial records	50
Printing insurance forms	33
Electronic billing	3
Clinical	
Test administration	25
Test scoring	11
Printing psychological profiles	22

[a]Adapted from Rosen (1995).

information systems' evoke images of computers, software discs, electrical cables and the like. To others ... it evokes imagines of machines and numbers, frustration and fear" (p. 43). Rosen and Weil (1995) identify three types of attitudes displayed by computer users: the "eager adopters" (10%), the "hesitant prove-its" (50%), and the "technology resisters" (40%). With specific respect to psychologists, about 30% rate themselves as moderately to highly technophobic, while 36% say they would rather not use the emerging technology unless they must. Interestingly, 54% want to wait until the new technology is "proven" before they decide to use it. These responses suggest that behavioral health professionals may be "behind the curve" when computerized information systems form the core of administrative and clinical operations in developing behavioral health care systems. Because the technology is emerging at a rapid rate, providers are well advised to become familiar with computers and application programs. The technology is here to stay and the impact promises to be far-reaching.

THE CHANGING ECOLOGY OF PROFESSIONAL PRACTICE

The use of computers in behavioral health care has evolved in a steady fashion over the last decade with a veritable explosion in technology the last few years. Early applications focused on the use of computers in psychological testing (Fowler, 1985), computer interviews (Erdman, Klein, & Griest, 1985), triage screening (Chang, 1987a), and in the development of rudimentary psychiatric records (Van Vort & Mattson, 1989). These applications were relatively simple in terms of functionality and clinical sophistication. Financial management systems, specifically billing systems, soon followed as more offices became computerized and behavioral clinicians became aware of the cost and time savings realized from such tools.

Farrell (1989) observed that three different psychware publications listed at least 150 different computer applications (mostly computerized assessment tools) available for behavioral health. Much more sophisticated systems now exist. Financial data can now be processed electronically with electronic transfer of funds from the payer to the bank account of the provider. Expert systems built on clinical logic and those that derive from complex algorithms are now available to predict the necessity for psychiatric hospitalization, to triage care in a continuum of behavioral health care services, and to predict the optimal time for discharge from outpatient services (Gray & Glazer, 1994). Chang (1987b) accurately predicted that market demands would force changes in record-keeping practices for behavioral clinicians. In the very near future, providers will store patient information in computerized patient records that will track care throughout highly integrated delivery systems.

This is the emerging picture. Providers, managed care organizations (MCOs), business-industry, and patients will be brought together using the new information technology. The next service delivery model is what could be referred to in the broadest sense as "participative care." The emerging behavioral health care system will become a "hospital without walls" where outpatient alternative treatment facilities compete successfully with psychiatric hospitals and psychiatric units in general and surgical hospitals. Diverse centers for outpatient treatment will proliferate. Patients in need of intensive care but not requiring costly hospitalization will attend specialty outpatient centers that will focus exclusively on treatment of specific disorders such as anxiety, depression, pain, geriatric behavioral health problems, and so forth. New administrative structures (e.g., physician equity practices, regional group practices, etc.) will emerge and managed behavioral health will increase focus at the community level. Behavioral health care providers will become partners in outpatient health networks, will own and manage outpatient centers of excellence, and will provide management, supervision, and research expertise to the emerging market.

National corporations will continue to contract with large MCOs. These MCOs will shrink in number as they consume one another for market share. Hospitals and provider groups will organize to form their own competitive outpatient behavioral health care systems. Networks that form partnerships with MCOs will profit not only from case management but also from the economies of scale derived from sound and centralized business management. Local networks will contract and capitate directly with private industry, traditional third party payers, and with health purchasing alliances (i.e., businesses merged together to negotiate quality service for a fair price).

Most providers will practice in organized groups or in integrated health care settings. A reorganization of behavioral health care resources will emerge to form the administrative structure that will manage the finances of health care and control the flow of patients through these systems. The need will exist for "a communication system that allows people to compile data and communicate with one another while enabling them to work together despite geographical dispersal" (Cagney & Woods, 1994, p. 43). Systems will be financially integrated but geographically distinct. Some providers will form their own networks or large groups to contract with various payers. Others will enter into management contracts with "full service" management service organizations (MSOs) that will market their services to various payers. Other providers will be absorbed by managed care entities and will become staff-level providers in health maintenance organizations (HMOs) or other similar entities. Some provider groups will become "anchor groups" for large managed care companies and will assume risk for capitated contracts and will essentially manage their own care through the use of sophisticated computer systems. Other providers will "sell" their practices to psychological health care companies, which will then both manage and "grow" the practices through competitive contracting. The constant will be the computer link that will tie these human systems together.

As the information structure develops within behavioral health, providers will find it necessary to change the way they work and the way they conduct business. Providers will face an increase in accountability. The structure of clinical practice will change. Cummings (1995) suggests that provider groups will form various partnerships and networks to address issues of quality, to define outcome standards, and to ultimately address issues that relate to quality of care.

Managed care companies are also aware of the "winds of change." They are beginning to broaden their goals to include measures of quality. Managed care organizations increasingly understand that "delivering on the promise" of meaningful quality and outcome data creates a marketing advantage. They are also integrating data collection into ongoing service delivery. Accountable cost centers will increasingly emphasize the collection of "convincing data on quality and outcomes" (Brown, Frazier, & Bendoraitis, 1995). What will close the loop between providers and sophisticated behavioral health care administrative systems will be the new information technologies that will allow the provider to take a more active role in case management and will allow the MCOs and other business entities to deliver cost-effective services and also reduce backroom expenses (i.e., claims processing and utilization management).

Enter the new information technology. Value will be defined as a function of both cost and effectiveness, rather than cost alone. The systematic evaluation of clinical outcome will shape the marketplace. Outcome-based reporting to business and industry will result in an increased level of sophistication on the part of the corporate consumer. Integrative data looking at "relevant business variables" such as medical cost offset, absenteeism, employee turnover, managerial effectiveness, and work unit efficiency will become critical evaluative dimensions to relate to treatment and clinical outcome data. These data will derive from electronic connectivity between payer/ administrator and the provider's office.

THE COMPUTERIZED PATIENT RECORD

Central to these developments is the need for an office information system that will do everything from scheduling patients for appointments, to compiling both assessment and treatment data, automatically preparing patient chart notes, processing financial information and collecting various types of outcome measurement (Meredith & Bair, 1995). These systems will have the advanced capability to analyze stored data to generate cost information, select level and type of care, download electronic treatment plans, evaluate patient improvement, and examine provider and organizational effectiveness. The trend will be toward "suite" software packages that integrate through relational databases commonly required functionality (Rosen & Weil, 1996). Of critical importance will be a mechanism to connect providers to multiple payers using one integrated system.

The systems will follow a client–server model where one primary computer

TABLE 2. Hardware Requirements for Office Practice

	Approximate expenses
Single provider model	
Pentium 233 32MB RAM 1 GIG HD	$1,200.00
Laser printer	$750.00
Group practice model	
Server: Pentium 233 64MB RAM 2 GIG HD Tape Backup	$2,400.00
Novell network	$1,500.00
Work stations: Pentium 233 32MB RAM 1 GIG HD	$1,000.00

loaded with all necessary programs will be networked to "work stations" for individual users. The computer systems will be relatively robust and fast IBM-compatible systems operating in a graphical interface using the popular Windows 95 (and Windows 98) operating systems. Table 2 details system specifications for a "typical" provider office. These systems will need to possess the following business requirements:

> Instantaneous system response time, capacity to operate multiple applications at one time, reliable and valid data base, high system reliability (24-hour availability), easily acquired user skills, single copy chart information, closed loop connectivity between provider, payer, facilities, reviewers, researchers, employers, regulatory powers, and one style of interface. (Fain, 1994, pp. 26–27)

What this translates to is the use of one interface (Windows), using a system that supports a clinical patient record with integrated clinical, management, and financial functionality with secure connectivity, that will be required to transmit information to various sites including payers, a behavioral health data bank and various treatment facilities (or providers) where the patient will be seen (hospitals, day treatment centers, outpatient provider offices, etc.). The point about single copy chart information is essential, as using separate systems that do not automatically reconcile databases will inevitably lead to data contamination [an enormous problem for large management information system (MIS) projects].

What else do we know about the future of the high-tech provider office? The availability of the new technology will affect the way practice is conducted and how care is delivered. For instance, the intake process will be automated by having patients complete computerized screening inventories and psychosocial histories. These will be administered either on-line or via paper-and-pencil with clerical support personnel entering data into the computer system.

Much more clinical and diagnostic information will be available to the clinician before the patient is seen for the first visit. Electronic telephone intake data will be downloaded to the provider at the time the initial appointment is scheduled. Fairly detailed information about presenting problems and complaints will be available along with information about history of treatment, level of risk, medications, medical problems, and the presence or absence of contributing chemical abuse problems. Initial evaluations will be entered into the computer systems to generate electronic treatment plans that will form templates that will guide subsequent treatment. Intake information will prompt the collection of further specialized information using a variety of specialized scales and measurement instruments. Target behaviors and treatment goals will be identified and tracked as one component of sophisticated multidimensional outcome measurement systems. Electronic treatment plans will be revised and updated from the emerging clinical record. On-line review (MCO's Select Software: Providers come On-line, 1995) by case managers or peers will provide an interactive method to encourage quality of service delivery. Treatment sessions will be automatically allocated and updated as computer systems sort and analyze downloaded information from provider offices.

Information sharing with patients will greatly improve the treatment process. For example, the new technology will combine the latest in computerized projection technology (LED panels) with armchair consoles so the provider can project on the office wall (i.e., screen) unlimited information about problems, disorders, treatments, and so forth, using prepackaged laser disks and CD-ROM technology. Interactive learning modules on topics such as assertiveness training (Assertiveness Training, 1996), self-esteem (Self-Esteem and Values, 1996), and stress management (Total Stress Management System, 1996) will guide patients through educational materials designed to facilitate treatment. Patients will be able to view and discuss computer-generated treatment trends plotted automatically by target behavior, method of intervention (psychotherapeutic or psychotropic), and date of service delivery.

Treatment will be more accountable and more information will be immediately available to the clinician about treatment alternatives. Prescriptive treatments and workbooks will be downloaded from commercial sites and/or from professional associations and managed care entities. The very latest information on treating specific disorders will be at the provider's fingertips. Information sharing between different types of providers (e.g., family physician and behavioral health care provider) in integrated health care systems will be conducted via secure internet domains and will facilitate the communication and decision-making process.

On-line forums with "expert" professionals will allow the provider to acquire or refine existing skills. On-line access to computer searches and published information will allow the practitioner to access the latest treatment or other clinical information and download these data to their laser printers for immediate review. Immediate access to pharmacological databases will alert the clinician to medication side effects and to possible drug interactions. Interactive programs will use animation and social models to demonstrate and teach more effective behavioral patterns. Computerized "exercises" will teach patients various cognitive and self-instructional skills to address particular problems. Virtual reality (Lanier & Biocca, 1992) will allow the clinician to simulate social interactions and exposure to various stimulus situations (e.g., phobic stimuli, conflict situation, etc.). Standardized stimulus material will become available through CD-ROM technology and will allow a much "closer to life" and more controllable exposure to stimulus situations than has heretofore been available through behavioral rehearsal or role-playing.

Assessment of treatment outcome will become an automatic and relatively inconspicuous part of ongoing care. Session-by-session data will complement patient satisfaction measures and posttreatment surveys. Much more emphasis on value will accrue as the methodology to measure outcome is dispersed to the provider community. As the point of diminishing returns in cost reduction is approached in behavioral health care, the variable that will distinguish various delivery systems will be quality as defined by standardized measures of outcome.

THE USE OF COMPUTER SYSTEMS IN DIAGNOSIS AND ASSESSMENT

ON-LINE WITH DSM-IV

The *Diagnostic and Statistical Manual of Mental Disorders*, 4th edition (DSM-IV) (American Psychiatric Association, 1994) is the recognized standard for classification of psychological and psychiatric disorders. Although the ICD continues to be used internationally, the DSM-IV system is more broadly accepted by the insurance industry in this country. This system uses a multiaxial schema that allows the clinician to classify patient characteristics across the following dimensions: primary clinical disorders, personality disorders/mental retardation, general medical conditions, psychosocial and environmental problems, and assessment of global functioning. Thus, the diagnostic system is a formal categorization system that also defines parameters relevant to assessment and treatment.

Various on-line products are available to facilitate the process of making an accurate and meaningful diagnosis. First, Gibbon, Williams, and Spitzer (1996a) have introduced an on-line Structured Interview for DSM-IV (SCID) for patients that generates both a summary and comprehensive diagnostic report. The report covers mood disorders, anxiety disorders, substance use disorders, somatoform disorders, eating disorders, and psychotic symptoms. A companion software package presented by First, Gibbon, Williams, and Spitzer (1996b), AUTOSCID II, covers Axis II diagnoses (personality disorders). This system likewise is an automated on-line system that is completed by either the patient or the clinician. All major personality disorders are screened and the program also provides clinical "pearls of wisdom" about each disorder. A complete diagnostic report is also included. A third diagnostic aid developed by First, Williams, and Spitzer (1996) is the DTREE: The DSM-IV Expert. The clinician follows screen prompts consisting of simple "yes" or "no" responses about the patient's presentation. The system uses a branching technology that reviews (or rules out) psychotic disorders, medical disorders, mood disorders, anxiety disorders, somatoform disorders, and substance use disorders, compiling a clinical diagnostic report. Similarly, a diagnostic software product is available for assessment of children that presents the Diagnostic Interview for Children and Adolescents on-line for completion by either the child (ages 6–12 and 13–18 years of age) or a parent (Reich, Welner, & Herjanic, 1996). The program examines 22 different diagnostic entities and produces a number of clinical reports, including a summary report, positive and negative symptoms, and a complete interview summary.

The American Psychiatric Association has released an Electronic DSM-IV (1996) for use with either IBM or McIntosh formats. The system includes the entire DSM-IV, word for word, and is fully searchable by diagnostic code, term, phrase, and number. It is hyperlinked to allow rapid movement through the system.

Another company, The Psychological Corporation (OPTAIO, 1999), has developed a software product for the DSM-IV that allows the user to easily navigate the system using electronic menus and hyperlinked text references. This system is integrated with a more elaborate practice management system and is not available for individual purchase. These advances allow the user to access specific diagnoses and then move quickly throughout the system, examining alternative diagnoses or related conditions.

One additional advance in computer diagnostics is predicted. Expect to see computerized checklists that allow the clinician to determine the similarity between observed or reported characteristics and diagnostic criteria. Presented on-line, clinicians will be able to determine in a quantitative fashion the "degree of fit" between their observations of a patient and the abstract diagnostic classification categories. Heretofore, formal psychiatric diagnoses have been seen as absolute entities that overlooked idiographic differences in favor of "commonalities of symptoms" that defined the diagnostic entity. Adding the capacity to quantify a range of pathology within a diagnostic class may contribute to a more meaningful, accurate, and useful nomenclature. Because diagnosis is integrally tied to medical reimbursement, those systems that share databases with billing systems will be the more desirable, although "stand alone" diagnostic systems will be very useful to the behavioral health care provider.

Computerized Test Administration, Scoring, and Interpretation

The use of computers for scoring and interpreting psychological assessment instruments represents an early application of computer technology to the practice of psychology (Fowler, 1985). The early programs, however, were relatively limited in terms of functionality. For example, many allowed only the entry of data from previously scored paper-and-pencil instruments, while some provided a "cookbookish" interpretation and stiff and inflexible written reports of results and findings.

This situation has changed greatly. *Psychware Sourcebook* (Krug, 1993) offers a comprehensive listing and analysis of available software for behavioral health. Additionally, it includes sample interpretative reports. Numerous instruments allowing for the automation of many facets of assessment are available to the clinician, including on-line administration, scoring, and interpretation. Automated reports that facilitate diagnosis and treatment planning are also reviewed. Software is also described that transforms paper-and-pencil inventories to on-line products along with software that produces comprehensive reports for virtually all categories of psychometric instruments. Products are differentiated on the basis of features–functionality: on-line administration–off-line administration, electronic scoring capability, automated interpretation, production of narrative reports, editing from word processing files, and so on.

Table 3 lists the general types of computerized assessment instruments available to the practitioner. The fully computerized office will include menus of frequently administered tests, scoring and interpretation programs, and report-generating software. Work flow in the provider's office will change to accommodate the flow of information that can be gathered and processed prior to treatment (intake, screening, history, baseline assessment for outcome), during treatment (special scales to investigate particular problems and intermediate measures of outcome to assess mid-point changes in presenting symptoms or other measures of outcome), and posttreatment assessment (to evaluate the effectiveness of the selected interventions).

Most of these instruments are available for IBM or IBM-compatible computers, which will be the standard in the industry. Many of these instruments can accommodate on-line administration, while some provide the versatility to also print paper-and-pencil forms for off-line administration. These various instruments also can be distinguished by the method of payment for repeated utilization. Some allow unlimited administration following purchase of the software, others allow a finite number of administrations with purchase of the software, and still others require mail-

TABLE 3. Computerized Assessment Instruments

Types of instruments	On-line administration	Electronic scoring	Narrative reports
Intake			
Telephone intake histories	Yes		Yes
Psychosocial histories	Yes		Yes
Screening inventories	Yes	Yes	Yes
Mental status evaluations	Yes	Yes	Yes
Problem behavior scales	Yes	Yes	Yes
Symptom checklists	Yes	Yes	Yes
Diagnostic systems			
DSM-IV	Yes		
Diagnostic formulations	Yes		Yes
Assessment of specific problems			
Anxiety	Yes	Yes	Yes
ADHD	Yes	Yes	Yes
Chemical dependency	Yes	Yes	Yes
Depression	Yes	Yes	Yes
Developmental assessment	Yes	Yes	Yes
Domestic violence	Yes	Yes	Yes
Eating disorders	Yes	Yes	Yes
Geriatric problems	Yes	Yes	Yes
Marital problems	Yes	Yes	Yes
Menstrual distress	Yes	Yes	Yes
Parenting skills	Yes	Yes	Yes
Self-concept scales	Yes	Yes	Yes
Stress assessment	Yes	Yes	Yes
Evaluation of risk			
Suicidality	Yes	Yes	Yes
Aggressiveness	Yes	Yes	Yes
Cognitive evaluation			
Intellectual assessment			Yes
Neuropsychological screening	Yes	Yes	Yes
Neuropsychological norms		Yes	Yes
Academic achievement		Yes	Yes
Personality evaluation			
Projective		Yes	Yes
Objective	Yes	Yes	Yes
Screening	Yes	Yes	Yes
Outcome measurement			
Patient satisfaction	Yes	Yes	Yes
Clinician ratings	Yes	Yes	Yes
Psychometric scales	Yes	Yes	Yes
Behavioral tracking	Yes	Yes	Yes
Utility programs			
Report writing programs			Yes
Scale conversion programs	Yes	Yes	Yes
Norm development programs	Yes	Yes	Yes

in or teleprocessing of raw test scores to produce interpretative narrative reports. Instruments requiring mail-in or teleprocessing promise rapid turn around and indeed are much faster than what was observed with early test services. Most of these instruments are supported by impressive psychometric properties. A caveat here for the user to be certain to examine the psychometric properties of these instruments. Computerized evaluative instruments can be very impressive in function and form but may lack strong empirical support.

Advantages of Computerized Assessment Instruments

New products offer rapid scoring, interpretation of test results, and report generation. They reduce professional time and effort. The psychometric properties of these instruments are in most cases well developed. The result is the capacity to quickly access reliable and valid behavioral data. Clerical time and expense is also reduced, especially with systems that use sophisticated report writing technology. Turnaround time for delivery of the product (e.g., report out of results) can be reduced from hours to minutes.

Computerized Interviews and Screenings

Farrell (1991) notes that one of the early uses of computers in behavioral health care was the structured interview. He reviews these developments noting specifically the Computerized Assessment System for Psychotherapy Evaluation and Research (CASPER) (McCullough, Farrell, & Longabaugh, 1986). CASPER is used to identify presenting problems, track these problems over time, and evaluate treatment outcome. Once particular problems have ben identified, then additional questions that further define the problem are presented for response. During subsequent interviews, the patient's problem list is accessed and additional ratings can be entered to reflect changes over time. This system has been subjected to psychometric evaluation and meets basic requirements for internal consistency, convergent validity, and discriminant validity.

Social and developmental histories (Rainwater & Coe, 1996), psychological–psychiatric status interviews (Honaker & Harell, 1996), developmental history reports (Rainwater & Slade, 1966), mental status checklists (Schinka, 1995a), on-line psychosocial histories (Giannetti, 1996), and personal history checklists (Schinka, 1995b) are examples of computerized intake instruments that will assist the clinician with accurate problem formulation and basic understanding of the clinical case. Additional computerized assessment products that might be of value to the clinician include symptom inventories such as the Brief Symptom Inventory (Derogatis, 1996) and the Symptom Checklist 90-Revised (SCL-90-R) (Derogatis, 1996), both of which produce computerized narrative reports describing presenting symptomatology.

Computerized Psychological Assessment

Computerized versions of a number of popular broad-based assessment instruments are also available. For example, software to score, interpret, and report projective test results (Rorschach) are available from a number of sources, including the Psychological Corporation [Rorschach technique (1996), Rorschach Interpretation

Assistance Program (1996), and the Exner Rorschach Scoring Program (1996)], Multi-Health Systems (MHS) (Hermann: The Rorschach Assistant, 1996) and Psychological Assessment Resources (PAR) (Rorschach Interpretation Program Version 3.1, 1996). Teleprocessing for both scoring and interpretation of the original Minnesota Multiphasic Personality Inventory (MMPI) is available through NCS. For the original MMPI, Western Psychological Services presents narrative reports based on actuarial data derived from the Marks system for both child/adolescent (Marks MMPI Report, 1996) and adult versions as well as a Marks actuarial report for the MMPI-2 (Marks MMPI & MMPI-2 Adult Clinical Report, 1996). The MMPI-2 is also available for on-line administration, scoring, and report generation from NCS (The Minnesota Report: Adult Clinical System—Revised Interpretative Report, 1996). A structural summary of prescored MMPI-2 profiles that provides summaries addressing test-taking attitude, factor scales, moods, cognitions, interpersonal relationships, and other problem areas is available from PAR (Minnesota Multiphasic Personality Inventory-2, 1996). MHS (Minnesota Multiphasic Personality-2, 1996) also provides a detailed interpretive summary of MMPI-2 scores.

Available from PAR (Minnesota Multiphasic Personality Inventory Adolescent Norms, 1996) are conversion norms for adolescent populations and an adolescent interpretative system. For the MMPI-A (Adolescent Version), PAR (Minnesota Multiphasic Personality Inventory—Adolescent, 1996a) provides a structural summary of scored protocols. MHS (Minnesota Multiphasic Personality Inventory—Adolescent, 1996b) provides a detailed summary derived from scored protocols that includes profile validity, presenting problems, probable symptoms, treatment issues and suggestions, diagnostic considerations, and configural interpretations. NCS (Minnesota Multiphasic Personality Inventory—Adolescent, 1996c) provides a system to administer, score, and provide narrative reports.

The Psychological Corporation also has developed software for scoring and report packages for the Million Index of Personality Styles (1996) and the Personality Assessment Inventory (1996). The California Psychological Inventory (1996) is available for on-line scoring or scanning of test data. Both provide narrative reports. The Eysenck Personality Inventory (1996) and the Meyers-Briggs Type Indicator (1996) are also available for computer analysis and report generation. NCS provides scoring, interpretation, and report-generating software for the Million Clinical Multiaxial Inventory—III (1996) and the Sixteen Personality Factor Questionnaire (1996).

A number of software programs are available to assess patient problems in specialized areas. These include "mood" software programs for several of Aaron Beck's scales, including the Beck Depression Inventory (1996), the Beck Hopelessness Scale (1996), Beck Anxiety Inventory (1996), and the Beck Scale for Suicide Ideation (1996). Two depression observer rating scales are from Integrated Professional Systems: one based on the Hamilton Depression Scale (Essan Depression Scale A, 1996) and the other based on the Depression Status Inventory (Essan Depression Scale B, 1996). Integrated Professional Systems also offers patient-rating versions of the same scales (Essan Self-Rating Depression Scale A, 1996; Essan Self-Rating Depression Scale B, 1996). A computerized version of the State–Trait Anxiety Inventory (1996) is available from MHS, while Integrated Professional Services offers observer rating scales for anxiety based on the Anxiety Status Inventory (Anxiety Scale A, 1996) and the Hamilton Anxiety Scale (Anxiety Scale B, 1996). Western Psychological Association presents a computerized version of the Endler Multidimensional Anxiety Scales

(1996), which provides a narrative report covering state anxiety, trait anxiety across four generic anxiety-provoking situations and allows for the assessment of the perception and intensity of anxiety in the immediate situation.

Several programs are available for the identification and evaluation of stress. Two measures of stress, one a screening instrument (Brief Computerized Stress Inventory, 1996) and the other a very comprehensive tool (Comprehensive Computerized Stress Inventory, 1996) that examines stress across 30 different lifestyle areas (e.g., work, family, time management, worrying, etc.), are available from Preventive Measures. The Coping Inventory for Stressful Situations (1996) examines different coping styles for stress and provides extensive normative data and a narrative report. The Jenkins Activity Scale (1996) explores the intensity and breadth of type A behavior in examining four scales: Speed/Impatience, Job Involvement, Hard-driving Characteristics, and Competitiveness. The Occupational Stress Inventory (1996) examines dimensions in the workplace (occupational stress, psychological strain, and coping resources) to produce both clinician and patient narrative reports.

Specialty scales are available for assessment of marital satisfaction (Marital Satisfaction Inventory, 1996), which compare the response of partners via a computerized report and one which compares the results of partner's Sixteen Personality Factor (1996) scores (Marriage Counseling Report, 1996) to generate a narrative report identifying interpersonal patterns and differences as well as suggestions about methods and approaches that might prove useful in treatment. Other software programs useful in the family setting include one that assesses child abuse potential (CAPSCORE 1.04, 1996) and another that assesses the risk of domestic violence (Domestic Violence Inventory, 1996).

Integrated Professional Systems provides three scales to evaluate degree of behavioral, social, and physical impairment with geriatric patients. These include one scale based on the Sandoz Clinical Assessment—Geriatric (Geriatric Clinical Assessment Scale, 1996), one based on the Plutchik Geriatric Rating Scale (Geriatric Rating Scale A, 1996), and the third based on the Crichton Geriatric Rating Scale (Geriatric Rating Scale B, 1996). Two software programs are available for the evaluation of pain: the Chronic Pain Battery (1996) and the Chronic Pain Administrator (1996), which combines a comprehensive assessment of pain with evaluation of other presenting symptoms.

Specialty assessment software programs are also available for assessment of various dimensions (Somatic, Negative Affect, Impaired Concentration, and Behavior Change) of menstrual-related distress (Menstrual Distress Questionnaire, 1996). Programs to assist with evaluation of eating disorders are available from PAR (Eating Disorders Inventory—2, 1996) and MHS (Eating Disorder Inventory, 1996). Other specialty instruments include those designed to assess suicidality (King & Lowalchuk, 1996).

Additional computerized products include interactive modules on attitudes and knowledge about alcohol use: "If You Drink" (Meier, 1996); and the Chemical Dependency Assessment Profile (Hanaker, Harrell, & Ciminero, 1996), which details drinking history, patterns of reinforcement, beliefs about chemical dependency, and self-concept and relationships. Horn, Wanberg, and Foster (1996) have developed the Alcohol Use Inventory, which measures a broad spectrum of factors related to problem drinking including benefits, styles, consequences, concerns, and subtle drinking attitudes. This instrument is normed in 1200 individuals treated in residential programs. Western Psychological Services offers the Alcadd Test (1996), which provides a computerized narrative report that addresses regularity of drinking, drinking preference, lack of controlled drinking, rationalization of drinking, and excessive emotionality.

Halstead–Reitan normative programs are available through both PAR (HBR Norms Program, 1996) and MHS (Comprehensive Norms for an Expanded Halstead–Reitan Battery, 1996), while Integrated Professional Systems offers the Russell, Neuringer, and Sparks scoring system to generate ratings, calculate test findings, and summarize various hypotheses in a narrative report (Halstead–Reitan Neuropsychological Battery, 1996). The Halstad–Reitan Hypothesis Generator (1996) is also available to automatically provide data interpretation based on keyboard entry of test scores. On-line administration and scoring of the Halstead Category Test (Category Test Computer Program, 1996) is available through MHS and Precision People (Halstead Category Test—A Computer Version, 1966). A program that scores and provides interpretation of the Luria–Nebraska Neurological Battery (1996) is available from the Western Psychological Services for use with children and adults. The Psychological Corporation also has made available an on-line version of the MicroCog: Assessment of Cognitive Functioning (1996), which measures a variety of cognitive skills including attention, memory, reasoning, spatial processing, reaction time, and other measures of cognitive efficiency. Two different aphasia screening instruments (Western Aphasia Battery, 1996; Boston Diagnostic Aphasia Examination, 1996) are available through the Psychological Corporation. Scoring and report generation programs are also available for all the Wechsler Scales through the Psychological Corporation (Scoring Assistant for the Wechsler Scales, 1996).

Several software programs to assist with neuropsychological screening have become available. These include the Bender Report (1996), the Bender Clinical Report (1996) and the Bender Report 4.0 (1996). PAR presents the Memory Assessment Scale (1996), which allows for comparison of memory functions with Wechsler scores, while Psychometric Software provides a scale-by-scale narrative for the Wechsler Memory Scale Report (1996). Additional software packages for assessment of child and adolescent problems are also available. A thorough review of these systems is provided by Meredith, Bair, Ford, and Morris (1998).

In an interesting industry development, both the Psychological Corporation and NCS have developed proprietary software programs to score and interpret the various tests that they distribute. By purchasing their software, the clinician is then able to score tests, analyze results, and produce narrative reports and/or summaries of a number of different types of scales. Packaged separately, these programs must be purchased from the distributer. In both cases test results can be typed into the system or scanned using scanning software and hardware. Both companies offer their proprietary products for free with a significant purchase of test materials.

In an effort to gain a foothold in the managed care arena, NCS is also offering a comprehensive package of assessment instruments that operate on their Microtest Q (1996) proprietary program. This series of instruments include the Brief Symptom Inventory (1996), the Health Status Questionnaire 2.0 (1996), the Inventory to Diagnose Depression (1996), the Inventory of Suicide Orientation-30 (1996), the Post Traumatic Personality Profile (1996) and the Quickview Social History (1996). Although additional software assessment packages are available commercially, this overview provides some sense of the range and diversity of products available. The fact that the major publishing houses are moving rapidly into this area further documents the trend toward facilitating clinical judgment using sophisticated assessment software programs, thus providing a cost-effective, rapid, and efficient means to examine a variety of patient data. Clearly the movement will be toward computer systems loaded with a variety of commonly used instruments that will become standard fare in the provider's office.

Utility Programs

Several utility programs are available that allow the practitioner to create computerized assessment instruments from paper-and-pencil forms. These programs create a rich versatility for the clinician, as they can convert intake, screening, and psychosocial historical information and a virtually unlimited range of questionnaires and rating scales to computer-accessible instruments. Other utility tools produce detailed reports for most of the major psychological and/or educational psychometric instruments [e.g., Wechsler Intelligence Scale for Children—III (WISC-III) (PPVT)]. Of the various utility tools allowing for the creation of computerized instruments, the Interactive Tester (1996) facilitates this process through interactive information input to produce an instrument that is computer driven in all facets (e.g., administration, scoring, profiling, and interpretation). A second tool, Q-Fast (1996), allows for the computerization of questionnaires, surveys, and interviews. Questionnaire entry is similarly menu-driven, producing an instrument that can be administered on-line, scored, and stored in a form compatible with other software. The MicroCAT Testing System (1996) contains separate subsystems that are sold separately or as a package. It features one subsystem allowing the added versatility of incorporating graphics or scanned images in test construction; a separate subsystem controlling on-line administration, scoring, and report generation; a subsystem capable of performing test development functions such as item analysis; and a subsystem allowing the user to build his or her own conventional test. Relative to the other test utility devices available, this system is clearly the most sophisticated and conductive to test generation and development, although its versatility and power may exceed the needs of most clinicians in private practice.

The second type of utility programs facilitate report generation and also differ in terms of sophistication. The Psych-Educational Report Writing System (1996) was designed for school psychologists. It generates comprehensive narrative reports according to school specifications for such widely used psychometric instruments as the Wechsler Preschool and Primary Scale of Intelligence (WOPSI) and Wide Range Achievement Test-Revised (WRAT-R). In addition, it is capable of producing two types of reports, one detailed and extensive and the second shorter and more concise. A second report-generating utility tool, RADAR PLUS (1996), represents an on-line psychological software library and delivery system connecting the provider with over 70 psychometric instruments, including tests, history-gathering devices, and checklists. Once loaded, RADAR PLUS guides the clinician through demographic information entry and then selection of instruments to be administered from a test menu. It then guides the client through all phases of assessment, including instructions and administration. Finally, RADAR PLUS scores all instruments interactively at a separate site through modern connection and produces printable results. A final report generation utility device is the Report Builder-Screentest (1996). The Report Builder-Screentest, which runs in conjunction with the Screentest Assessment and Data Manager (1996), allows the user to build customized narrative report formats for assessment center results, attitude surveys, and performance appraisal forms. It creates the overall definitions for individual reports, which can then be printed, displayed on screen, or sent to a word processing program for further editing. Attention should be paid to avoid copyright violation and to be aware of the psychometric properties of various instruments that are employed.

Observational Data

Computers have been used to collect both self-monitoring data and observational data. Two interesting systems are presented by Farrell (1991), one showing the application of computers (Tombari, Fitzpatrick, & Childress, 1985) in monitoring compliance and a second illustrating how an obesity training program can be monitored using computers (Agras, Taylor, Feldman, Losch, & Burnett, 1990). Repp, Harman, Felce, Acker, and Karsh (1989) describe a software program for a portable computer that recorded observational data on 43 different target behaviors and automatically prepared summary statistics. These are representational of the way computer technology will be used to help behavioral clinicians monitor and change single behaviors or more complex behavioral patterns. As the technology develops so that smaller and more portable computers are available, this type of measurement will be greatly facilitated in not only data collection but also data reduction.

On-Line Analysis of Psychophysiological Data

Psychophysiological measures, including electroencephalography (EEG), electrodermal activity (EDA), and cardiovascular activity (CVA), have been applied in a variety of clinical settings since the early 1980s. EEG technology, for example, has been used to identify early cortical abnormalities in low-birth-weight infants that place them at increased risk of speech and language disorders (Cone-Wesson, Kurtzberg, & Vaughan, 1983). On-line EEG measurement is also critical in the diagnosis and monitoring of patients with epilepsy (Novelly, 1992), and in the diagnosis and treatment of sleep disorders. Measures of electrodermal activity, including skin conductance levels (SCLs), have been utilized in the treatment of anxiety disorders (Lader & Noble, 1975), as well as learning disabilities (Mangina & Beuzeron-Mangina, 1988). On-line measurement of cardiovascular activity, including heart rate and blood pressure, through ambulatory monitoring, also has proved to be a useful tool in the clinical management of patients with panic disorder (Taylor, Telch, & Havvik, 1983), in the diagnosis and management of individuals with essential hypertension (Perloff, Sokolov, & Cowan, 1983), in stimulant drug monitoring with attention deficit disorder (Solanto & Conners, 1982), and in monitoring the effects of shock treatment for severe psychotic depression (Noble & Lader, 1971). With the recent availability of software allowing for the reduction and/or on-line assessment of these measures, what could once be assessed only in the laboratory now can be assessed by the clinician in private practice, offering a powerful and immediate source of direct data for such clinical conditions as pervasive developmental disorders and mental retardation, learning disabilities, attention deficit disorder, anxiety and depressive disorders, medical conditions with psychological sequelae, such as epilepsy and hypertension, and in monitoring response to stress.

Two examples are illustrative of the available technology in this area: ambulatory

CVA monitors and polysomnography software, allowing for the reduction and analysis of previously scored sleep records. First, sophisticated measurement of cardiac function is now available with the use of portable (ambulatory) monitors that can provide treatment personnel a record of fluctuations in moment-to-moment cardiovascular response. Most of these monitors are capable of collecting and storing up to 48 hours of continuous heart rate and/or blood pressure readings, thereby providing an invaluable source of in vivo data to the clinician and aiding in the diagnosis, treatment, and medication monitoring in such conditions as anxiety disorders and essential hypertension (e.g., Accutracker II, 1996). In addition, data can then be downloaded to the personal computer for data reduction, analysis, and printout. Similar advances in measurement and data reaction are noted with EEG and EDR technologies. In EEG, even very complicated data from sleep laboratories are now easily reduced to meaningful clinical information by computer programs (MORPHEUS Version 3.0, 1996). Following initial hand scoring of the sleep record, the sleep technician enters the raw data by keyboard. MORPHEUS then generates a summary report including information on sleep staging, respiratory (apnea) events and duration, as well as additional information such as number of awakenings and limb movement. This information is printed out both in the form of tabular text as well as in graphical displays.

THE USE OF COMPUTER SYSTEMS IN RECORD KEEPING

Two office systems are available that assist the clinician in providing documentation of care. MHS offers a system called "The Perfect Chart" (1996), which records demographics, historical information, and biological factors, and handles some managed care and insurance information. It utilizes a popular word processing program to assist the clinician in generating social histories and clinical notes. It includes ready-made forms, letters, and prescription templates for psychotropic medication, as well as provides diagnostic, treatment, and other specialized clinical information. The Psychological Corporation offers QuickDoc for Windows (1996), which generates intake reports, progress notes, and discharge summaries. In addition, the system will record several measures of outcome and track several types of financial data useful in the managed care industry. MHS also markets both a session summary program (Honaker, 1996a) and a termination–discharge summary program (Honaker, 1996b), which produce automated narrative notes that can be extracted to a word processing program for modification or editing. These programs assist the clinician by creating a well-documented patient database and a standardized computer record of care and outcome. Meredith and Bair (1990) provide a detailed summary of considerations for using electronic records in clinical practice.

OFFICE BILLING SYSTEMS

A wide variety of software systems are available to meet the general billing requirements of the typical provider office. Many of these systems share common elements that have become "industry standards" for behavioral health. All programs include documentation of patient demographics, insurance and fee information, diagnostic information and specific information about a given point of service delivery. The programs print the necessary billing forms including bills for patients and for insurance carriers including the standard health insurance claim forms. Programs will document accounts receivables by provider/office, provide aging reports (how long the debt has been owed), generate patient statements and mailers, provide superbills that detail patient claim-filing information, generate referral reports and accurately track payments by time and source of payment, and so forth. Some programs will provide integrated electronic office schedule and some will provide electronic billing capabilities, whereby patient claims are sent either to clearing houses or payers for payment. In some cases electronic deposits can be made to the provider's office. Billing programs are becoming more sophisticated in response to managed care industry needs and many now have the capacity to track allocated sessions, set differential fees by insurer or MCO, and to provide summary reports and data that will allow the practice or group to determine if they are "on-task" in meeting managed care capitation requirements (e.g., average cost per session, average cost per client, average duration of care, etc.). Typically these programs do not include a general ledger to handle payables, although some of the systems have begun to incorporate this functionality. Few of these programs provide any type of actual claims processing but should interface in standard ways to allow for electronic data transmission to clearing houses or payers. Programs are largely differentiated by the level of customer support provided by the company, the ease of use and "feel" of the system, and the relative cost of the product. In this time of increased accountability, it is imperative that the provider office have the capacity to accurately track financial information and relate these data to clinical outcome. The current environment demands that systems be in place to generate reports for examination of complex cost issues in behavioral health care delivery. Rosen and Weil (1996) provide a detailed overview of various billing programs available to the practitioner.

MANAGEMENT INFORMATION SYSTEMS FOR BEHAVIORAL HEALTH

The latest development in behavioral health care is the development of robust and complex systems that provide connectivity between provider offices and other administrative entities (e.g., MCOs, networks, integrated health networks, health care purchasing alliances, etc.). The provider piece typically consists of a complete office management system including recordkeeping capabilities, electronic schedule, fully integrated billing systems, and some form of outcome measurement system. This system forms a computerized patient record that details patient demographic data, insurance information, provider credentials, diagnostic information, and information related to treatment or intervention (both behavioral and psychotropic). These systems also may include utilization management technology and electronic treatment plans and formulas, a well as a host of resident applications that produce telephone intake evaluations, psychosocial histories, psychological report capabilities, risk evaluation, and evaluation of a number of variables which may impact treatment (e.g., history of health care treatment, history of chemical abuse, medical problems, and associated treatments). These systems may provide automated chart note capabilities and may provide for multiple levels of assessment of patient outcome.

The host functionality may include advanced case management tools, financial processing to certify and pay claims, and automated "clinical decision-making" technology to assist with triage, level of care, risk, and optimal length of treatment. These systems operate in a fashion so that the entire patient chart is resident at the host with electronic copies available to appropriate providers for review throughout the networked systems. These systems operate with various types and levels of security to protect the integrity of the data and to protect the confidentiality of the patient. Some transmit data via fax, dedicated telephone lines, or through commercial carriers, while others will employ secure internet domains to route patient information to various payers and host administrative entities. Some of these systems have elaborate psychopharmacological databases that automatically report medication side effects and alert providers to negative drug interactions. Sophisticated diagnostic systems are available with on-line access to the DSM-IV. These systems provide for electronic mail within the networks and through internet sites. Table 4 lists those companies that have introduced these products into the market within the last 2 years. Because of the complex nature of these systems, they must be individually evaluated for applications in each specific clinical and administrative setting. It is of critical importance that the system selected have the capability to provide connectivity to multiple host sites and payers, as offices will tend to organize their business activities around these systems and the users will not want either the expense or the inefficiency of running multiple management information system programs.

THE USE OF COMPUTER SYSTEMS IN TREATMENT FORMULATION

Electronic Treatment Plans

Effective treatment starts with an organized conceptualization of the presenting problems, identification of treatment goals/targets, and a choice of intervention method(s). Hammond and Munnecke (1984) developed an early prototype of the automated treatment plan. The system was structured around menu-selected items that were merged to form narrative text. Free-form text could be inserted at any point

Table 4. Management Information Systems for Behavioral Health

Company	Product	Mailing address
Care Computer Systems	The TresCARE Computer System	P.O. Box 1408 Bellevue, Washington 98009
Community Sector Services	PsychAccess	700 Fifth Avenue Suite 5500 Seattle, Washington 98104
Compulink Business Systems, Inc.	The Psych Advantage	31348 Via Colinas Suite 103 Westlake Village, California 91362
Medipay, Inc.	Medipay Systems	620 Southwest Fifth Avenue Suite 610 Portland, Oregon 97204-1421
OMS	Touched	P.O. Box 661 Nevada City, California 95959
Synergistic Office Solutions, Inc.	SOS Case Manager	Suite 208 P.O. Box 1677 Melbourne, Florida 32903-1677
The Psychological Corporation	OPTAIO	555 Academic Court San Antonio, Texas 78250

in the data input process. The authors noted that the computer used to develop the software system was a $70,000 Digital Equipment PDP 11 3/4 equipped with a 10 megabyte disk. They further noted that a similar configuration could be implemented on MUMPS-compatible microcomputers equipped with a hard disk costing at that time about $20,000.

The concept was on target and ahead of the times. Currently, a number of automated treatment plans are available for use with personal computers at a fraction of the cost. One product, TP Write (Reason House, 1996), has recently been reviewed by Schlosser (1992). TP Write is currently a DOS-based program that allows the user to make selections from menu screens that produce narrative text that can be edited by a word processor program. The system covers both patient and provider data as well as diagnostic information, reason for treatment, description of treatment, functional impairment, mental status, psychological test results, previous treatment, treatment modalities, goals, and treatment progress. It produces a number of reports including initial treatment plans, treatment plan updates, and clinical progress notes, mental status reports, and generates reports for referral sources. Importantly, the user can create "custom" report formats for his or her own unique purposes.

Another approach to automated treatment plans is offered through Caldwell Report (1996). This model uses the MMPI-2 and generates specific treatment information categorized by prognosis (baseline suicidal risk, potential for chemical dependency, likely acting out behaviors, and possible psychopharmacological interventions), pitfalls (transference problems, defensiveness and denial, and interfering psychological styles), and positive interview intervention (specific points of focus, consideration as to significant other involvement, and beneficial directions for treatment to proceed). This system uses expert logic in producing individually tailored treatment planning information.

A third approach to treatment planning is the electronic treatment plan and the electronic treatment plan formulary developed by The Psychological Corporation (1999) for its Notewriter product line. This system allows users to develop step-by-step treatment plans specifying a host of relevant parameters (e.g., provider, diagnosis, type of treatments, target behaviors, type of medication, type of assessment, number of authorized sessions, review cycle, and outcome measures to be employed), which are then integrated into a comprehensive computerized patient record that subsequently directs the treatment process. Once signed off by a managed care company or payer, the treatment plan electronically scrubs the claim so that when it reaches the MCO, the claim is ready for review without human intervention. The treatment plan formulary allows for the generation of modal treatment plans based on data developed through repeated trials of patients with given symptoms or disorders. These plans can be downloaded automatically by the host site and reviewed by the user. Electronic mail allows for an ongoing dialogue between the practitioner and the case reviewer to establish the parameters of treatment for a given case. In this way the electronic treatment plan becomes a guide to treatment based on aggregate data collected from many different clinicians seeing similar patients.

Computer-Driven Evaluation Models in Clinical Care

Due to increased demands for accountability, a growing trend has been the development of standardized treatment protocols that are designed as specific interventions for specific clinical problems. These protocols often follow very circumscribed workbooks that detail the treatment process. Deriving from the clinical laboratory, these techniques are often the most well researched and empirically supported interventions for a given problem. Although strongly buttressed by research support, these treatments have come under critical attack as being biased in favor of short-term treatment approaches, overly represented by behavioral approaches that lend themselves to ease of treatment specification, focusing primarily on circumscribed problems, embracing a nomothetic approach disregarding the idiographic nature of clinical problems, and reflecting a subtle science-centric bias (Levant, 1995). Although definite problems exist in how "prescriptive treatments" have been construed, the concept of relatively well-defined interventions for particular disorders has much to offer, especially in standardization of treatment protocols for clinical investigation. Computer technology provides a method to help define various interventions employed and a way to track outcome to evaluate the effectiveness of particular treatment methods or packages. The technology, however, will not be of significant value until research models evolve that are acceptable to the clinical community and that simultaneously meet basic standards for experimental investigation.

Assessing value in psychotherapy is complicated by how the process is approached by the various participants. An ongoing controversy (Stricker & Trierweiler, 1995) exists between the view of "clinical scientists" and "clinical practitioners" concerning the relevancy of particular types of outcome studies and the meaningfulness of results that derive. It should be noted, however, that behavioral science has no corner on this dispute. As Beutler, Williams, Wakefield, and Entwistle (1995) note:

> In virtually every discipline in which the usual access to knowledge is through the scientific method, scientists have lamented that practitioners are inadequately trained, are insensitive to the value of scientific findings, and fail to read the right journals. Conversely, practitioners are dismayed because scientists offer too little, are consumed by irrelevant questions, and fail to appreciate the knowledge that arises from practice. (p. 985)

The current "scientific trend" in the behavioral sciences is most clearly away from a broad-stroke evaluation of psychotherapy and toward treatment specification. The tradition of research on psychotherapy has focused on either highly controlled experimental conditions that lend themselves to little or no generalizability (Persons, 1991) or more loosely defined studies of more generic approaches that were relatively vague in definition and description of subject variables, therapeutic variables, and experimental conditions. Those favoring the "clinical scientist model" have contributed a fairly narrow definition of "empirically validated" treatment techniques. It is not surprising, given that most clinicians do little or no research, that initial developments in prescriptive treatments and treatment guidelines have originated more from the clinical laboratory than from the field. The questions asked from the clinical scientist model typically take the form of: What type of treatment, for what type of problem, at what duration, as assessed by what measurements is efficacious relative to appropriate control conditions? From the clinical scientist model, the belief that all forms of psychotherapy are effective for all problems is clearly not a very convincing standard for assessing value.

Alternatively, clinical practitioners are typically more interested in asking broad, pragmatic, and generic questions such as: Is this treatment effective for this general disorder as provided by clinicians in the field? Stricker and Trierweiler (1995) have discussed what they refer to as the "local scientist model," which is an attempt to articulate how the application of scientific thought and behavior can guide and shape decision making in the clinical setting. Seligman (1995) has strongly argued for a more open view of clinical research that places a higher premium on the results of field studies. In his review of *Consumer Reports*'s psychotherapy outcome study (Mental Health: Does Therapy Help? 1995), Seligman (1995) speaks to the issues that have frustrated both clinicians and clinical scientists. Efficacy studies of outcome are by definition highly controlled and lead to strict definition of treatment variables but do not necessarily impact the behavior of the provider community. Critics point out that such treatments do not reflect the moment-to-moment decision points of "actual therapy" nor do they provide the clinician with the flexibility to change goals or interventions based on client issues or idiosyncratic responses to the intervention. Concern has been raised by practitioners at the possibility that only certain empirically validated treatments that have rigorous empirical support will ultimately be included in lists of reimbursable services. Seligman (1995), however, argues for the value of clinical field studies that approximate more closely the conditions faced by practitioners in the clinical arena. Thus, he advocates a role for effectiveness studies that look at the outcome of psychotherapy for less rigorously defined patient groups treated by less standardized interventions. Herein lies the value of computer technology as multiple providers within an integrated system can routinely collect standardized outcome data to begin to amass a data set from which clinical effectiveness can be evaluated.

The issue becomes more complicated when payer groups enter the discussion. Business and industry, the primary purchaser of behavioral health services, have recently demanded outcome data to document value. Predictably, they are concerned with the cost of intervention and tend to favor briefer, less expensive treatment approaches. The questions asked by business and industry have little to do with professional arguments about efficacy versus effectiveness. The questions asked by payer groups tend to be: What is the relative cost of a behavioral health product (i.e., intervention)? Who should provide it? What is the benefit of the service to the employee? How does it affect the bottom line? For business and industry, the bottom line speaks more to productivity and associated variables (e.g., absenteeism, "burn out," level of performance, cost, medical cost offset, etc.) and less to concerns about the employee's general state of well-being, although this too is important to many companies. Concern about the definition of the appropriate dependent variable (i.e., enhanced productivity versus symptom reduction) and issues related to relative cost more clearly define the agenda of payer groups.

Professional guilds have also begun to respond to the challenge for convincing outcomes by establishing standards of care and practice guidelines. The result is a general move toward increased accountability where the relevant question has been defined as: Is the psychotherapeutic treatment supported by replicable research demonstrating efficacy as compared to psychopharmacological intervention, placebo, or to an already proven and well supported method of intervention (Barlow, 1994). The American Psychiatric Association has published two clinical practice guidelines, one for eating disorders and one for mood disorders (Barlow, 1994). Not surprisingly, the guidelines for treating major depression call for the use of medication as the first-line intervention.

Division 12 (Clinical) of the American Psychological Association has established a task force, Task Force for the Promotion and Dissemination of Psychological Procedures, to develop models for identifying "efficacious" treatments and disseminating these empirically validated treatments to the provider community (Chambless, 1995). Sanderson (1995) lists 25 empirically validated treatment techniques that derive from the work of the Division 12 task force. Of these 25 empirically validated treatments, all but four were either behavioral, cognitive, or cognitive–behavioral in description, leading to concern about possible bias toward a particular method or approach (Levant, 1995; Kovacs, 1996).

The role of computer technology in prescriptive treatment will be prominent. The availability of sophisticated computerized patient records will allow clinicians in diverse settings to utilize standardized assessment and outcome measures to evaluate the effectiveness and cost associated with clinically standardized treatments for specifically defined diagnoses, problems, or behavioral targets. The definition of clinically standardized treatments will result from on-line session ratings by clinicians of specific in-session behaviors, methods, and general procedures. Computer technology provides a way for the clinician in the field to accurately report what they do session to session. Heretofore, practitioners have not really developed a workable model for collecting clinical treatment or outcome data. The mechanism to collect and store objective clinical outcome data was simply not available. With the advent of powerful personal computer systems with relational databases, clinicians will soon have tremendous tools for generating a strong empirical base for commonly employed procedures. These systems will make it possible for clinicians in the field to participate in large-scale field trials and to connect on-line to various research-oriented databases to share standardized data. Research protocols will be delivered on-line, informed patient consent will be obtained, and outcome data will be forwarded automatically for critical review. Once large databases have been established, specific questions will be asked of the anonymous data that can be used to define more effective treatment approaches. In this fashion, some of the historical friction between clinical researchers and practitioners may dissipate as the results of rigorous controlled studies from the laboratory can be further scrutinized by examination of similar treatment data stored in the computerized database. In this fashion science can more directly support and guide clinical practice and the local clinical scientist (Stricker & Trierweiler, 1995) will be able to generate further data to stimulate new research questions for more rigorous evaluation in the controlled laboratory setting.

With the availability of large standardized databases on treatment outcome, computer technology will be invaluable in disseminating information on clinically effective treatments to practitioners. Furthermore, interactive technology will be available to provide on-line training in the delivery of these services. The potential for sophisticated on-line training forums with associated continuing education credits and specialized credentialing is also a realistic possibility. On-line credentialing agencies will support these training programs and will disperse provider information regarding qualifications to appropriate payer groups. In this fashion technology will advance clinical practice and clinical practice will help define further technological advances as systems emerge to serve the clinician in developing an empirical data base. Empirically validated treatments may originate from the clinical laboratory where care and precision can be embraced to define relevant parameters, but will ultimately have to pass the test of real world outcomes.

Accurately assessing the current trends, Therapy Works (1999) was introduced by The Psychological Corporation, a major publisher of psychological assessment and training materials, has recently announced the release of a number of prescriptive treatment programs including units on the treatment of panic disorder, agoraphobia, generalized anxiety disorder, phobias, and major depressive disorder. The package of products includes client workbooks/guides, therapist treatment manuals, client videotapes, and various assessment instruments. Programs for future release include treatment of female assault victims, addictive behaviors, sexual arousal problems, major depression, eating disorders, obsessive–compulsive disorder, social phobia, shyness and social anxiety for children, and school refusal behavior. These treatment programs have been developed by leading researchers and in all cases are supported by outcome data. The next logical step is the computerization of these protocols and the testing of these treatment programs by clinicians in the field who will doubtlessly add their own knowledge base and unique clinical nuances to these standardized treatments. The technology is now available for large relatively well-controlled field studies to be performed to convert these empirically validated treatments into a consumer-sensitive context as clinically effective treatments.

The introduction of these types of products on the market further reinforce the concept of making assessment and treatment information available to practitioners interested in using the emerging computer technology. More and varied treatment modules will be developed and in a rather short time frame will be available for downloading to office systems. Although many of these products will be proprietary, it would seem reasonable that professional associations also might help to disseminate these types of materials to clinicians in the field at modest charges or as a part of an association shareware program whereby the information is disseminated without charge.

Computerization and Psychoeducational Treatments

Pipal (1995) has correctly charged that behavioral science is not in the purest sense a medical profession. She argues that due primarily to a desire for third-party reimbursement, behavioral practitioners now find themselves embroiled in the medical–economic issues of the time. Like Albee (1968) many years earlier, she suggests that our identity as a profession is more closely allied with education (and religion) rather than with medicine per se. Interestingly, some realignment with education may help behavioral practitioners compete more successfully in the medical marketplace. Behavioral practitioners may be especially well prepared to develop educational materials that can be used to decrease costs associated with treatment of behavioral disorders.

At the heart of the managed care movement is the goal of reducing cost of care per session. Cost containment with traditional psychotherapeutic models of care will only go so far before a diminishing return (e.g., outcome) will force the development of alternative modes of treatment. Especially promising are group-oriented treatments where a larger number of participants can avail themselves of professional support and assistance at a fraction of the cost for traditional individual therapy models. Most large managed care companies are now thinking in terms of a continuum of care that will provide a wider range of services than psychiatric hospitalization and outpatient psychotherapy. A specific example is the emergence of outpatient structured day programs to complement expensive psychiatric hospitalization. It is likely that outpatient educational services will be developed to complement traditional psychotherapy in much the same fashion. For example, Seligman (1995) reports favorable outcome for problem drinking for those who attend Alcoholics Anonymous meetings. Long established and fairly well structured, these voluntary programs offer emotional and spiritual support, structure, an alternative worldview, a prescription for success, and an ongoing follow-up and maintenance system. Given the nature of most problems in living (Szasz, 1960), it would seem that educationally oriented treatment programs could be developed to teach specific skills and to address specific deficiencies in a group format.

Computer technology is especially adaptive to these types of group interventions, as the new technology allows an untapped flexibility for automating and standardizing educational materials to facilitate group discussions and to prompt modeling and behavioral rehearsal. Conceivably, prepackaged psychoeducational units covering a variety of subjects soon will become available to augment the clinical interventions and skill of practitioners. Examples might include units on developing social skills, reducing aggressive behavior, modifying eating problems (anorexia and bulimia), reducing anxiety through cognitive techniques, understanding and changing depressive mode, overcoming shyness, developing assertive skills, and so on. The use of LED projection panels allow computers to drive wall-sized multimedia presentations of educational materials for large group presentations.

Computerized patient records will provide for the recording of measures of change with relative ease across large numbers of patients, thereby creating a database to evaluate the effectiveness of these interventions. Standardized formats would allow for assessment of outcome and clinical replication of successful programs. Packaging of programs as self-contained units would facilitate program evaluation. Psychoeducational treatment packages might augment ongoing therapy or replace individual therapy modalities for certain disorders depending on the results of clinical field studies.

One company, Quinco Behavioral Health Systems (1995), is presently offering a series of standardized group treatments for a number of disorders including depression, adolescent issues, victims of abuse, and so on. These types of products would seem to fit very well with the predicted trend of delivering more clinical services through group psychoeducational modalities. Although these specific programs are not yet computerized, this appears to be the next logical step, as many of these materials could be released through CD-ROM and multimedia technology.

COMPUTERIZED DECISION-MAKING MODELS

The area of intellectual modeling to develop "smart models" to make accurate decisions about placement, triage, risk, and level of care are potentially fertile areas for ongoing research and development. Research by Kopta, Lowry, and Beutler (1994) suggests that recovery from psychological symptoms occurs in stages. Specifically, chronic distress symptoms (e.g., phobic anxiety, obsessional symptoms, and depression) remit most rapidly, with 60–86% of the patient sample achieving remission at 52 sessions. Characterological symptoms (e.g., hostility, paranoid ideation, and psychoticism) respond the slowest, with less than 59% of the patients showing clinically significant recovery at 52 sessions. Acute distress symptoms show the highest average percentage of patients recovered across doses (68–95%). Overall, these data suggest that a typical outpatient required about a year of psychotherapy to have a 75% chance of symptomatic recovery. These findings also suggest that recovery is a multidimensional process, cutting across both symptoms and patients, with some symptoms and/or patients remitting faster relative to others. These findings highlight the need for more advanced decision-making tools utilizing diagnostic, symptom, psychometric, and other patient demographic, historical, and functional variables to facilitate clinical decision making. Such efforts promise dividends for maximizing cost-effectiveness of treatment and also selection of the optimal level and intensity of care for a given patient to facilitate multidimensional recovery.

Early decision-making models (e.g., Flynn & Henisz, 1975; Costello, Dulcan, & Kalas, 1991) were largely developed in the private sector to allow clinicians to make decisions about the need for psychiatric hospitalization. These models, developed in the late 1960s and early 1970s, represented an advancement in reducing clinician-derived variability in decision making, but as a whole suffered from inadequate psychometric qualities (Gray & Glazer, 1994). These scales were typically employed for retrospective chart review to validate the judgments of inexperienced workers and to justify decisions for hospitalization. In most cases these early tools were not utilized as prospective predictors for level of care decisions.

These scales were largely developed for adult psychiatric settings with one notable exception, Costello and co-workers' (1991) checklist of criteria for hospitalization of children. This scale, a modification of the Flynn and Henisz (1975) scale of criteria for adult hospitalization, included differentially weighted items sampling such domains as patient aggressiveness, mental status, physical condition, family functioning, and clinician's concern (e.g., acute or chronic nature of the condition). This 12-item scale, designed for use with children under the age of 12, was shown to predict correctly in over 95% of the cases whether the child was hospitalized or treated in an outpatient setting. In addition, a shortened 6-item factor-derived checklist was only slightly less accurate in making these predictions, predicting treatment level in over 94% of these cases. This scale is thus notable not only in its application to psychiatric decision making with children but in its psychometric properties, with interrater reliability found to be in the .68 to .79 range. This scale suffered from the same limitations inherent to its predecessors. It was not capable of facilitating decision making in continuous care environments that included treatment options less restrictive than hospitalization (e.g., partial hospitalization). It also was not computerized, and thus did not have the power to more easily manage and manipulate broad-based assessment data for prescriptive treatment planning. It was a promising first step, however, in the development of a sophisticated computerized instrument capable of utilizing a large clinical database to facilitate sophisticated decision making (e.g., level of care).

In contrast to these early checklists, currently available or soon-to-be-available computerized tools will assist clinicians in making rapid, empirically based treatment decisions. These tools promise to greatly enhance the clinician's ability to rapidly and accurately make clinical decisions about all aspects of treatment management, including assessment, treatment planning, the monitoring of therapeutic effect, and tracking of behavioral targets and outcome. These tools will allow the clinician to balance the competing demands of clinical and therapeutic integrity with cost-effectiveness of treatment. Using these models, clinicians will be better able to make decisions about clinically effective treatments, including specifics about appropriate level of care, dosage, and optimal therapeutic strategies for a given patient. In addition, these tools will enable the clinician to accurately assess on-line session-to-session changes in patient functioning. This capability allows for a continuous reevaluation of treatment decisions, including considerations about type of intervention (psychotherapeutic or psychopharmacological) and associated parameters (level of care and appropriate dosage). Specifically, these tools will assist the clinician in making accurate diagnostic decisions on-line and will consider critical patient, therapist, and environmental variables in determining the appropriate care for a given patient (Beutler & Williams, 1995).

Computerized decisional tools fall into two broad categories: (1) models based on clinical logic to aid diagnostic, patient placement, and level of risk decisions, and (2) those based on computer-generated algorithms derived from actuarially derived clinical data to make treatment-planning decisions. Among currently available or soon-to-be-available tools falling in the first category are computerized branching assessment instruments and instruments useful for gross treatment assignment decisions based on baseline screening of patient functioning. Tools using sophisticated algorithms are the Systematic Treatment Selection model of Beutler and Clarkin (1990) and PsychPro, developed by Gray and Glazer (1994), both of which convert weighted clinician-based assessment ratings of patient functional status into level of care decisions.

Among models based on clinical logic, several are currently available that utilize computer technology to assist with diagnostic choice (First et al., 1996c). Such instruments as the DTREE use branching logic, whereby a patient, parent, or provider can answer questions on-line about presenting symptoms and problems. The system guides the user through response choices to the point of arriving at approximate diagnoses or disorders to be ruled out. Using this technology, vast amounts of information can be processed quickly, leading to faster and often more accurate diagnostic decisions.

A second instrument utilizing clinical logic to assist treatment decisions is the Outcome Questionnaire (OQ-45.1), developed by Lambert, Lunnen, Umphress, Hansen, and Birlingame (1994). Designed primarily for purposes of monitoring progress in outpatient psychotherapy, rather than for diagnostic purposes, the OQ 45.1 can also be used as a baseline screening instrument for purposes of treatment placement decisions. Based on Lambert's (1983) multidimensional conceptualization of patient functioning, the OQ-45.1 contains 45 items in the areas of symptom distress, social role functioning, and interpersonal relationships. Using the OQ-45.1, a patient's overall functioning, as well as his or her functioning in each of these areas, is rated at baseline, during therapy, and at termination, allowing for a session-to-session assessment. Each item is scored on a 5-point Likert scale, yielding a total score range of 0 to 180. Change from session to session is assessed with reference to this total score, with changes from baseline greater than or equal to 12 points considered to be clinically meaningful. The OQ-45.1, available in a Windows application, has separate undergraduate and multiple patient (e.g., community mental health setting) norms and possesses impressive psychometric properties while remaining brief enough to be clinically useful. The multidimensional nature of the OQ-45.1 is a strength in monitoring change in psychotherapy, particularly in light of research (Howard, Leuger, Maling, & Martinovish, 1993), suggesting that such change occurs in a stepwise pattern of recovery across symptoms such as subjective distress, social and interpersonal functioning, and work functioning.

A third example of expert clinical systems is the OPTAIO Practice Manager (1999) Behavior Outcome Measurement System. This system, which is one feature of a comprehensive behavioral health care management information system, allows the clinician to select target behaviors from a table-driven menu of over 1300 different behaviors derived from the various DSM-IV diagnostic entities. These target behaviors are clinician rated using operationally defined anchors forming one idiographic component of the OPTAIO assessment system. Nomothetic ratings across various outcome variables (both Likert scales and psychometric instruments) are also collected. Similarly, patient ratings of outcome by session can also be collected. These data are then automatically plotted by intervention, medication, and time, compiling graphic depictions of the treatment process for review and comparison. This system further allows the clinician to assess risk of suicide and aggressive behavior using comprehensive theoretical, clinical, and epidemiological models to identify relevant predictor variables (Bongar, 1992; Truscott, Evans, & Mansell, 1995). OPTAIO Practice Manager (1999) uses sophisticated intellectual models to produce a treatment plan formulary that automatically reviews treatment decisions and patient progress to generate routine treatment decisions (e.g., to extend treatment, to recommend consultation, to collect specific types of data, to require a formal case review, etc.) using data derived from relational databases. This type of system is designed to assist providers and payers to more accurately evaluate outcome and to support clinical decision making.

Computer systems also store and integrate multidimensional data from which to derive treatment decisions using computer-generated algorithms. Two commercially available clinical decision-making tools are PsychPro (Gray & Glazer, 1994) and the systematic treatment selection system (Beutler & Clarkin, 1990). PsychPro uses sophisticated decision-making models utilizing actuarially derived clinical data to predict level of requisite care. Its developers sought to design a tool that could go beyond the dichotomous nature (e.g., admit–not admit) of early decision-making checklists to allow for decisional support along a continuum from most (e.g., inpatient) to least (e.g., outpatient) restrictive treatment setting with various intermediate options, including day treatment.

Gray and Glazer identified five clinical dimensions that were thought to be critical to clinical decision making. These dimensions included occurrence of dangerous behavior, social performance, and availability of social resources, along with provider opinion regarding risk of dangerousness and/or relapse as well as risk of medical complications due to ongoing substance abuse. A patient is rated on each of these dimensions using a three-point scale, with a "3" consistent with inpatient treatment, a "1" consistent with standard outpatient treatment and a "2" consistent with diversion care, such as day treatment or other outpatient alternatives. Behavioral anchors are provided to facilitate these ratings. These scores contribute to a weighted clinical profile that predicts intensity and requisite level of care. Psychometric properties for PsychPro are promising, with interrator reliability in the .73 to .80 range. Early validation studies support the clinical usefulness of the computer model compared with expert clinical judgments.

Like PsychPro, the systematic treatment selection (STS) model of Beutler and Clarkin (1990) utilizes computer-generated algorithms, based on empirically derived data, to facilitate treatment selection decision making. Unlike PsychPro, which is designed to support level of care and substance abuse treatment decisions, STS was designed to generate a comprehensive functional assessment to assist in clinical decision making across many aspects of outpatient treatment, including level of care, dosage, intensity, and even choice of treatment techniques. STS integrates assessment and treatment planning by guiding and prompting the clinician for critical information, including diagnostic, background, clinical impression and standardized test score input (Beutler & Williams, 1995). STS then uses computer-generated algorithms for purposes of prescriptive treatment planning. It differs from the diagnostic branching tools in that patient functional status (in nine broad areas), rather than diagnosis, is the basis for treatment planning decisions.

These nine broad areas, each with several decisional branches, include considerations such as assessed need for a restrictive setting, variations in the chronicity and complexity of the problem, variations in patient motivation, the patient's openness to the therapist's suggestions, patient demographics, and the role of various therapist factors. Algorithms based on these factors, along with entry of scores from psychometric assessment instruments, such as the Beck Depression Inventory and the MMPI, are used to compile specific prescriptive treatment determinations presented in a comprehensive report. The report includes suggestions regarding therapist style of interaction and the strategies and techniques that may be most helpful given the characteristics of the patient (Beutler & Williams, 1995).

The STS model is noteworthy in several regards:

1. It represents a hybrid of a theoretically based assessment instrument that also utilizes actuarially based data to make prescriptive treatment decisions. In addition, the database is continuously updated with each new data entry.
2. It is a multimedia instrument available in Windows offering audio and video presentation of screen images.
3. Numerous concurrent validation studies are being conducted by Beutler and his colleagues (i.e., using the STS for treatment planning with couples in which alcoholism is a focus of treatment).

This instrument is illustrative of the power of computer-based systems that utilize theoretical constructs and a strong empirical base from which to guide clinical decision making.

These computerized decision-making tools represent the potential of the marriage between strong clinical and theoretical constructs with computer systems using relational databases from which to build empirical models for assessment and treatment. Several potential advantages derive from these types of models. First, these tools represent a significant change in clinical decision-making capability as clinician judgment is augmented and refined by the virtually unlimited capability of computer systems to quickly integrate vast amounts of multidimensional data into useful empirical decision support. Second, these tools offer the capability of reducing provider-derived variability in decision making. Clinicians will have immediately available to them continuously updated and clinically accurate information to assist/guide their decision making in the areas of diagnosis, risk, and treatment (optimal intensity, level, and dosage of care). Third, these systems offer the functionality to monitor session-to-session changes in therapy through on-line entry of clinician ratings, patient ratings, and patient response to psychometrically sound outcome instruments.

Soon, electronic treatment templates will be developed corresponding to successful treatment outcome results for specific problems or difficulties. Electronic treatment plans will incorporate these trends to match patients to treatment recommendations. These treatment plans will document multiple dimensions of care and help direct the clinician to more effective treatment choices. Providers will communicate electronically with case managers or peer reviewers to blend clinical sophistication with empirical predictive data. Providers will be evaluated based on their effectiveness compared with empirically derived standards of care. Review of care will be in real time and will largely end the "paper process" of endless forms to be completed on demand by various administrative entities.

Clinically effective care will be rewarded with less stringent oversight of providers and more liberal practice standards. Much of the management of care will migrate to the community level where provider groups will utilize the emerging decision-making models to assist them in providing clinically meaningful and cost-effective care. Providers will develop their own data systems and will contract with various business entities marketing their track record of clinical effectiveness.

What will separate these groups? Groups and individual providers that flourish will be those that are electronically connected to various administrative entities that will secure contracts, evaluate outcome, and provide claims processing. Those that have sophisticated computer applications will have a decided advantage in the capability to empirically support their treatment decisions and in generating various data-based reports for business and industry. The key will be the integration of outcome data and financial data to form a blend of value more acceptable to providers and patients.

THE EVALUATION OF OUTCOME

As Schlosser (1995) correctly points out, many semantic issues revolve around the issues of assessment of clinical outcome. As Seligman (1995) has noted, differences exist between clinical scientists and "clinical practitioners" in how they define adequate measurement of outcome. A recent survey of brief therapies (Steenbarger, 1994) suggested that measurement of outcome is a multidimensional problem involving such complex variables as patient capacity for attachment, involvement, patient expectations about duration of care, therapist degree of influence, the therapist–patient capacity for relatedness, patient–therapist match along multiple dimensions, and posttherapy environmental stress and level of social support. Steenbarger (1994) further suggests that outcome may be associated with different degrees of patient readiness to deal with different stages of the therapy process (e.g., problem identification, therapy work, and consolidation).

Persons (1991) suggests that psychotherapy research models for outcome studies do not reflect current models of therapy. She argues for a case formulation model in which the idiographic nuances of a clinical case are examined in a theory-rich fashion that integrates assessment and treatment. From this model she notes that each patient could have a different set of idiographic measures for assessing outcome that reflect the specific theoretical school of thought. The dependent measures she describes include mean pre- to postchange scores for ratings of clinical problems (converted to mean proportion of change over all problems identified) for each patient, proportion of patients in experimental groups reaching the "nondeviant" range for all identified problems, and mean improvement in daily functioning. As can be seen, Persons (1991) is arguing for an approach that focuses on the idiographic characteristics (behavior) of a given patient, while also allowing for examination across different schools of thought or different types of therapeutic intervention.

Eckert (1994) has borrowed concepts from industrial quality improvement research [i.e., the Deming–Shewhart cycle (Deming, 1986)] in proposing that both the process and outcome be evaluated simultaneously. He argues that process can be better understood through standardization including such concepts as use of practice guidelines, formulation of standardized treatments, use of treatment manuals, and even standardized psychotherapy training for behavioral health graduate students. He states: "Greatest effectiveness may be achieved when process standardization is closely linked with multidimensional outcome measurement" (Eckert, 1994, p. 6). He is careful to note, however, that "the purpose of standardization is not to eliminate the legitimate exercise of clinical judgement" (p. 6). Eckert (1994) also notes that "value is optimized at the level of quality yielding the greatest possible degree of *long-term* cost containment" (p. 6). Schlosser (1995) argues for a patient-centric view of outcome that places a premium on patient experience and level of functioning.

Review of health care payers yields yet another set of priorities. Bilbrey and Bilbrey (1995) note that private and public payer groups were significantly interested in customer satisfaction data but were also interested in cost-benefit data and in data that would assist in selection of providers. Responding tongue-in-cheek, Williams (1995) reports on how his practice would change if he managed his practice by catering solely to patient satisfaction.

The picture that emerges is one of very different attitudes and priorities advanced by different players in the outcome assessment arena. Schlosser (1995) cautions to be aware of "turf and political issues." Questions posed include: Who decides what types of measures will be employed? When will they be administered? Who will provide outcome data (e.g., patients, providers, business managers, etc.). How are results analyzed and disseminated? To whom should data be released and for what purpose? How does the patient fit into the picture? These are complex and difficult questions that are answered in different ways by each of the participants.

In keeping with the local scientist model, it is proposed that providers are in the best position to define relevant outcome variables that are sensitive to both patients and to the needs of business and industry. Computer systems will be central to this evolution of concepts. Computer systems are needed that will collect a broad spectrum of reliable and valid information including data on patient variables, therapist variables, and treatment variables. Multidimensional outcome assessment models need to be developed that examine both idiographic and nomothetic measures and that call for repeated measurement over time. Immediate and summary feedback to providers and patients involved in the treatment process should be a function included in these systems. The technology must be affordable to clinicians so they can actively participate in the outcome evaluation process. By systematically collecting computerized data, providers will be able to transmit data to research databases where it can be analyzed and disseminated to providers, networks, and to payer groups.

Prototypes of comprehensive computerized patient records currently are being developed and tested clinically (The Psychological Corporation, 1999). They will be available in the very near future, first to large provider groups affiliated with specific payers, and ultimately to professional associations (Newman, 1995) and providers

(Meredith & Bair, 1995). These systems will allow clinicians to participate in active research protocols while performing routine clinical activities. With one-step data entry, clinicians will enter financial and treatment information quickly and efficiently following the provision of a clinical service. With patient authorization, these data will be used to shape the emerging industry.

THE DATA SET

Behavioral health care systems have begun to struggle with what constitutes the most appropriate data set for evaluation of outcome. Stated more scientifically, what is it that should be measured and what are the most reliable and valid methods to generate such data? As the American Psychological Association notes (1993), the dearth of outcome information inhibits payers, providers and patients. Managed care entities that are moving in the direction of emphasizing value as a primary product that are also interested in data such as utilization, cost effectiveness, cost by type and unit of service, rate structure and cost per consumer treated, and data related to specific (and relative) provider effectiveness might be added to this list (Bilbrey & Bilbrey, 1995).

Several guidelines must be addressed to satisfy the scientific community. Measures first must be psychometrically sound. Measurement sophistication and quality should not be sacrificed in the face of increasing demand by business and industry for "data." This area creates a rich focus for psychometric research designed to quickly and accurately measure various patient characteristics and to design sensitive outcome instruments. Instruments used must be relatively simple, quick to administer, and designed for low-cost administrations.

What type of clinical outcome data will be collected within these systems? Outcome data fall roughly into five categories. The first type of information and by far the most rudimentary and widely employed are various posttreatment paper-and-pencil satisfaction inventories sent to patients to report on their treatment experiences. These ask the patient to rate improvement and also request information about the qualitative aspects of care, for example, attitudes of personnel, accessibility and general satisfaction, and so forth.

The second level of outcome data derives from periodic clinician ratings of change. These ratings may be idiographic in nature (rating of specific behaviors or problems for a given patient) or may be nomothetic, creating a standardized data set for comparison across different patients or patient groups. These too can be paper and pencil, but increasingly they are becoming available on-line with data entry at the computer terminal. These data sets must pass the test of different schools of thought so that relevant comparisons can be made across different types of interventions. Sophisticated systems now exist that automatically plot treatment outcome by session across time and by method of intervention (The Psychological Corporation, 1999). Thus, graphic depictions of patient progress across any number of relevant dimensions are immediately available to the clinician.

The third type of data supports complex algorithms that drive decision-making models to assist with the development of treatment plans or in some cases with triage of patients to the most cost-efficient level of care. These systems may be either paper and pencil or on-line and can involve patient self-report and/or clinician ratings (see section on computerized decision-making models).

The fourth type of primary data involves the patient's ongoing evaluation of their own treatment. As Ball (1995) stated: "The major variable being left out of medical information systems is the patient." Using computerized technology, it is a very easy and quick task to request patient feedback and report to the patient's provider comments about goals, level of satisfaction, attitudes about treatment, and so on. Certainly these data are not without problems and can reflect both positive and negative biases dependent on a number of issues including transference, personality type, or type and degree of pathology. A growing awareness, however, suggests that patients will have increased input into these emerging outcome systems (Schlosser, 1995), but that these types of data should be buttressed by other measures of change including ratings by clinicians and/or other observers (e.g., parents and teacher). Although specific data about session-to-session observations and impressions will be important, more general measures of daily functioning also will be useful in documenting the type of change that is of interest to payer groups.

The fifth type of data currently being collected deals less directly with the process of treatment but instead relates treatment to function in the workplace. Increasingly, business/industry is willing to provide data on patients such as absenteeism, work attitudes, accidents in the workplace, medical costs, performance evaluations, and so on. In the not to distant future, a markedly different type of data relating to employee job performance and related variables (e.g., general health) will enter the pool of other types of outcome information. Certainly, these movements champion the "value" issue in therapy, as "benefit" may be more broadly defined than cost savings alone.

Dosage and Clinical Treatment

Effective therapy may not always be brief therapy, although this has been the model advocated by some payers and some therapeutic schools of thought. With collection of both clinical outcome data and financial data across time, an accurate understanding of treatment by time interactions will result. For example, certain disorders might respond well to longer, more supportive or "uncovering" therapies, and might prove to be more rather than less cost-effective when compared to repeated episodes of brief therapy. On the other hand, some disorders may respond to an optimal number of treatment sessions, with no evidence to support a clinical advantage for longer durations of treatment. The scientific study of the "dosage model" (Howard et al., 1993) for psychotherapy offers promise in uncovering the difficulties associated with treating the relatively small percentage of patients who receive the majority of financial resources. Using computer models to triage patients to the most appropriate but least expensive level of care also will become a significant development as the profession struggles with providing optimum levels of care/optimum dosage.

The Evaluation of Providers

Provider Profiling

Increasingly, pressure is being applied by payers, consumers, governmental bodies, and accreditation agencies for documentation of provider effectiveness. Patient ratings and ratings by peer reviewers of practitioner case management skills presently are being used to assess provider performance. Hiatt and Hargrove (1995) reported on a detailed study of therapists in a managed care setting. Results of their investigation essentially confirmed results of better-controlled laboratory studies of the role of therapist variables in clinical outcome (Beutler, Crago, & Arizemdi, 1986; Lambert, Shapiro, & Bergin, 1986). They found a significant and positive relationship between patient ratings of satisfaction and peer ratings of case management skill. They concluded from their work that therapist characteristics associated positively with outcome were empathy and the use of active techniques. Highly effective therapists were significantly more likely to be seen as "understanding" and "to have developed an active plan to promote problem resolution."

Historically, "provider profiling" too often consisted primarily of "cost profiling" (Brown et al., 1995). Both cost of care and clinical effectiveness need to be examined. Providers doubtlessly will be profiled in terms of clinical trends and attitude. Systems will be designed to constantly upgrade clinical standards. Providers will be able to participate in the development of assessment methodologies and approaches, thereby removing some of the threat associated with increased accountability deriving from the immediate availability of on-line clinical outcome data.

As more powerful systems develop to assess provider characteristics, credentials, and performance, the industry will attempt to identify "effective providers." Potential abuses can occur in this process if payers begin to selectively contract based on provider profiles. By participating actively in the evaluation development process and actively contributing to computer data banks, providers will amass their own set of data to use in approaching payers and business/industry.

Rather than discipline providers through elimination from panels, a more enlightened process will be the identification of provider strengths and weaknesses accompanied by the development of training programs to enhance provider skills and effectiveness. Providers with "sterling records" or those who develop the requisite skills to meet the new accountability standards will receive more autonomy and enjoy more freedom to exercise their best clinical judgment. Those providers who develop good working relationships with patients and who treat disorders fairly efficiently will receive the majority of referrals in this more accountable system. Quality will become an important standard and will be reflected in marketing efforts by behavioral practitioners at the local, regional, and national level.

PARTICIPATIVE CARE

Patients will be brought actively into the process. Central to the concept of "participative care" is that the patient will be an active participant not only in the treatment process but also in evaluating the results of treatment. To date, post hoc patient satisfaction data are the primary example of this emerging trend. Much more is to come. Increasingly patients will be asked to evaluate treatment sessions and to assess their ongoing progress along relevant dimensions. Patients will have input into choice of treatment goals and will receive regular feedback as to their level of progress. The level of scrutiny of providers will increase not only from administrative systems but also from patients more actively involved in their own change process. Triage decisions related to intensity and frequency of care will reflect the patient's attitude, motivation, and responsiveness to care as variables examined through new statistically derived predictive models.

Advantages to Providers

The information revolution occurring in mental health promises to create a number of advantages and benefits for the practitioner. Introducing information technology to the typical practice will add a new dimension to the provider's armamentarium that can potentially provide a competitive edge. Information will be the name of the game. For the first time, providers will participate in large-scale standardized evaluation of "clinical effectiveness" in the field setting. Computerized patient records will greatly reduce time demands by creating an on-line chart that is automatically uploaded to the host site. Presently, too much time is spent in financially unproductive information gathering, retrieval, and dissemination. Record keeping will be simplified, rapid, and comprehensive. Sophisticated systems will allow the clinician to enter clinical/financial data and to update treatment plans and write clinical notes with the same operation. Administrative efficiency will be greatly enhanced. Information systems will create the conduit that will connect the practitioner electronically to the payer and to various administrative systems. Information systems will allow the clinician to bill electronically and to receive rapid turnaround on electronic payments to their personal bank accounts. Data-based reports will assist marketing efforts by provider groups and networks. Credentialing will be on-line with rapid updates and confirmation by legitimate sources requiring such information (e.g., hospitals, networks, etc.). Outcome data will stimulate continuing education units programs to assist providers with acquiring information about the latest techniques and trends in behavioral health.

Providers will have available to them much more specific data to evaluate their treatment interventions. On-line clinical management information, data-based treatment guidelines, and educational forums will facilitate the delivery of efficacious clinical services without being intrusive to the clinician's judgment or expertise.

Advantages to Business and Industry

Business and industry will enter the process as consumers of value-added services. New information systems will provide data-based reports for companies where they can objectively evaluate the products they are purchasing. Though change will come slowly and corporate America may in some cases resist the concept of "value" in behavioral health services, they will find it easier to respond to empirical data that address their concerns about levels of productivity and bottom-line profitability. The new technology will provide an integrated database that examines both financial and treatment outcome information. In time, data on medical cost offset and performance enhancement will provide business and industry with the information to make sound decisions affecting their employees and dependents. With a strong empirical database, behavioral health care will gain acceptance and will make meaningful contributions to both management and to employees and their families. The new technology will be a driving force in this evolution in thought.

Advantages to Consumers

The clinical needs of the consumers should once again become a primary concern of behavioral health care. Although economics have driven the process during the last few years, there is much optimism that the focus on value will highlight the needs of the consumer. Certainly, there have been historical financial abuses in the behavioral health care delivery system. Too often benefit plans defined therapeutic need. Likewise, in recent years errors of restrictive care have been observed. As Karon (1995) notes about managed behavioral health care: "There are legitimate ways to save money without impairing the quality of care, but they take careful thought and research" (p. 6). Heretofore, little data-based literature was available to recommend one course of treatment over another. Gradually, empirical studies supporting clinically effective treatments will emerge. For example, Howard et al. (1993) demonstrated that different levels of psychotherapy resulted in very different outcomes. If the goal was for patients to report feeling better, as little as three sessions were sufficient. Symptom change took longer: as much as 20 to 50 sessions. If a change in work efficiency was the desired goal, then 100 sessions might be required.

These numbers seem grossly excessive to most MCOs used to thinking in terms of rapid stabilization/symptom reduction. The information technology will address different levels of change and will begin to answer and empirically address such issues as dosage level of psychotherapy for particular problems or difficulties. It may demonstrate that most patients resolve their difficulties in the oft-quoted eight sessions or less. Likewise, it may prove that when specific goals are defined, treatment duration and cost vary with the selected goals. The information technology promises to take the guesswork and dogma out of behavioral health care decision making. As standards are set to measure value and empirical data derive to address these issues, a much greater likelihood exists that more patients will receive the care they need, by the level of provider best equipped to deliver that care, and in the setting most suitable for the patient and his or her particular problem.

NATIONAL CLEARINGHOUSE FOR BEHAVIORAL HEALTH DATA

Systems designed properly will interface with multiple administrative structures, allowing the provider to be credentialed and to communicate electronically with a variety of entities. Herein lies the possibility of an integrated database from which to develop national normative data to support various clinical care models. Each major payer (e.g., MCO) will create their own proprietary outcome measures and decision formulas to operate their particular businesses. A step beyond the present proprietary developments, however, is a national clearinghouse for behavioral health data where data from diverse patient groups can be aggregated for analysis and dissemination through data-based reports for government, business and industry, MCOs, professional associations, networks, and providers. Industrywide collaboration regarding large-scale studies of outcome in behavioral health will address the cost–quality issues that characterize the current behavioral health care industry. Addressing such issues as employee productivity and medical cost offset on a large scale will bolster arguments for parity with medicine in terms of benefit design and structure. The development of generic psychometrically sophisticated measurement instruments that can be added to the proprietary protocols of MCOs and distributed widely to practitioners and patients will greatly facilitate the development of clinically effective treatments.

CONNECTIVITY: CLOSING THE LOOP

The picture emerges where providers are electronically linked to treatment sites and to MCOs or other administrative structures. Data flow both ways. Going upstream from the provider will be sophisticated clinical and financial data. Coming back will be treatment authorizations, provider feedback and evaluations, as well as referrals and detailed referral information. Assessment will be an ongoing process and treatment evaluation will commence with the initiation of treatment. What happens to data once they are captured at the host site? For the first time in the history of behavioral health, large-scale field studies can be conducted to examine the relative efficacy of various treatment modalities (e.g., medication versus psychotherapy plus medication), to isolate treatment components that work effectively for specific clinical problems and difficulties and to develop predictor variables to assist with triage and treatment programming. As the data and systems mature, so too can provider education and feedback. Business and industry can be brought into the loop to understand more concretely how behavioral health issues affect the work place and the impact of emotional and behavioral problems on the bottom line. Patients will gain a voice in helping define what goals are important to them and what techniques, practices, and methods serve to address their problems most effectively. Providers are likely to regain some control over their practices through community and regional-based partnerships with various organizational entities and through the systematic collection of computerized data measuring outcome and provider effectiveness. Providers will gravitate to new jobs in the emerging behavioral health field as they assume important roles in clinical system design, research, information system design and implementation, supervision of lesser-skilled professionals, and administration of more complex behavioral health care businesses. Skilled, dedicated, and experienced psychotherapists will continue to see patients and deliver highly beneficial assistance in an environment that creates a host of new clinical decision-making tools to guide and facilitate clinical care and that will structure and organize clinical data in innovative and helpful ways. Clinical decision making will be supported by a variety of information sources made available through the developing computer technology.

REFERENCES

Accutracker II [Computer software]. (1996). Raleigh, NC: Suntech Medical Instruments, Inc.

Agras, W. S., Taylor, C. B., Feldman, D. E., Losch, M., & Burnett, K. F. (1990). Developing computer-assisted therapy in the treatment of obesity. *Behavior Therapy, 21,* 99–109.

Albee, G. W. (1968). The uncertain future of clinical psychology. *American Psychologist, 23,* 317–320.

Alcadd Test [Computer software]. (1996). Los Angeles, CA: Western Psychological Services.

American Psychiatric Association. (1994) *Diagnostic and statistical manual of mental disorders* (4th ed.). Washington, DC: Author.

American Psychological Association. (1993). *Setting the stage for outcome measurements.* Washington, DC: Author.

Anxiety Scale A [Computer software]. (1996). Youngstown, OH: Integrated Professional Systems.

Anxiety Scale B [Computer software]. (1996). Youngstown, OH: Integrated Professional Systems.

Assertiveness Training. [Computer software]. (1996). San Diego, CA: Psychological Psoftware Company.

Ball, M. (1995). *Where are we headed? Visioning the computer-based patient record.* Keynote address presented at the meeting of Behavioral Informatics Tomorrow, San Diego, CA.

Barlow, D. H. (1994). Psychological interventions in the era of managed competition. *Clinical Psychology: Science and Practice, 1*(2), 109–122.
Beck Anxiety Inventory [Computer software]. (1996). San Antonio: The Psychological Corporation.
Beck Depression Inventory [Computer software]. (1996). San Antonio: The Psychological Corporation.
Beck Hopelessness Scale [Computer software]. (1996). San Antonio: The Psychological Corporation.
Beck Scale for Suicide Ideation [Computer software]. (1996). San Antonio: The Psychological Corporation.
Bender Clinical Report [Computer software]. (1996). Jacksonville, FL: Precision People, Inc.
Bender Report [Computer software]. (1996). North Tonawanda, NY: MHS.
Bender Report 4.0 [Computer software]. (1996). Melborne, FL: Psychometric Software, Inc.
Beutler, L. E., & Clarkin, J. (1990). *Systematic treatment selection: Toward targeted therapeutic interventions.* New York: Brunner/Mazel.
Beutler, L. E., & Williams, O. B. (1995, July/August). Computer applications for the selection of optimal psychosocial therapeutic interventions. *Behavioral Healthcare Tomorrow, 4*(4), 66–68.
Beutler, L. E., Crago, M., & Arizemdi, T. G. (1986). Therapist variables in psychotherapy process and outcome. In S. L. Garfield & A. E. Bergin (Eds.), *Handbook of psychotherapy and behavior change* (3rd ed., pp. 257–310). New York: John Wiley & Sons.
Beutler, L. E., Williams, R. E., Wakefield, P. J., & Entwistle, S. R. (1995). Bridging scientist and practitioner perspectives in clinical psychology. *American Psychologist, 50*(12), 984–994.
Bilbrey, J., & Bilbrey, P. (1995, July/August). Judging, trusting, and utilizing outcomes data: A survey of behavioral healthcare payors. *Behavioral Healthcare Tomorrow, 4*(4), 62–65.
Bongar, B. (1992). Effective risk management and the suicidal patient. *Register Report, 18*(6), 1, 3, 21–27.
Boston Diagnostic Aphasia Examination [Computer software]. (1996). San Antonio: The Psychological Corporation.
Brief Computerized Stress Inventory [Computer software]. (1996). Lawrence, KS: Preventive Measures, Inc.
Brief Symptom Inventory [Computer software]. (1996). Minneapolis, MN: NCS.
Brown, G. S., Frazier, J. B., & Bendoraitis, T. M. (1995, January/February). Transforming the future: The coming impact of cis. *Behavioral Health Management, 15*(1), 8–12.
Cagney, T., & Woods, D. R. (1994). Clinician update: Clinical mis. *Behavioral Healthcare Tomorrow, 3*(1), 43–45.
Caldwell Report [Computer software]. (1996). Los Angeles, CA: Caldwell Report.
California Psychological Inventory [Computer software]. (1996). Palo Alto, CA: Consulting Psychologists Press, Inc.
CAPSCORE 1.04 [Computer software]. (1996). Los Angeles, CA: PSYTECK.
Category Test Computer Program [Computer software]. (1996). North Tonawanda, NY: MHS.
Chambless, D. L. (1995). Training in and dissemination of empirically validated psychological treatments. *The Clinical Psychologist, 48*(1), 3–24.
Chang, M. (1987a). Clinician-entered computerized psychiatric triage records. *Hospital and Community Psychiatry, 38*(6), 652–656.
Chang, M. (1987b). In reply. *Hospital and Community Psychiatry, 38*(12), 1341.
Chronic Pain Battery [Computer software]. (1996). Durham, NC: Pain Resource Center, Inc.
Chronic Pain Battery Administrator [Computer software]. (1996). North Tonawanda, NY: MHS.
Comprehensive Computerized Stress Inventory [Computer software]. (1996). Lawrence, KS: Preventive Measures, Inc.
Comprehensive Norms for an Expanded Halstead–Reitan battery: Demographic corrections, research findings, and clinical applications [Computer software]. (1996). North Tonawanda, NY: MHS.
Cone-Wesson, B., Kurtzberg, D., & Vaughn, H. G., Jr. (1983). *Detection of auditory system dysfunction in very low birthweight infants.* Paper presented at the meeting of the Society for Ear, Nose, and Throat Advance in Children, San Diego, CA.
Coping Inventory for Stressful Situations [Computer software]. (1996). North Tonawanda, NY: MHS.
Costello, A. J., Dulcan, M. K., & Kalas, R. (1991). A checklist of hospitalization criteria for use with children. *Hospital and Community Psychiatry, 42*(8), 823–828.
Cummings, N. A. (1995). Impact of managed care on employment and training: A primer for survival. *Professional Psychology: Research and Practice, 26*(1), 10–15.
Deming, W. E. (1986). *Out of the crisis.* Cambridge, MA: Massachusetts Institute of Technology, Center for Advanced Engineering Study (CAES).
Demuth, P. (1984). Eliza and her offspring. In M. D. Schwartz (Ed.), *Using computers in clinical practice: Psychotherapy and mental health applications* (pp. 321–327). New York: Haworth Press.
Derogatis, L. R. (1996a). Brief Symptom Inventory [Computer software]. Minneapolis, MN: NCS.

Derogatis, L. R. (1996b). SCL-90-R [Computer software]. Minneapolis, MN: NCS.
Domestic Violence Inventory [Computer software]. (1996). Phoenix, AZ: Risk & Need Assessment, Inc.
Eating Disorder Inventory [Computer software]. (1996). North Tonawanda, NY: MHS.
Eating Disorders Inventory—2 [Computer software]. (1996). Odessa, FL: Psychological Assessment Resources, Inc.
Eckert, P. A. (1994). Cost control through quality improvement: The new challenge for psychology. *Professional Psychology: Research and Practice, 25*(1), 3–8.
Electronic DSM-IV [Computer software]. (1995). Washington, DC: American Psychiatric Association.
Endler Multidimensional Anxiety Scales [Computer software]. (1996). Los Angeles, CA: Western Psychological Services.
Erdman, H. P., Klein, M. H., & Griest, J. H. (1985). Direct patient computer interviewing. *Journal of Consulting and Clinical Psychology, 53,* 760–773.
Essan Depression Scale A [Computer software]. (1996). Youngstown, OH: Integrated Professional Systems.
Essan Depression Scale B [Computer software]. (1996). Youngstown, OH: Integrated Professional Systems.
Essan Self-Rating Depression Scale A [Computer software]. (1996). Youngstown, OH: Integrated Professional Systems.
Essan Self-Rating Depression Scale B [Computer software]. (1996). Youngstown, OH: Integrated Professional Systems.
Exner Rorschach Scoring Program [Computer software]. (1996). San Antonio: The Psychological Corporation.
Eysenck Personality Inventory [Computer software]. (1996). San Diego, CA: Educational and Industrial Testing Service.
Fain, E. (1994, January/February). Today's or tomorrow's computer systems. *Behavioral Healthcare Tomorrow, 3*(1), 25–31.
Farrell, A. D. (1989). Impact of computers on professional practice: A survey of current practices and attitudes. *Professional Psychology: Research and Practice, 20*(3), 172–178.
Farrell, A. D. (1991). Computers and behavioral assessment: Current applications, future possibilities, and obstacles to routine use. *Behavioral Assessment, 13,* 159–179.
First, M. B., Gibbon, M., Williams, J. B., & Spitzer, R. L. (1996a). Mini-scid [Computer software]. North Tonawanda, NY: MHS.
First, M. B., Gibbon, M., Williams, J. B., & Spitzer, R. L. (1996b). AUTOSCID II [Computer software]. North Tonawanda, NY: MHS.
First, M. B., Gibbon, M., Williams, J. B., & Spitzer, R. L. (1996c). DTREE: The DSM-IV Expert [Computer software]. North Tonawanda, NY: MHS.
Flynn, H. R., & Henisz, J. E. (1975). Criteria for psychiatric hospitalization: Experience with a checklist for chart review. *American Journal of Psychiatry, 132,* 847–850.
Fowler, R. D. (1985). Landmarks in computer-assisted psychological assessment. *Journal of Consulting and Clinical Psychology, 53,* 748–759.
Geriatric Clinical Assessment Scale [Computer software]. (1996). Youngstown, OH: Integrated Professional Systems.
Geriatric Rating Scale A [Computer software]. (1996). Youngstown, OH: Integrated Professional Systems.
Geriatric Rating Scale B [Computer software]. (1996). Youngstown, OH: Integrated Professional Systems.
Giannetti, R. A. (1996). Quickview Social History [Computer software]. Minneapolis, MN: NCS.
Gray, G., & Glazer, W. (1994, January/February). Psychiatric decision making in the 90s. *Behavioral Health Tomorrow, 3*(1), 47–54.
Halstead Category Test—A Computer Version [Computer software]. (1996). Jacksonville, FL: Precision People, Inc.
Halstead–Reitan Hypothesis Generator [Computer software]. (1996). Jacksonville, FL: Precision People, Inc.
Halstead–Reitan Neuropsychological Battery [Computer software]. (1996). Jacksonville, FL: Precision People, Inc.
Hammond, K. W., & Munnecke, T. H. (1984). A computerized psychiatric treatment planning system. *Hospital and Community Psychiatry, 35*(2), 160–163.
Hanaker, M., Harrell, T., & Ciminero, A. (1996). Chemical Dependency Assessment Profile [Computer software]. North Tonawanda, NY: MHS.
HBR Norms Program [Computer software]. (1996). Odessa, FL: Psychological Assessment Resources, Inc.
Health Status Questionnaire 2.0 [Computer software]. (1996). San Antonio: The Psychological Corporation.
Hermann: The Rorschach Assistant [Computer software]. (1996). North Tonawanda, NY: MHS.

Hiatt, D., & Hargrove, G. E. (1995, July/August). The characteristics of highly effective therapists in managed behavioral provider networks. *Behavioral Healthcare Tomorrow, 4*(4), 19–21.

Honaker, L. M. (1996a). Session Summary [Computer software]. North Tonawanda, NY: MHS.

Honaker, L. M. (1996b). Termination/Discharge Summary [Computer software]. North Tonawanda, NY: MHS.

Honaker, L. M., & Harell, T. (1996). Psychological/Psychiatric Status Interviews 2.0 [Computer software]. North Tonawanda, NY: MHS.

Horn, J. L., Wanberg, K. W., & Foster, F. M. (1996). Alcohol Use Inventory [Computer software]. Minneapolis, MN: NCS.

Howard, K. I., Lueger, R., Maling, M. S., & Martinovich, A. (1993). A phase model of psychotherapy outcome: Causal mediation of change. *Journal of Consulting and Clinical Psychology, 61*, 678–685.

Interactive Tester [Computer software]. (1996). Los Angeles, CA: PSYTEK.

Inventory of Suicide Orientation-30 [Computer software]. (1996). Minneapolis, MN: NCS.

Inventory to Diagnosis Depression [Computer software]. (1996). Minneapolis, MN: NCS.

Jenkins Activity Survey [Computer software]. (1996). San Antonio, TX: The Psychological Corporation.

Karon, P. (1995). Provision of psychotherapy under managed care: A growing crisis and national nightmare. *Professional Psychology: Research and Practice, 26*(1), 5–9.

King, J. D., & Lowalchuk, B. (1996). Inventory of Suicide Orientation–30 [Computer software]. Minneapolis, MN: NCS.

Kopta, S. M., Howard, K. I., Lowry, J. L., & Beutler, L. E. (1994). Patterns of symptomatic recovery in psychotherapy. *Journal of Consulting and Clinical Psychology, 62*(5), 1009–1016.

Kovacs, A. L. (1996, Winter). We have met the enemy and he is us. *AAP Advance*, 6, 19, 22.

Krug, S. (1993). *Psychware sourcebook: A reference guide to computer-based products for assessment in psychology, education, and business*. Champaign, IL: Metritech, Inc.

Lader, M., & Noble, P. (1975). The affective disorders. In P. H. Venables & M. J. Christie (Eds.), *Research in psychophysiology* (pp. 259–281). New York: Wiley.

Lambert, M. J. (1983). Introduction to assessment of psychotherapy outcome: Historical perspective and current issues. In M. J. Lambert, E. R. Christensen, & S. S. DuJulio (Eds.), *The assessment of psychotherapy outcome* (pp. 3–32). New York: John Wiley & Sons.

Lambert, M. J., Lunnen, K., Umphress, V., Hansen, N. B., & Burlingame, G. M. (1994). *Administration and scoring manual for the outcome questionnaire (OQ45.1)*. Salt Lake City: IHC Center for Behavioral Healthcare Efficacy.

Lambert, M. J., Shapiro, D. A., & Bergin, A. E. (1986). The effectiveness of psychotherapy. In S. L. Garfield & A. E. Bergin (Eds.), *Handbook of psychotherapy and behavior change* (3rd ed., pp. 157–212). New York: John Wiley & Sons.

Lanier, J., & Biocca, F. (1992). An insider's view of the future of virtual reality. *Journal of Communication, 42*(4), 150–172.

Levant, R. F. (1995). Outcomes measurement and empirically validated treatments: What's all the fuss about? *Psychotherapy Bulletin, 30*(3), 20–22.

Luria–Nebraska Neurological Battery [Computer software]. (1996). Los Angeles, CA: Western Psychological Services.

Mangina, C. A., & Beuzeron-Mangina, J. H. (1988). Learning abilities and disabilities: Effective diagnosis and treatment. *International Journal of Psychophysiology, 6*, 79–90.

Marital Satisfaction Inventory [Computer software]. (1996). Los Angeles, CA: Western Psychological Services.

Marks MMPI Report [Computer software]. (1996). Los Angeles, CA: Western Psychological Services.

Marks MMPI & MMPI-2 Adult Clinical Report [Computer software]. (1996). Los Angeles, CA: Western Psychological Services.

Marriage Counseling Report [Computer software]. (1996). Champaign, IL: Institute for Personality and Ability Testing, Inc.

MCO's select software; providers come on-line. (1995). *Practice Strategies, 1*(4), 1–2.

McCullough, L., Farrell, A., & Longabaugh, R. (1986). The development of a microcomputer-based mental health information system: A potential tool for bridging the scientist-practitioner gap. *American Psychologist, 41*, 297–314.

Meier, S. (1996). If you drink [Computer software]. North Tonawanda, NY: MHS.

Memory Assessment Scale [Computer software]. (1996). Odessa, FL: Psychological Assessment Resources, Inc.

Menstrual Distress Questionnaire [Computer software]. (1996). Los Angeles, CA: Western Psychological Services.

Mental health: Does therapy help? (1995, November). *Consumer Reports*, 734–739.
Meredith, R. L., & Bair, S. L. (1990). Computer generated client record keeping. *Register Report, 16*(3), 15–19.
Meredith, R. L., & Bair, S. L. (1995). Myrt rides the superhighway. *Register Report, 21*(2), 1, 14–17.
Meredith, R. L., Bair, S. L., Ford, G. R., & Morris, R. J. (1998). Integrating behavioral informatics into the practice of child therapy. In T. R. Kratochwill & R. J. Morris (Eds.), *The practice of child therapy* (pp. 471–509). New York: Plenum Press.
Meyers-Briggs Type Indicator [Computer software]. (1996). Palo Alto, CA: Consulting Psychologists Press, Inc.
MicroCAT Testing System [Computer software]. (1996). St. Paul, MN: Assessment Systems Corporation.
MicroCog: Assessment of Cognitive Functioning [Computer software]. (1996). San Antonio: The Psychological Corporation.
Microtest Q [Computer software]. (1996). Minneapolis, MN: NCS.
Million Clinical Multiaxial Inventory—III [Computer software]. (1996). Minneapolis, MN: NCS.
Million Index of Personality Styles [Computer software]. (1996). San Antonio: The Psychological Corporation.
Minnesota Multiphasic Personality Inventory [Computer software]. (1996). Minneapolis, MN: NCS.
Minnesota Multiphasic Personality Inventory Adolescent Norms [Computer software]. (1996). Odessa, FL: Psychological Assessment Resources.
Minnesota Multiphasic Personality Inventory–2 [Computer software]. (1996b). North Tonawanda, NY: MHS.
Minnesota Multiphasic Personality Inventory—Adolescent [Computer software]. (1996a). Odessa, FL: Psychological Assessment Resources.
Minnesota Multiphasic Personality Inventory—Adolescent [Computer software]. (1996b). North Tonawanda, NY: MHS.
Minnesota Multiphasic Personality Inventory—Adolescent [Computer software]. (1996c). Minneapolis, MN: NCS.
The Minnesota Report: Adult Clinical System—Revised Interpretative Report [Computer software]. (1996). Minneapolis, MN: NCS.
MORPHEUS Version 3.0 [Computer software]. (1996). Birmingham, AL: Martin Software and Consulting.
Newman, R. (1995, May/June). The American Psychological Association's response to the outcome challenge. *Behavioral Health Management*, 17–19.
Noble, P., & Lader, M. (1971). Depressive illness, pulse rate and forearm blood flow. *The British Journal of Psychiatry, 119*, 261–266.
Novelly, R. A. (1992). The debt of neuropsychology to the epilepsies. *American Psychologist, 47*(9), 1126–1129.
Occupational Stress Inventory [Computer software]. (1996). Odessa, FL: Psychological Assessment Resources, Inc.
OPTAIO Practice Manager [Computer software]. (1999). San Antonio: The Psychological Corporation.
The Perfect Chart [Computer software]. (1996). North Tonawanda, NY: MHS.
Perloff, D., Sokolow, M., & Cown, R. (1983). The prognostic value of ambulatory blood pressures. *Journal of the American Medical Association, 249*, 2792–2798.
Personality Assessment Inventory [Computer software]. (1996). San Antonio: The Psychological Corporation.
Persons, J. P. (1991). Psychotherapy outcome studies do not accurately represent current models of psychotherapy. *American Psychologist, 46*(2), 99–106.
Pipal, J. E. (1995). Managed care: Is it the corpse in the living room? An expose. *Psychotherapy, 32*(2), 323–332.
Post Traumatic Personality Profile [Computer software]. (1996). Minneapolis, MN: NCS.
Psych-Educational Report Writing System [Computer software]. (1996). Newport Beach, CA: Planet Press.
Q-Fast [Computer software]. (1996). Tulsa, OK: Statsoft.
QuickDoc for Windows [Computer software]. (1996). San Antonio: The Psychological Corporation.
Quickview Social History [Computer software]. (1996). Minneapolis, MN: NCS.
Quinco Behavioral Health Systems. (1996). *Life-work products* [Brochure]. Columbus, IN: Corporate.
Rainwater, G., & Coe, D. (1996). Psychological/Psychiatric Status Interview 2.0 [Computer software]. North Tonawanda, NY: MHS.
Rainwater, G., & Slade, B. (1996). Developmental History Report 4.0 [Computer software]. North Tonawanda, NY: MHS.
Reason House. (1996). *TP write* [Brochure]. Towson, MD: Corporate Author.
Reich, W., Welner, Z., & Herjanic, B. (1996). Diagnostic Interview for Children and Adolescents—Revised

(for DSM IV) Computer Program: Child/Adolescent Version and Parent Version [Computer software]. North Tonawanda, NY: MHS.
Report Builder—Screentest [Computer software]. (1996). Berkshire, England: Nelson Publishing Company.
Repp, A. C., Harman, M. L., Felce, D., Acker, R. V., & Karsh, K. G. (1989). Conducting behavioral assessments on computer-collected data. *Behavioral Assessment, 11*, 249–268.
Rorschach Interpretation Assistance Program [Computer software]. (1996). San Antonio: The Psychological Corporation.
Rorschach Interpretation Program Version 3.1 [Computer software]. (1996). Odessa, FL: Psychological Assessment Resources, Inc.
Rorschach Technique [Computer software]. (1996). San Antonio: The Psychological Corporation.
Rosen, L. (1995). Cruising the info-ban: Psychologists relish computer opportunities. *The National Psychologist, 4*(4), 14–15.
Rosen, L., & Weil, M. (1995, Fall). Tips for mental health professionals to merge on-line. *Treatment Today*, 48–49.
Rosen, L., & Weil, M. (1996). *Technology for today's mental health practitioner*. Orange, CA: Byte Back Technology and Consultation Services.
Saeman, H. (1995, March/April). "Physician equity model" will dominate by 2000. *The National Psychologist*, 10–11.
Sanderson, W. C. (1995, March). Which therapies are proven effective? *American Psychological Association Monitor, 4*, 3.
Schinka, B. (1995a). Mental Status Checklists—Adult: Computer Report [Brochure]. Odessa, FL: Psychological Assessment Resources, Inc.
Schinka, B. (1995b). Personal History Checklist—Adult: Computer Report [Brochure]. Odessa, FL: Psychological Assessment Resources, Inc.
Schlosser, B. (1992). Computer-assisted practice: The laws of natural selection. *The Independent Practitioner, 12*(4), 146–149.
Schlosser, B. (1995). Clinical outcomes assessment: A "patient-centric" perspective. *The Independent Practitioner, 15*(3), 131–133.
Scoring Assistant for the Wechsler Scales [Computer software]. (1996). San Antonio: The Psychological Corporation.
Screentest Assessment Data Manager [Computer software]. (1996). Berkshire, England: Nelson Publishing Company, Ltd.
Self-Esteem and Values [Computer software]. (1996). San Diego, CA: Psychological Psoftware Company.
Seligman, M. E. P. (1995). The effectiveness of psychotherapy. *American Psychologist, 50*(12), 965–974.
Sixteen Personality Factor Questionnaire [Computer software]. (1996). Minneapolis, MN: NCS.
Solanto, M. V, & Conners, C. K. (1982). A dose–response and time action analysis of autonomic and behavioral effects of methylphenidate in attention deficit disorder with hyperactivity. *Psychophysiology, 19*, 658–667.
State–Trait Anxiety Inventory [Computer software]. (1996). North Tonawanda, NY: MHS.
Steenbarger, B. N. (1994). Duration and outcome in psychotherapy: An integrative review. *Professional Psychology: Research and Practice, 25*(2), 111–119.
Stricker, G., & Trierweiler, S. J. (1995). The local clinical scientist. *American Psychologist, 50*(12), 995–1002.
Szasz, T. S. (1960). The myth of mental illness. *American Psychologist, 15*, 113–118, 541.
Taylor, C. B., Telch, M. J., & Havvik, D. (1983). Ambulatory heart rate changes during panic attacks. *Journal of Psychiatric Research, 17*, 261–266.
Therapy Works (1999). Psychological Assessment and Intervention Catalogue.
Tombari, M. L., Fitzpatrick, S. J., & Childress, W. (1985). Using computers as contingency managers in self-monitoring interventions: A case study. *Computers in Human behavior, 1*, 75–82.
Total Stress Management System [Computer software]. (1996). San Diego, CA: Psychological Psoftware Company.
Truscott, D., Evans, J., & Mansell, S. (1995). Outpatient psychotherapy with dangerous clients: A model for clinical decision making. *Professional Psychology: Research and Practice, 26*(5), 484–490.
Van Vort, W., & Mattson, M. (1989). A strategy for enhancing the clinical utility of the psychiatric record. *Hospital and Community Psychiatry, 40*(4), 407–409.
Wechsler Memory Scale Report [Computer software]. (1996). Melborne, FL: Psychometric Software, Inc.
Western Aphasia battery [Computer software]. (1996). San Antonio: The Psychological Corporation.
Williams, M. H. (1995). Patient satisfaction therapy. *The Independent Practitioner, 15*(1), 34–35.

5

Quality Improvement

Current Research in Outcome Management

MICHAEL J. LAMBERT, JONATHAN C. HUEFNER, AND CURTIS W. REISINGER

At the core of ensuring quality treatment is the assessment of changes in patients following interventions—so-called "outcome research." This area of research is central to quality improvement because the scientific study of patient change tempers the undocumented and often overstated consequences of psychological and medical practitioners. We attempt here a brief summary of research on psychosocial interventions and its implications for quality management. This research summary examines outcome and process research as they apply both to the individual patient as well as to the delivery system in which the outcome of larger populations becomes an overriding concern. We first review outcome in its historical context, followed by issues of matching patients with treatments and selecting therapists to maximize positive outcomes.

OUTCOME RESEARCH— WHAT WE KNOW FROM PAST STUDIES OF TREATMENT EFFECTS

OVERALL EFFECTS

Overwhelming evidence exists documenting the positive impact of psychotherapy on patient improvement (Lambert & Bergin, 1994). A graphic depicting this literature is presented in Fig. 1. This figure suggests that treated patients who received 14 to 20 sessions of therapy do better than both untreated controls and patients who get minimal support or placebo interventions.

The general conclusion that therapy is effective is based on research spanning over five decades, including thousands of clients and therapists and a multitude of intervention strategies. This research, based mainly on the results of clinical trials with

MICHAEL J. LAMBERT • Department of Psychology, Brigham Young University, Provo, Utah 84602. JONATHAN C. HUEFNER • Magellan Behavioral Health, Salt Lake City, Utah 84070. CURTIS W. REISINGER • Department of Psychiatry, Hackensack University Medical Center, Hackensack, New Jersey 07601, and Department of Psychiatry, UMDNJ-New Jersey Medical School, Newark, New Jersey 07103.

Handbook of Quality Management in Behavioral Health, edited by Stricker *et al.* Kluwer Academic / Plenum Publishers, New York, 2000.

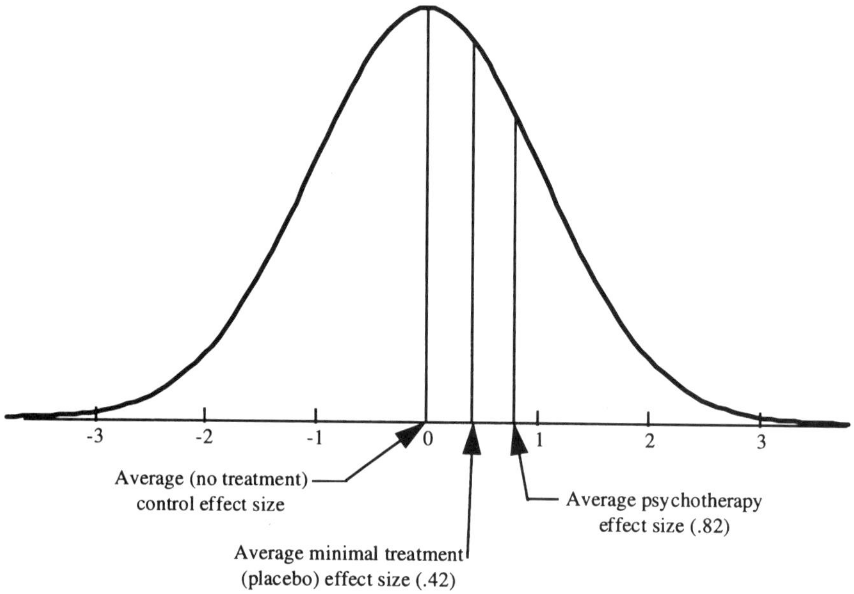

FIGURE 1. Comparison of placebo and psychotherapy effects in relation to no-treatment control. Reprinted by permission of Lambert and Bergin (1994).

random assignment and appropriate experimental controls, has clear implications for the management of patients. Managing the care of those with behavioral disorders cannot be properly accomplished without making certain that patients are treated with systematic, theory-driven psychosocial treatments.

Lasting Effects

An important question is whether the beneficial effects of psychotherapy last over time. Although there is no reason to believe that a single course of psychotherapy should permanently inoculate a person from psychological disturbance, reviews of the research show that many patients who undergo treatment achieve healthy adjustment over long periods of time (Nicholson & Berman, 1983). Several recent reviews have even suggested that some patients continue to improve after termination of treatment (Jorm, 1989). Lasting relief can occur even for patients who have a long history of recurrent problems. At the same time, there is clear evidence that some patients do relapse. Importantly, relapse occasionally has been shown to be related to the number of therapy sessions patients receive (Shapiro et al., 1995). Problems that have been shown to be particularly prone to reoccurrence include drug addictions, alcohol abuse, smoking, obesity, and possibly depression. The use of "booster sessions" to maintain treatment gains with periodic therapy sessions after formal treatment is completed may delay relapse but does not prevent it. A major factor in maintaining positive results is the degree to which patients recognize that changes are related to their own effective efforts (Lambert & Bergin, 1994).

Length of Therapy and Outcome

How long someone stays in treatment is significantly related to their eventual improvement. Historically, psychotherapy has been considered a long-term process, in many cases taking up to several years. In today's current health care environment, where much of the payment for psychotherapy comes from third-party sources, there is an increasing emphasis on cost-effectiveness. Brief therapies have developed and become the standard form of therapy practiced under our third-party systems of payment. Clearly, a therapy designed to bring about the same degree of beneficial change in 10 sessions rather than 20 is preferable. If this same result can be achieved in five sessions, so much the better. Research has shown that psychotherapy can bring about change quite rapidly. Howard, Kopta, Krause, and Orlinsky (1986) reported a meta-analysis of several studies showing that approximately 50% of patients were measurably improved by the eighth session and 75% by the 26th. In their analysis the subjects were outpatients with a variety of diagnoses, including a small percentage with personality disorders. The therapists were experienced professionals engaged in psychodynamically oriented, time-unlimited therapies.

Kadera, Lambert, and Andrews (1996) studied self-ratings of patients prior to their weekly meeting with therapists. These researchers found less rapid recovery in their sample of patients than were observed by Howard et al. (1986). Figure 2 presents the dose–effect curves for both studies.

The main difference between the methods of these studies is that Kadera et al. (1996) actually measured change at every session, while Howard et al. (1986), who did not have weekly ratings, based their estimate of change on a mathematical formula. The Kadera data places estimates for improvement of patients at 22% after 8 sessions and 75% at 26 sessions. The patients were from an outpatient training clinic and were diagnosed with a variety of mood and anxiety disorders. The therapists, under supervision, were trainees in clinical psychology and social work who offered a variety of therapeutic interventions. Almost all therapy was terminated by the 20th session. Both studies suggest rapid recovery for the majority of outpatients.

A recent survey of consumer satisfaction also sheds some light on the relationship

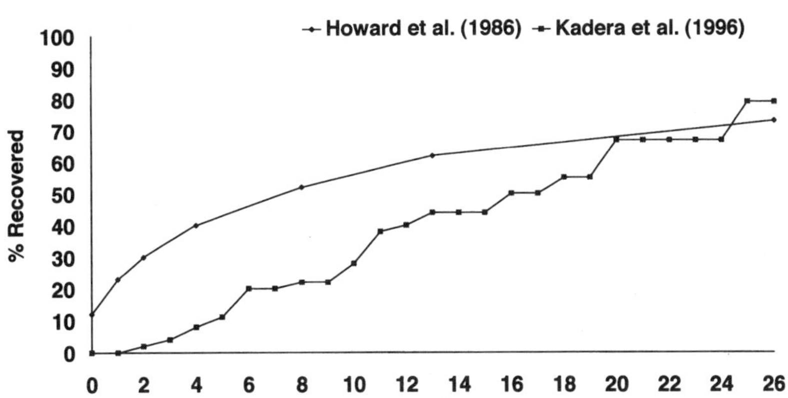

Figure 2. Dose–effect estimates calculated from 45 dysfunctional patients receiving psychotherapy (squares) from Kadera et al. (1996) compared with dose–effect estimates of Howard et al. (1986) (diamonds).

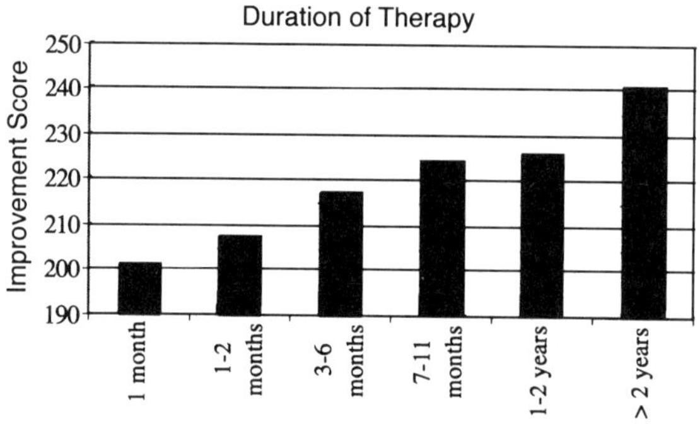

FIGURE 3. The relationship between duration of therapy and client satisfaction ($N = 2,846$). The 300-point scale is derived from the unweighted sum of responses to three 100-point subscales. The subscales measured specific improvement (i.e., how much treatment helped with problems that led to therapy), satisfaction with therapist, and global improvement (i.e., how respondents felt at time of survey, compared with when they began treatment). Reprinted by permission from Seligman and the American Psychological Association (1995).

between duration of treatment and improvement. Unlike the prospective study by Kadera et al. (1996), the consumer satisfaction study published by *Consumer Reports* (1995) and Seligman (1995) asked patients to look back at their therapy experience and rate its helpfulness. Figure 3 summarizes therapy data related to time in treatment and the degree of helpfulness. Those who received long-term therapy rated themselves as more improved than those who had short-term therapy. Improvement was related to specific symptoms that led to therapy and also in ratings of general functioning, coping, and ability to relate to others.

Seligman (1995) also reports contrasts between patients reporting more than and patients reporting less than six months of therapy. These two groups showed significant differences in work performance and social behavior. The difference between these time frames was as follows: 30% of respondents having more than 6 months of treatment indicated they were "a lot better," while only 15% of respondents receiving less than six months of treatment reported they were "a lot better."

Research has provided support for the effectiveness of brief therapies for some problems, but casts doubt on their value for others. Shapiro et al. (1995), for example, found a significant relationship between severity of depression and duration of treatment required to yield improvement. Clients with mild and moderate depression did as well with 8 sessions as they did with 16; in contrast, clients with severe depression improved more during 16 sessions than during 8. Knowing which disorders require more or less treatment allows practitioners and payers to better allocate resources. The research suggests that mental health care cost containment measures should be based on patient severity ratings rather than on arbitrarily determined limits so that services covered are sufficient for individual patients to derive a benefit.

Due to its practical, economic, and ethical consequences, continued research on duration of treatment and change in psychotherapy is highly important, if not an urgent need. Future research will depend on the availability of large databases before the relationship between number of sessions and improvement can be determined. This research must take into account the most relevant patient variables if the standard of quality care is applied to all persons who seek help.

Psychotherapy versus Pharmacotherapy

While psychotherapy may be significantly more effective than no treatment, it is not the only intervention available to treat most disorders. Psychotherapeutic medication is used as a treatment of choice as often as verbal therapy. Indeed, there is some belief that these drugs are used too often (see, for example, *The Wall Street Journal*, 1995). When comparative effectiveness between pharmacological and psychological treatments has been studied, many researchers have found the effect of psychotherapy to be equal to or greater than that of medication (Antonuccio, Danton, & DeNelsky, 1995; Lambert & Bergin, 1994). In this regard, no study is more important than the National Institutes of Mental Health (NIMH) Collaborative Depression study conducted in the early 1980s. This was a multisite endeavor examining the comparative outcomes of a standard medical treatment for depression (imipramine, a commonly prescribed drug for depression, plus clinical management defined as weekly meetings between psychiatrist and patient in which support as well as medication are offered) with two psychotherapies (cognitive–behavioral therapy and interpersonal psychotherapy). These three treatments were contrasted with a control group receiving a drug placebo combined with weekly clinical management.

This NIMH study is important for several reasons. It was the first direct comparison of two psychotherapies, both of which had been shown in previous research to be specifically effective with depression. The study typifies improving research strategies involving "ideal" or pure forms of therapy. It employed manuals and competency ratings of therapists rather than examining therapy as usually practiced. The use of manuals that provided treatment guidelines and defined how a therapy was to be practiced and included goals, tasks, and the sequence of procedures was critical. It enabled researchers to ensure that the therapies (as well as the drug management) were carried out in a consistent manner by monitoring therapists' adherence to the protocols defined in the manuals.

Findings of this study showed that over two thirds of the patients were symptom free at the end of treatment and all patient groups improved. Surprisingly, little evidence was found for the superiority of the psychotherapies over the placebo combined with clinical management. When patients were categorized into two levels of severity, however, interpersonal psychotherapy and medication appeared to be equally effective. Further, both methods appeared more effective than the placebo and cognitive–behavioral treatments on some measures (Elkin et al., 1989; Imber et al., 1990; Ogles, Lambert, & Sawyer, 1995).

Other studies have found the effects of psychotherapy to be equal to or better than the effects of a variety of antidepressant medications. Since antidepressant medication is often considered the treatment of choice for depression, the finding that some psychotherapies produce comparable effects are of significant importance (Robinson, Berman, & Neimeyer, 1990; Steinbrueck, Maxwell, & Howard, 1983).

Reviews of the treatment of agoraphobia (fear of open places) and panic disorder show results similar to those on depression. That is, the psychotherapies that have been tested with these disorders often have been shown to be equal to or more effective than pharmacotherapeutic interventions, especially when follow-up data are considered. This is because relapse rates are typically higher for medication-only treatment. For an exception, see de Beuirs, van Balkom, Lange, Koele, and van Dyck (1995). On the other hand, research on the comparative effectiveness of psychotherapies and pharmacotherapy for schizophrenia and similar disorders generally indicates the greater value of medication for alleviating symptoms.

Differences between Therapies

While psychotherapy can produce effects equal to or above that of medication, the relative effectiveness of different psychotherapies is still debatable. The variants of psychotherapy have proliferated to such a degree that one review made reference to over 400 kinds (Kazdin, 1986). This enormous variation is a serious obstacle to conclusive research. Most studies have focused on the major schools: behavioral, cognitive, humanistic, and psychodynamic. These reviews generally find little difference in the success among these four approaches (Lambert & Bergin, 1994). When differences have been found, they often support the superiority of cognitive treatments over humanistic and psychodynamic treatments.

Behavioral and cognitive treatments have been shown to have significant success with a number of specific problems such as panic, phobias, health-related problems, and a wide variety of childhood disorders. The treatment of choice for panic, for example, seems to be a cognitive–behavioral therapy "package" including relaxation, breathing retraining, cognitive restructuring, and simulation of the sensations of panic within the session to practice coping (Barlow, 1988; Michelson & Marchione, 1991). Continued research on the most effective treatment for specific disorders will enhance the ability of practitioners to more efficiently bring about positive outcomes. At the same time, there is some evidence that some managed behavioral health care companies are moving too rapidly toward embracing specific therapies for specific disorders without sufficient empirical justification. The research suggests that treatment guidelines advocating particular treatments are premature.

The modest differences in overall outcomes for highly diverse therapies have had a significant effect on the professional theoretical orientations of those practicing psychotherapy. The number of mental health professionals claiming to adopt an eclectic approach, with no strong allegiance to a particular theory or school, has increased. One study has reported 68% of professionals identify themselves with such an approach (Jensen, Bergin, & Greaves, 1990). An eclectic approach supposedly allows the professional to match the therapy best suited to the patient's needs. There are, however, drawbacks to this approach. Because eclecticism does not represent any systematic view, research on the effectiveness of such an approach is difficult if not impossible to conduct. Bergin and Garfield (1994) have argued that eclecticism may be a stage in the growth of psychotherapy toward a more integrated discipline. Whether or not this is true, the adoption of eclecticism (or integration of diverse theories and techniques) among mental health professionals has given them greater freedom to adapt their approaches to interventions that have higher success rates with the disorders being treated.

Selecting Patients for Brief Therapy

The increasing use of brief therapy in employee assistance programs (EAPs) and other managed care products makes it more critical than ever to ensure that patients are carefully selected for these treatments. There are risks in assigning a patient to short-term treatment. There is less time to correct both diagnostic errors and the treatment plans on which they are based. There is less time to overcome resistance. If the problem is truly one that requires long-term treatment, unrealistic expectations for cure may be raised, leading to impatience and eventual disappointment for both parties (Binder, Henry, & Strupp, 1987).

Careful selection of patients for brief therapy is critical. A number of authors have made this point. Malan (1976) and Marmor (1979) have asserted that the selection process is every bit as important as the therapeutic technique itself. Schneider and Pinkerton (1986) have stated that selection is the cornerstone of successful short-term therapy. Sifneos (1979) attributed most of his treatment failures to improper selection procedures.

Lambert and Anderson (1996), in a review of selection criteria for brief therapy, identified the following factors (in descending order of citation frequency) as important: severity of disturbance, motivation for treatment, capacity to relate to others (including the therapist), ego strength, psychological-mindedness, specificity of presenting problem, and response to trial therapy. These factors are similar to those listed in previous reviews of this literature (Barber & Crits-Christoph, 1991; Demos & Prout, 1993; Koss & Shiang, 1994; Lambert, 1979).

The exclusion of severely disturbed individuals from brief therapy was recommended by the majority of the therapists surveyed by Lambert and Anderson (1996) and appears to have the most empirical support. A variety of diagnoses have been included in these groups. Specifically, patients with active psychoticism; those with either a history of psychotic decompensation or potential for it; severe personality disorders; intense dependency needs, especially when these are unrecognized by the patient; rigid reliance on immature defenses such as denial, withdrawal, externalization, and projection; predominantly psychosomatic complaints; substance-related disorders, particularly when such addictions are chronic; impulse control disorders (especially when acting out is the predominant problem or when it is severe and persistent); entrenched negativism and hostility; severe mood disorders including bipolar and severe major depression; and organic brain damage or severe cognitive deficits.

A task of considerable importance in improving systems of managing patient care is further research into patient selection criteria. To date, there is an abundance of opinion and a rather short supply of systematic empirical study. Management of patient treatment length is a task that managed care corporations seem eager to take upon themselves, but in the absence of more data on selection decisions, judgments remain little more than guesses.

Common Factors across Treatments

The lack of consistent differences in the overall success rates of varied therapies and therapists with different training (Seligman, 1995) has spurred research on factors found to be common across all therapies. It has been argued that common factors in therapies account for substantial degrees of improvement in psychotherapy patients (Lambert & Bergin, 1994). Common factors can be viewed as originating from the patient as well as the therapist (Strupp, 1980). Together, the patient and therapist create a cooperative working endeavor. The patient's increased sense of trust, security, and safety, along with a decrease in tension, threat, and anxiety, lead to changes in conceptualization of problems. Ultimately, the patient acts differently by refacing fears, taking risks, and working through problems in interpersonal relationships.

Among the factors most frequently studied are those identified by the proponents of humanistic and client-centered orientations. They list empathy, positive regard, nonpossessive warmth, and genuineness as factors that are necessary for change (Lambert, DeJulio, & Stein, 1978). Reviewers are virtually unanimous in their opinion that the therapist–patient relationship is critical to positive patient outcome. Research on empathy provides a good example of the importance of this relationship. Therapist empathy is highly related to beneficial outcomes, even for behavioral techniques aimed at helping problem drinkers control their alcohol intake (Miller, Taylor, & West, 1980). Examples of the effect of the relationship are plentiful. For example, Lafferty, Beutler, and Crago (1991) found that less effective trainee therapists had lower levels of empathic understanding. The authors state, "The present study supports the significance of the therapist's empathy in effective psychotherapy. Patients of less effective therapists felt less understood than did patients of more effective therapists" (p. 79).

Psychodynamically oriented researchers have generated research on the importance of the therapeutic alliance—the degree to which patient and therapist are able to develop a collaborative relationship. Some components that are measured include: (1) the patient's affective relationship to the therapist, (2) the patient's capacity to work purposefully in therapy, (3) the therapist's empathic understanding and involvement, and (4) patient–therapist agreement on the goals and tasks of therapy (Gaston, 1990). Although there are instances where the therapeutic alliance fails to predict or has little association with outcome, a strong therapeutic alliance is one of the most important common factors leading to a positive outcome (Safran & Muran, 1995).

Another approach to studying the common factors involved in outcomes is the use of client checklists, which rate clients' perceptions of therapists in various areas. Clients who view their therapist as understanding and accepting also have higher self- and therapist-rated improvement (Lorr, 1965; Cooley & LaJoy, 1980). A study in which clients generated a list of curative factors revealed that talking to someone and receiving advice correlated most highly with good outcome. Patients frequently attribute their success in treatment to the personal qualities of the therapist. Across studies, these qualities bear a striking resemblance to each other. Patients clearly believe that the personal qualities of therapists are more important than specific technical aspects of treatment. The implications for quality improvement in managed care are clear: assess and retain providers with those qualities and attitudes, make training available to those who are falling short, and periodically assess these qualities via patient ratings or encourage therapists to do this on their own. An example of these types of assessments for quality care has been provided by Hargrave and Hiatt (1995). These researchers found a clear relationship between patient satisfaction, relationship ratings, and ratings of therapist compliance with treatment standards and guidelines.

Effect of Training and Experience on Outcome

The effects of psychotherapy offered by experienced clinicians have been contrasted with the effects of helping efforts on the part of lay therapists, paraprofessionals, and inexperienced clinicians. On the one hand, the research findings in this area have been highly debated due to contradictory results. On the other hand, Hattie, Sharpley, and Roger (1984) indicated that clients who seek help from paraprofessionals are more likely to achieve resolution of their problems than those who consult professionals! Several subcomparisons suggest, however, that the most effective therapists were those who were currently undergoing training or had just completed it, and that experienced paraprofessionals were superior to less experienced paraprofessionals. Some research suggests that more experienced clinicians obtain outcomes superior to those obtained by less experienced clinicians. Experienced professionals appear to do better overall across the widest range of age groups and problems, particularly when dropout rates are considered (Stein & Lambert 1995; Weisz, Weis, Alicke, & Klots, 1987). Other studies have noted that, while a failure to detect an overall difference between professionals and paraprofessionals might be unsettling, a more thoughtful consideration of the findings shows that in almost all studies, paraprofessionals were selected, trained, and supervised by professionals in techniques designed by professionals (Weisz et al., 1987). Many of these studies, however, have been cited for conceptual problems and frequently seem to be observing improvements in the morale of patients due to attention and support. If this is true, it reemphasizes the role of common factors, like attention and support, in positive outcomes. It suggests that these factors can be used effectively by paraprofessionals and clinicians who have the lowest levels of professional training such as social workers, marriage and family therapists, and addiction counselors.

Causes of Deterioration

Some patients are worse as a result of psychotherapy. Understanding the causes of such deterioration is important for ethical as well as scientific reasons. In addition, the extent to which negative changes occur obviously moderates overall success rates. Negative effects are, of course, impossible to study in an experimentally induced manner because of the resulting harm inducing them would cause patients. Researchers have looked instead at those studies that have reported negative outcomes.

The worsening of some patients is not necessarily due to therapy itself. Some patients may be on a progressive decline that no therapeutic effort can stop. A causal link between negative outcomes and therapeutic activities has been suggested, however, particularly with specific kinds of clients (Lambert, Bergin, & Collins, 1977; Mohr, 1995). For example, more severely disturbed patients are more likely to have negative outcomes. In addition, several diagnostic types, such as schizophrenia and borderline personality, have a disproportionate number of negative outcomes. This is sometimes because of the disorder itself but it also may be because there is less margin for therapeutic errors with such patients.

In group treatment, a widely quoted study reported that variables such as low involvement in the group, low level of self-esteem, low positive self-concept, and greater anticipation of or need for fulfillment were positively related to deterioration (Lieberman, Yalom, & Miles, 1973).

Therapist errors also have been linked to negative outcomes. Examples include failure to structure or focus the therapy time, failure to address a patient's negative attitudes toward either the therapist or the therapy, the passive acceptance of problematic aspects of the patient's behavior such as resistance or evasiveness, and the use of inappropriate or poorly timed interventions (Sachs, 1983). The values therapists hold also correlate with poor outcome. For example, therapists who place emphasis on values such as "having a comfortable and exciting life" were not as effective as therapists who place significantly more emphasis on intellectual values (Lafferty et al., 1991).

Examining types of group therapy in an inpatient setting, Beutler, Frank, Schieber, Calvert, and Gaines (1984) found that expressive–experientially focused therapy, which emphasized emotional expression, breaking down defenses, and emotional release, outscored two other therapies in the numbers of negative outcomes. This led the authors to express caution about using such treatments. Research also has been reported on the growing number of nonprofessional programs that foster an emotionally intense pressure for disclosure and conformity. Doherty, Lester, and Leigh (1986) reported that one in eight couples who had undergone a "marriage encounter" weekend were strongly affected by the encounter. Of these, approximately 50% were helped and 50% were negatively affected. Similar rates of negative effects have been reported in other studies (Lambert & Bergin, 1994). Unrealistic expectations for help by some participants, combined with coercive group norms for openness and intimacy, should lead the professional clinician away from the use of these techniques. As the emphasis in managed care moves more toward less expensive group treatments, managed care organizations need to encourage the use of screening and matching criteria to ensure positive outcomes in group interventions. A reasonable guideline at this point would seem to be that the more disturbed the patient, the more the group intervention should be structured and aimed at skill enhancement rather than self-exploration (Fuhriman & Burlingame, 1995).

Conclusion

Many psychotherapies have been subjected to empirical study and have been shown to have meaningful positive effects. Psychotherapy both speeds up the natural healing process and often provides additional coping strategies and methods for dealing with future problems. Psychologists, psychiatrists, social workers, and marriage and family therapists, as well as patients, can be assured that a broad range of therapies are likely to result in appreciable gains for the patient when offered by skillful, wise, and stable therapists. Research continues to provide information on the amount of time needed for meaningful changes to take place, suggesting brief therapies are effective for some problems but not for others. Research also has shown that the effects of therapy tend to last over time, with some patients continuing to make appreciable gains after treatment has concluded.

Although there is little firm evidence for the superiority of one form of psychotherapy over another, behavioral and cognitive methods appear to be significantly more effective than other strategies in treating certain specific problems. Psychotherapy has effects that are equal to that of medication in most instances. There is also significant research that supports the role of common factors, such as empathy and support, in creating a beneficial outcome. It should be no surprise that helping people deal with depression, inadequacy, anxiety, and inner conflicts, as well as helping them form viable relationships and develop meaningful directions for their lives, can be greatly facilitated in a therapeutic relationship characterized by trust, warmth, acceptance, and human wisdom.

Research suggests that clients would be wise to pick therapists on the basis of their ability to relate. Recognition of the important role a therapist's relationship skills and related nontechnical skills play in producing positive change, however, should not be construed as suggesting that technical proficiency has no unique contributions to make. The use of manuals to guide the practitioner in implementing psychotherapies is an important development that will enable more reliable research and practice to be carried out. Paraprofessionals, who in many cases are selected, trained, and supervised by professional therapists, are sometimes able to be as helpful as practicing clinicians. They are especially useful in providing social support and in offering structured treatment programs under supervision.

While the foregoing statements about psychotherapy can be made with more confidence than ever before, it is still important to point out that some patients do get worse. These outcomes are instructive and should not be dismissed. Knowing empirically what kinds of treatments are inappropriate for a particular patient is crucial.

THE USE OF OUTCOMES IN CLINICAL QUALITY MANAGEMENT

While the outcome of individual patients traditionally has been the central focus of outcome research, it is also valuable to look at clinical outcomes within the broader perspective of health care systems. In this broadened viewpoint, issues such as satisfaction, accessibility to treatment by large populations, and cost of services must be considered. There is an increasing awareness in managed behavioral health care companies that measuring outcomes is an important accountability requirement. To limit the use of clinical outcomes to accountability alone, however, does not do justice to their full utility. We see this broader application of outcome as a quality management effort. The following system illustrates how outcomes are being used at one managed behavioral health care company: Human Affairs International (HAI), as a quality management tool.

QUALITY AND OUTCOME

The schematic pictured in Fig. 4 illustrates the relationship between outcome assessment and quality care at HAI. There are two levels to this process: the first, and more fundamental, enables providers to use outcomes to manage the efficacy of their therapeutic interactions; the second allows HAI to manage its provider network and evaluate the efficacy of its programs.

Provider Feedback

Any system of measuring outcomes that does not provide immediate feedback to the provider about the current status of the client fails to realize the tremendous potential of outcomes measurement. One productive means of providing this feedback is shown in Fig. 4. The section above the double line shows the provider–outcomes feedback dynamic.

When a client initiates treatment, an initial assessment is made (1). This assessment in essence is a pretest on the clinical outcome measure, but it also provides the clinician with an index of initial severity on a standardized scale. A client's initial

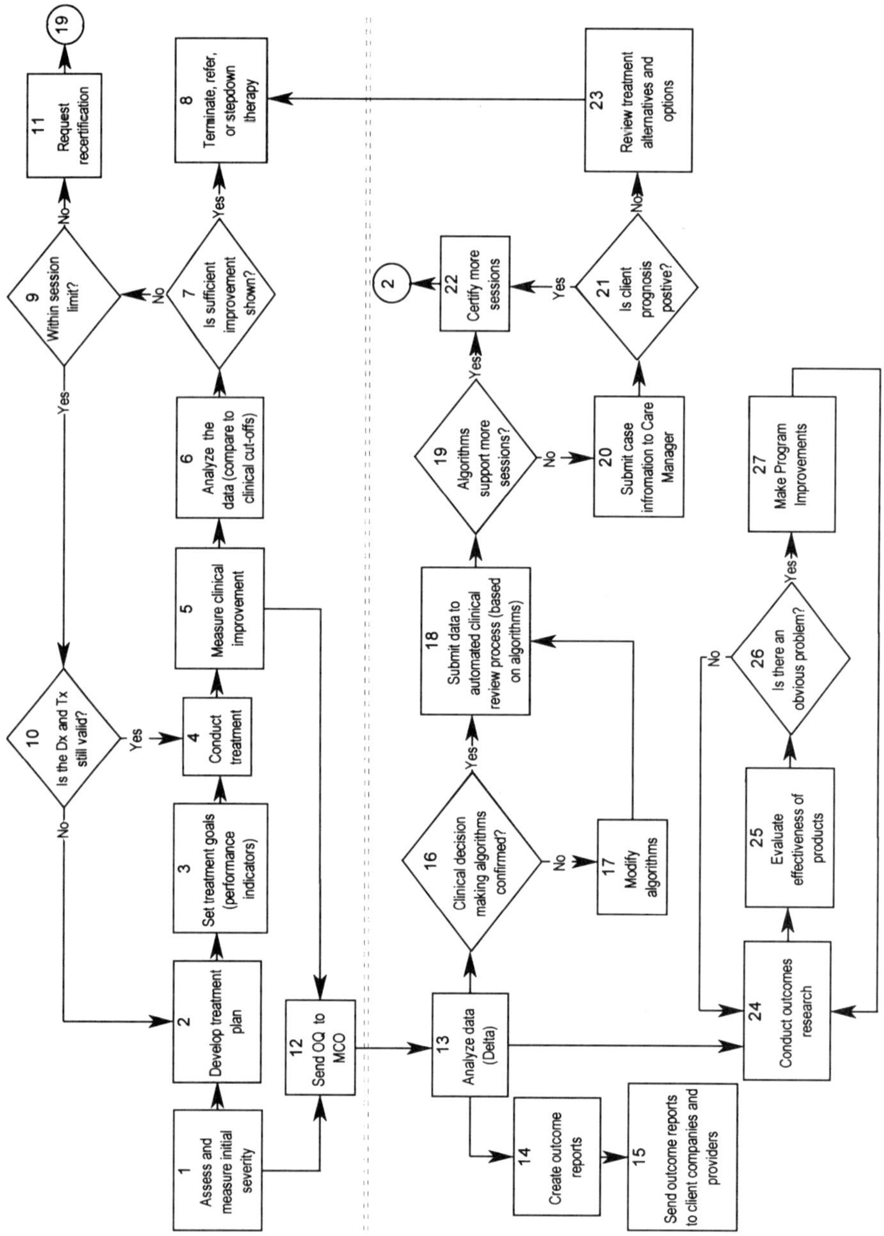

FIGURE 4. Outcomes work flow in a managed behavioral health care company.

symptom severity can play a significant role in the development of the treatment plan, including an estimate of treatment length (2). Additionally, the client's response to individual items on the questionnaire may be relevant to setting specific treatment goals (3).

At the beginning of the next session, the client is again given the clinical outcome measure in order to assess both current status and clinical improvement (5). The client's score is compared to standardized clinical cutoffs (6). The clinical cutoff score indicates whether the client's level of distress and symptomatic state has been reduced to "normal" levels. The outcome measure is combined with the clinician's judgment in determining whether the client has improved sufficiently to terminate treatment (7). If the client has improved sufficiently, therapy can be terminated or the client can be moved into an appropriate, less intensive level of care (8) (e.g., 12-step programs, group therapy, etc.).

If the client still requires continued therapy, two questions need to be answered. The first is whether clients still have sessions available to them from the initial certification of care (9). If not, clinicians can potentially bolster their assessment of the need for more care with the use of the score from the outcome measure (11). If the session limit has not been met, clinicians can use the outcome measure to determine whether the client is making sufficient progress (10). This evaluation can lead either to continuing with the same course of treatment (4) or reevaluating the diagnosis and/or treatment plan to better meet the client's needs (2).

This illustrates the use of outcomes in a dynamic feedback loop. Such a strategy should increase treatment efficacy by allowing providers to evaluate their clients on a standardized measure as well as using their own professional judgment. Using a standardized outcome measure during the entire course of treatment increases the likelihood that providers will require and deal with lack of patient progress or outright patient worsening, if such exists.

Behavioral Health Care Company Feedback

The section of Fig. 4 below the double line shows the ways in which outcomes feedback is or can be used at HAI. Every time a client completes an outcome measure, the instrument is sent to HAI (12). Large amounts of data are analyzed and used to three ends: reporting, algorithms, and research.

First, reporting client outcomes allows HAI to be accountable for the services it is providing. Currently, data are only being reported for clinical services in general. As the size of the database increases, however, it is anticipated that the reports will be generated (14) and sent to companies who have purchased behavioral health care for their employees and to providers as an element of provider profiling (15). Companies who pay a significant amount of their benefit dollars for behavioral health care for their employees want evidence that the services they purchase are having the desired effect. Without demonstrable outcomes, companies will stop paying for behavioral benefits and the vast majority of employees who need these benefits will be unable to afford them.

Provider profiling will allow HAI to manage its provider network. It is also a way for providers to manage themselves. It should be emphasized that the correct use of provider profiling requires case mix adjusting—recognizing and adjusting outcome ratings based on differences in case load. After differences in case load are accounted for, reports allow both parties to recognize specific needs and provide or obtain relevant training.

Second, HAI is using outcome measures to develop clinical decision-making algorithms (16). These algorithms will allow HAI's clinical managers to set session limits that are based on empirical, real-life data rather than on arbitrary standards. Continually feeding outcome data into the system and refining the algorithms (17) allows for increasingly accurate predictions of how much therapy will be needed and what kinds of clinicians and interventions are most effective.

Clinical algorithms also will allow HAI to more efficiently conduct business. In cases where client progress is normal and further sessions are warranted, the algorithms will automatically authorize more sessions (19, 22). In special situations, where the data fall outside the norms for automatic recertification, the case will be sent to a care manager (20). After discussing the case with the provider, more sessions will be certified if the prognosis is positive (21). If the prognosis is not positive, however, treatment alternatives will be discussed (23), and a new treatment decision made (8).

Third, outcome research allows HAI to evaluate the efficacy of existing products (e.g., EAPs, health maintenance organizations) as well as new, innovative approaches to treatment. This research does not take the form of a discrete study, where each has a clear beginning and end. Rather, it is itself a part of quality management, which is an ongoing effort to monitor product quality. Using outcomes in this process allows HAI to make the client's clinical improvement a central metric for evaluation. This perspective enhances the likelihood that cost containment will come at the expense of quality care.

Conclusion

The most efficacious use of outcome data is its integration into a strong quality management effort. This requires fully integrating outcomes into the way one does business. Anything less fails to realize the full potential of outcome measurement. This chapter presented one such approach, which emphasizes both clinicians and the managed behavioral health care company using outcomes to improve the quality of the services provided.

Clinicians can use outcomes to evaluate treatment efficacy with each individual client and make treatment adjustments as required. Managed behavioral health care companies can use outcomes to demonstrate accountability, provide general feedback to providers, develop treatment guidelines based on empirical data, and evaluate the efficacy of treatment programs in general. In short, consistent use and evaluation of client outcomes can do nothing but improve the value of services offered. There is little doubt that outcome research as practiced within the managed care environment will make a valuable contribution to the patients who are being treated and the pool of scientific knowledge aimed at understanding the process of effectively helping people.

REFERENCES

Antonuccio, D. O., Danton, W. G., & DeNelsky, G. Y. (1995). Psychotherapy versus medication for depression: Challenging the conventional wisdom with data. *Professional Psychology: Research and Practice, 26*, 574–585.

Barber, J. P., & Crits-Christoph, P. (1991). Comparison of the brief dynamic therapies. In P. Crits-Christoph & J. P. Barber (Eds.), *Handbook of short-term dynamic therapy* (pp. 323–356). New York: Basic Books.

Barlow, D. H. (1988). *Anxiety and its disorders: The nature and treatment of anxiety and panic*. New York: Guilford.

Bergin, A. E., & Garfield, S. L. (1994). *Handbook of psychotherapy and behavior change* (4th ed.). New York: Wiley.

Beutler, L. E., Frank, M., Schieber, S. C., Calvert, S., & Gaines, J. (1984). Comparative effects of group psychotherapies in a short-term inpatient setting: An experience with deterioration effects. *Psychiatry, 47*, 66–76.

Binder, J. L., Henry, W. P., & Strupp, H. H. (1987). An appraisal of selection criteria for dynamic psychotherapies and implications for setting limits. *Journal of Psychiatry, 50*, 154–166.

Consumer Reports. (1995, November). Mental health: Does therapy help? 734–739.

Cooley, E. F., & LaJoy, R. (1980). Therapeutic relationship and improvement as perceived by clients and therapists. *Journal of Clinical Psychology, 36*, 562–570.

de Beuirs, E., van Balkom, A. J. L. M., Lange, A., Koele, P., & van Dyck, R. (1995). Treatment of panic disorder with agoraphobia: Comparison of fluvoxamine, placebo, and psychological panic management combined with exposure and of exposure in vivo alone. *American Journal of Psychiatry, 152*, 683–691.

Doherty, W. J., Lester, M. E., & Leigh, G. K. (1986). Marriage encounter weekends: Couples who win and couples who lose. *Journal of Marital and Family Therapy, 12*, 49–61.

Elkin, I., Shea, M. T., Watkins, J. T., Imber, S. D., Stosky, S. M., Collins, J. F., Glass, D. R., Pilkonis, P. A., Weber, W. R., Docherty, J. P., Fiester, S. J., & Parloff, M. B. (1989). National Institute of Mental Health treatment of depression collaborative research program: General effectiveness of treatments. *Archives of General Psychiatry, 46*, 971–982.

Fuhriman, A. J., & Burlingame, G. M. (1994). *The handbook of group psychotherapy: An empirical and clinical synthesis*. New York: Interscience.

Gaston, L. (1990). The concept of the alliance and its role in psychotherapy: Theoretical and empirical considerations. *Psychotherapy, 27*, 143–153.

Hargrave, G. E., & Hiatt, D. (1995). Analysis of outpatient psychotherapy: Quality improvement indicators. *Managed Care Quarterly, 3*, 72–75.

Hattie, J. A., Sharpley, C. F., & Rogers, H. F. (1984). Comparative effectiveness of professional and paraprofessional helpers. *Psychological Bulletin, 95*, 534–541.

Howard, K. I., Kopta, S. M., Krause, M. S., & Orlinsky, D. E. (1986). The dose-effect relationship in psychotherapy. *American Psychologist, 41*, 159–164.

Imber, S. D., Pilkonis, P. A., Sotsky, S. M., Elkin, I., Watkins, J. T., Collins, J. F., Shea, M. T., Weber, W. R., & Glass, D. R. (1990). Mode-specific effects among three treatments for depression. *Journal of Consulting and Clinical Psychology, 58*, 352–359.

Jensen, J. P., Bergin, A. E. & Greaves, D. W. (1990). The meaning of eclecticism: New survey and analysis of components. *Professional Psychology: Research and Practice, 21*, 124–130.

Jorm, A. F. (1989). Modifiability of trait anxiety and neuroticism: A meta-analysis of the literature. *Australian and New Zealand Journal of Psychiatry, 23*, 21–29.

Kadera, S. W., Lambert, M. J., & Andrews, A. A. (1996). How much therapy is really enough? A session-by-session analysis of the psychotherapy dose–effect relationship. *Journal of Psychotherapy Research and Practice, 5*, 132–151.

Kazdin, A. E. (1986). Comparative outcome studies of psychotherapy: Methodological issues and strategies. *Journal of Consulting and Clinical Psychology, 54*, 95–105.

Koss, M. P., & Shiang, J. (1994). Research on brief psychotherapy. In A. E. Bergin & S. L. Garfield (Eds.), *Handbook of psychotherapy and behavior change* (4th ed., pp. 664–700). New York: Wiley & Sons.

Lafferty, P., Beutler, L. E., & Crago, M. (1991). Differences between more and less effective psychotherapists: A study of select therapist variables. *Journal of Consulting and Clinical Psychology, 57*, 76–80.

Lambert, M. J. (1979). Characteristics of patients and the relationship to outcome in brief psychotherapy. *Psychiatric Clinics of North America, 2*, 111–123.

Lambert, M. J., & Anderson, E. M. (1996). Assessment for the time-limited psychotherapies. *Annual Review of Psychiatry, 15*, 23–47.

Lambert, M. J., & Bergin, A. E. (1994). The effectiveness of psychotherapy. In A. E. Bergin & S. L. Garfield (Eds.), *Handbook of psychotherapy and behavior change* (4th ed., pp. 143–189). New York: John Wiley & Sons.

Lambert, M. J., Bergin, A. E., & Collins, J. L. (1977). Therapist induced deterioration in psychotherapy patients. In A. S. Gurman & A. M. Razin (Eds.), *Effective psychotherapy: A handbook of research* (pp. 452–481). New York: Pergamon.

Lambert, M. J., DeJulio, S. S. & Stein, D. M. (1978). Therapist interpersonal skills: Process, outcome, methodological considerations, and recommendations for future research. *Psychological Bulletin, 85,* 467–489.

Lieberman, M. A., Yalom, I. D., & Miles, M. B. (1973). *Encounter groups: First facts.* New York: Basic Books.

Lorr, M. (1965). Clients' perceptions of therapists. *Journal of Consulting Psychology, 29,* 146–149.

Malan, D. H. (1976). *The frontier of brief psychotherapy.* New York: Plenum Press.

Marmor, J. (1979). Short-term dynamic psychotherapy. *American Journal of Psychiatry, 136,* 149–155.

Michelson, L. K., & Marchione, K. (1991). Behavioral, cognitive, and pharmacological treatment of panic disorder with agoraphobia: Critique and synthesis. *Journal of Consulting and Clinical Psychology, 59,* 100–114.

Miller, W. R., Taylor, C. A., & West, J. C. (1980). Focused versus broad-spectrum behavior therapy for problem drinkers. *Journal of Consulting and Clinical Psychology, 48,* 590–601.

Mohr, D. C. (1995). Negative outcome in psychotherapy: A critical review. *Clinical Psychology Science and Practice, 2,* 1–27.

Nicholson, R. A., & Berman, J. S. (1983). Is follow-up necessary in evaluating psychotherapy? *Psychological Bulletin, 93,* 261–278.

Ogles, B. M., Lambert, M. J., & Sawyer, J. D. (1995). Clinical significance of the National Institute of Mental Health treatment of depression collaborative research program data. *Journal of Consulting and Clinical Psychology, 63,* 321–326.

Pollack, E. J. (1995, Dec. 1). Side effects: Managed care focus on psychiatric drugs alarms many doctors. *The Wall Street Journal,* p. A1.

Robinson , L. A., Berman, J. S., & Neimeyer, R. S. (1990). Psychotherapy for the treatment of depression: A comprehensive review of controlled outcome research. *Psychological Bulletin, 108,* 30–49.

Sachs, J. S. (1983). Negative factors in brief psychotherapy: An empirical assessment. *Journal of Consulting and Clinical Psychology, 51,* 557–564.

Safran, J., & Muran, J. C. (1995). Special issue on the therapeutic alliance. *In Session: Psychotherapy in Practice, 1,* 3–8.

Schneider, W. J., & Pinkerton, R. S. (1986). Short-term psychotherapy and graduate training in psychology. *Professional Psychology: Research and Practice, 17,* 574–579.

Seligman, M. E. P. (1995). The effectiveness of psychotherapy: The Consumer Reports study. *American Psychologist, 50,* 965–974.

Shapiro, D. A., Rees, A., Barkham, M., Hardy, G., Reynolds, S., & Startup, M. (1995). Effects of treatment duration and severity of depression on the maintenance of gains of cognitive-behavioral and psychodynamic interpersonal psychotherapy. *Journal of Consulting and Clinical Psychology, 63,* 378–387.

Sifneos, P. E. (1979). *Short-term dynamic psychotherapy.* New York: Plenum Press.

Stein, D. M., & Lambert, M. J. (1995). Graduate training in psychotherapy: Are therapy outcomes enhanced? Special section: The case for training in the provision of psychological therapy. *Journal of Consulting and Clinical Psychology, 63,* 182–186.

Steinbrueck, S. M., Maxwell, S. E., & Howard, G. S. (1983). A meta-analysis of psychotherapy and drug therapy in the treatment of unipolar depression with adults. *Journal of Consulting and Clinical Psychology, 51,* 856–863.

Strupp, H. H. (1980). Success and failure in time-limited psychotherapy: Comparison I. *Archives of General Psychiatry, 37,* 595–603.

Weisz, J. R., Weis, B., Alicke, M. D., & Klots, M. L. (1987). Effectiveness of psychotherapy with children and adolescents: A meta-analysis for clinicians. *Journal of Consulting and Clinical Psychology, 55,* 542–549.

6

Provider Profiling as a Quality Improvement Tool

SHARON A. SHUEMAN AND NANCY E. LANE

Accountability in health services is increasingly about answering one seemingly simple question: Is the consumer or payer getting value for money? We use the word value, rather than quality, to emphasize that "value" includes economic factors as well as the more traditionally defined "quality." Admittedly, there are important discussions that must occur at a societal level concerning the appropriate weighting of quality and cost in health care decisions. In the practical present, however, payers and health care systems are routinely making decisions regarding providers and their involvement in emerging systems that have an impact on the careers of many. Payers and the general public are demanding that providers and health care systems be accountable for both the quality and the cost of their services.

As is discussed elsewhere in this volume, calls for accountability in health services have a relatively short history. Accountability is sometimes viewed as synonymous with quality assurance, especially from the perspective of health care professionals. Providers have long histories of involvement in activities such as credentialing, continuing education, peer review, and similar activities. From their perspective, these constitute assurances that the services they provide are accountable to widely shared opinions of other professionals about acceptable quality. While accountability is strongly correlated with quality, it expands to include the perspective of payers and consumers in its definition. Including the opinions and values of third and even fourth parties is a relatively new development in health care. Consequently, technologies for demonstrating accountability and value are not well developed, even though demands for them increase every day. This is particularly true in behavioral health services where the often subjective nature of disorders, the lack of uniformity and even clear definition in approaches to treatment, and the unwillingness of providers to accept the need for accountability to a third party have made the evaluation of treatment outcome significantly more difficult than in general medical care. Further difficulties arise from the limitations in generalizing treatment approaches and expectable outcomes from current research literature. For most practicing clinicians, there may be little relevance to the general population they serve of research conducted

SHARON A. SHUEMAN • Shueman Troy Associates, Pasadena, California 91106. NANCY E. LANE • Massachusetts Behavioral Health Partnership, Boston, Massachusetts 02110.

Handbook of Quality Management in Behavioral Health, edited by Stricker *et al.* Kluwer Academic / Plenum Publishers, New York, 2000.

according to the clinical trials model in university settings. For managed care companies and payers, there are further difficulties in extrapolating the results of such research to settings where the focus of attention is on the treatment response and functional status of a population of patients that can number in the hundreds of thousands.

PROFILING: A TOOL FOR ENABLING SYSTEMS OF CARE

One of the technologies believed to have promise for enabling systems of care to demonstrate accountability is that of provider profiling of both individual providers and provider groups. As technologies, profiling and other systemwide evaluation strategies are examples of growing opportunities for population-based research approaches to be developed and used to improve overall system effectiveness. The ability to organize large data sets into effective evaluation approaches may well be one of the lasting contributions of the current generation of managed care systems to the understanding of behavioral health treatments as they are currently deployed in real-world settings. This chapter offers a definition of provider profiling, its place in the assessment of overall quality of a health care plan, a discussion of issues both conceptual and practical to be considered in the development of a model of profiling, and a discussion of the ways in which this activity may be used to monitor and improve the value of services delivered through organized systems of care. Since the authors are most familiar with systems of profiling used within managed behavioral health care organizations, this is the focus of the chapter. The same principles, however, are applicable to any organized service delivery system employing multiple providers and having the capability to collect, aggregate, and report clinical and administrative data. Similar principles also may be applied to services delivered by programs or facilities. Special considerations in applying these concepts to groups of providers, to facilities, and to situations where providers must profile themselves are discussed.

The chapter is written to be more conceptual than technical. While it deals to some extent with principles of measurement and analysis, the primary objective is to help the reader understand the higher-level issues related to the development and implementation of a provider profiling activity.

PROVIDER PROFILING: WHAT IS IT?

Provider profiling refers to a process of data analysis and reporting that describes a practitioner's performance on selected clinical and administrative indicators relative to benchmarks or norms. *Benchmarks* are levels of performance determined by judgments or an empirical process to reflect excellence in or a desired level of performance. Typically, they are aspirational and constitute targets for provider performance. *Norms* are observed levels of performance of providers in an appropriate reference group. The use of norms allows one provider to be compared to a (norm) group of his or her peers. The norm may or may not represent a high or desired level of performance.

Within organized health care systems, evaluation and quality assurance are increasingly targeted to systemwide measures. These measures cluster around the general categories of assessing cost, satisfaction (payers, patients, providers), success (functional outcomes), and ease (lack of administrative burden–provider cooperation with administrative procedures). Within each category, multiple measures are developed to answer specific questions that are of interest to multiple stakeholders. Provider profiling approaches draw from each of these categories to construct composite evaluative snapshots of provider performance. At its most ideal, provider profiling constitutes a measure of overall provider effectiveness that is used interactively with providers and other stakeholders to increase the overall clinical and cost effectiveness of health care systems.

Specific Purposes of Profiling

In the current health care market environment, it is virtually a necessity for systems of care to possess some mechanism for formally evaluating the performance of their provider network. It is expected, therefore, that a managed care organization will maintain some type of provider profiling system. The models in existence vary in sophistication, scientific rigor, and comprehensiveness, but they all share a common evaluative purpose. Profiling activities may be used within service systems to understand provider behavior, to influence or change provider behavior, and to meet other specific needs of the system, both operational and evaluative.

Understanding or Describing Behavior

In practice, a profile is nothing more than a reflection of an individual provider's performance on variables or indicators considered important by the organization or some other stakeholder. Some common types of indicators (and examples) are as follows:

- Outcomes (e.g., patient improvement on clinical measure; patient satisfaction).
- Utilization patterns (e.g., average number of outpatient sessions per treatment episode).
- Cost patterns of services provided (e.g., cost per episode of treatment).
- Quality concerns raised relative to the provider (e.g., patient- or case manager-initiated concern).
- Clinical process measures including areas such as patterns of collaboration with other providers (e.g., consulting with primary care physician when there is a coexisting medical problem relevant to the behavioral disorder), completeness of discharge planning, and effective referral and follow-up through multiple levels of care.
- Other combined clinical indicators (e.g., patient relapse or recidivism; frequency of referral to free or low cost community services).
- Compliance with administrative requirements (e.g., completing and returning forms).

Profiles based on indicators such as these allow the organization to determine how providers, individually and collectively, are performing. Based on profiling information, the organization may choose to eliminate deficient providers from the network, or it may target corrective actions toward the areas where performance is inadequate. In the special case of providers being viewed at a group or facility level, additional factors may include items such as sufficiency of the provider's internal quality assurance structures, compliance or adherence to professional accrediting body expectations, ability to effect staff performance, sufficiency of information systems, and ability to track and monitor outcomes or other indicators.

A difficult challenge for any organization that conducts provider profiling is to be certain that descriptions of provider performance are meaningfully extended to the understanding of that performance. A first pass at descriptions of providers according to preselected levels of performance may well identify a small group of providers who are well outside the boundaries of expected performance. Before this finding can be transformed into an action plan, possible reasons for an extreme variance need to be explored, often in collaboration with the providers themselves. (Any indications, however, of fraudulent or unethical patterns uncovered through profiling activities should be investigated apart from an organization's profiling programs.) This distinction helps both providers and payers understand what is being asked and given and for what purpose. This is essential if providers are expected to be willing participants in profiling; that is, to supply information and work to improve performance based on feedback received from profiling activities.

Influencing Provider Behavior

Profiles may be used at the individual provider or facility level as a feedback mechanism on performance so practitioners may attempt to improve their performance relative to the selected indicators. An assumption is that, once informed, the provider will have the capacity for self-improvement. This may or may not be a valid assumption. For example, it may be a simple matter for a provider to improve the timeliness of form submission but a much more challenging task to improve clinical effectiveness (e.g., effect increased patient change or patient satisfaction with treatment).

Based on the assumption that performance among providers on any indicator is normally distributed and that there is significant random variation on measurement outside of the laboratory, providers are typically expected to perform within "bands" of acceptable practice. In fact, there may be quite a large difference between the highest and lowest "acceptable" values on a given indicator. For example, data may reveal that for 90% of providers the mean number of sessions required to complete an outpatient episode of care is between five and ten sessions. Providers whose averages fall outside this band would be among the first to be scrutinized.

In sharing profiling information with providers, managed care companies will differ in their expectations for change. They also will differ widely in the kinds of support and direction they supply to effect that change. Expectations may involve reaching or maintaining a certain level of performance in order to become or stay a preferred provider. To achieve these expectations, some managed care entities will request action plans, while others will expect primarily to monitor successive levels of performance, leaving the methods for improvement largely in the hands of the providers. Additionally, some managed care entities will offer technical or conceptual assistance to providers willing to engage in collaborative efforts to improve performance.

Other Uses of Profiling Data

The primary purpose of profiling from the system's perspective is to ensure an adequately performing provider network. Besides being used to identify practitioners for removal from the network or to help providers understand the areas of performance in which they need to improve, profiling information may be used as a basis for giving preferential referrals or financial incentives to better-performing providers. A common question in requests for proposals for large managed care accounts is the extent to which on-line provider profiling results are available to those making referrals to network providers. Profiles may also help determine which providers should be subject to more intensive monitoring or case review by case management staff.

In managed care systems where providers accept capitation arrangements, provider profiling plays an important role in the ongoing monitoring of quality outcomes. Whether capitation is held by a managed care entity or by providers themselves (either directly or via subcapitation arrangements), high-quality, cost-effective performance of providers is an immediate and pressing concern in such environments to assure that resources are most effectively deployed in the interest of patient care.

Payers also are becoming increasingly interested and involved in holding managed care companies accountable for the performance of their contracted provider networks. Here, the managed care company itself must produce summary statistical descriptions of the performance of its network(s) and can be rewarded or penalized depending on aggregate performance.

A profile (or a "report card") of an individual provider or of a provider group, if made public, allows a potential consumer to make more informed judgments about which provider to choose. Payers and purchasers may use profiles to determine which providers they should encourage the managed care organization to use [this happens more often in context of employee assistance programs (EAPs) than in context of general managed behavioral health care programs]. If profiles are made available for public consumption, two things must be ensured. The first is that the data reported must be relevant to the person reading them. The second is that the data are presented in a form and format the reader can understand. There is evidence, for example, that if consumers do not understand the information in a profile (or report card), they tend to dismiss it as unimportant. This will happen even if the data reflect an important measure of quality (Hibbard & Jewett, 1997).

INFORMATION USED TO CREATE PROFILES

Serious thought must be given to the number of variables and types of data included in a model of provider profiling. The range of variables potentially related to the underlying construct of quality in context of a service system requires that any model be multivariate. A simplified example demonstrates why this is so:

> Dr. Smith is a clinical psychologist and contracted member of the network of Acme Behavioral Care (ABC). For all outpatients referred to her by ABC in 1996, Dr. Smith's mean for an episode of care was 6 sessions. The mean for all clinical psychologists on the ABC network was 8.5 sessions. At the same time, Dr. Smith reported that 50% of her patients left treatment (dropped out) without completing the agreed upon treatment plan. The average for all

providers was 15%. Further, the rate at which Dr. Smith's patients returned to ABC to request additional services was 27%, while for all ABC outpatients it was 12%. Her patients reported high levels of satisfaction with her care, moderate levels of symptom reduction, and small levels of improvement in functional status.

Were ABC evaluating outpatient providers strictly in terms of average number of sessions, Dr. Smith would probably be rated quite high and as a consequence might be given preference for referrals. It appears as though this may not be a wise decision on the part of ABC, however. Although she may be working quickly, it does not appear that Dr. Smith is working effectively. From the system's perspective, Dr. Smith might be a very costly provider. She also might be producing satisfied but not improved patients. This example demonstrates the importance of taking a multivariate approach to evaluating provider performance in context of the development of a network of providers (Mayhugh & Shueman, 1994).

It should be noted that much of the early activity aimed at profiling providers focused on utilization data, primarily as found in claims files (Eskow, 1991). One major reason for this was that little was available other than claims data. Current systems have progressed significantly, and managed care organizations (MCOs) create comprehensive databases including a range of data such as described below.

Sources of Data

As with any measurement activity, consideration must be given to both objective and subjective data. While objective data may have more appeal (i.e., it may appear more "scientific"), the nature of behavioral health services dictates that some subjective measures be employed. These typically include patient satisfaction or evaluation of treatment; providers' assessments of patient change, progress, disposition, or prognosis; and case managers' judgments about the quality of providers' clinical interventions or their responsiveness to administrative requests.

In an accountable health care system, it is not enough that providers be clinically effective. They also must operate effectively and efficiently as part of a service delivery system. For example, providers must respond in a timely way to requests from case managers for clinical information and they must be willing to consult with other providers when necessary. They also must be willing to assure that consumers can easily access all needed levels of care. As a consequence, both clinical and administrative data should be considered relevant indicators of a provider's performance within a system of care.

Profile data typically originate with any of five sources. These include the MCO's internal information systems, the MCO's staff, providers themselves, consumers and their families, and payers–purchasers.

MCO Information Systems

MCOs maintain a number of separate information bases which may contribute data to a profiling activity. These include:

1. Applications for network membership (e.g., provider specialties; number of years experience; participation in quality improvement activities).

2. Authorization* and utilization (claims) data sets (e.g., number of referrals received from the company; range and average number of outpatient sessions).
3. Quality management database (e.g., patient, family member, or case management staff complaints specifically related to quality of the provider's services).
4. Patient satisfaction data sets.
5. Clinical outcomes systems, when available (e.g., posttreatment score on standardized clinical instrument, patient or provider evaluation of outcome).

MCO Staff Evaluations

Most MCOs maintain formal databases reflecting staff evaluations of the quality of provider performance on clinical and administrative variables. These data constitute a critical component of profiles, despite shortcomings, discussed below, since staff interactions with providers about clinical issues or administrative matters are often the most direct evidence the MCO has concerning providers' general level of competence and professionalism. Typically, two categories of employees provide this type of data: clinical staff (case managers and physician advisors) who deal with providers about case-specific issues of necessity and appropriateness, and provider relations staff who are responsible for ensuring that providers comply with various aspects of their contract. It is essential that MCOs structure how these data are gathered to assure reliability and fairness in MCO staff assessments of providers. Also, MCOs must maintain open channels for providers to share concerns about the performance of MCO staff, as well.

Data Generated by Providers

In most MCOs providers themselves regularly submit data reflecting their evaluations of patient progress and outcome. These data are potentially limited in their usefulness because of some providers' propensity to respond in socially desirable ways (i.e., to affirm that the treatment was a success). At the same time, if used in a multidimensional profiling model where other indicators, such as patient perceptions of the same aspects of treatment, can play a validating role, these data become critical to the profiling process. The lack of universally accepted and adopted systems for both defining and measuring optimal treatment outcomes is a major stumbling block at this time.

Data Generated by Consumers

Patients contribute data about providers in several ways. The most common is through patient satisfaction surveys. These surveys provide useful data if they are provider specific and if response rates are sufficient to allow generalization to all of a practitioner's patients. Also useful are surveys reflecting perceptions of treatment outcome such as progress, goal achievement, and termination status. Patients and

*An authorization is a promise of payment for a practitioner/facility to provide designated services to a given patient for a specified number of sessions or days or period of time.

their family members also may submit compliments or complaints about any aspect of provider behavior, and these may be quantified and considered in a profile.

Data Generated by Payers

Payers may play a role in evaluating the performance of providers, particularly in context of EAPs. Employers may make direct referrals of their employees to practitioners on an EAP network. These referrals often result in direct contact between the employer's representative (i.e., human resources professional) and the practitioner, and the employer frequently forms an opinion of the "quality" of the practitioner from these interactions. Corporate payers also can generate information about how the patients of various providers fare in terms of time lost from work, entry to higher levels of care from the EAP setting, and movement into disability status.

THE QUALITY OF DATA

Three factors potentially threaten the quality (reliability, validity, and utility) of data typically used in provider profiling. These include (1) social desirability affecting the validity of data submitted by providers and patients; (2) lack of objectivity of consumers, payers, MCO staff, or clinical consultants making subjective evaluations of providers; and (3) lack of relevance of the data to the underlying concept of quality. Also, providers typically cite confidentiality concerns as a reason for carefully monitoring and filtering data to be provided to payers. Finally, there is concern about how data are combined into meaningful composite descriptions. As the number of variables combined increases, there can be a tendency to ascribe more "power" to a numeric description of a provider than the quality of the data can meaningfully support.

Social Desirability

This threat is a direct function of the willingness and ability of practitioners to provide information that objectively reflects a clinical situation. For example, practitioners are regularly asked to provide information about their patients and the treatment plans. Some of these data, most often severity indicators and evaluations of improvement or goal achievement, may be used for profiling. The practitioner who is aware that he or she is being evaluated on clinical competence may not be motivated to report honestly. That is, he or she may describe symptoms as more severe than they in fact are or describe progress more positively. There is a companion, but contradictory, social desirability pressure from patients who may wish their conditions to be seen and reported as less severe or disabling than they actually may be. This is most common in areas such as substance abuse, domestic violence, or psychotic or bipolar disorders. In systems where data are supplied directly by patients, this can be a major source of variation.

Lack of Objectivity

Just as providers may hesitate to report data that reflects poorly on them (e.g., the patient dropped out of treatment or did not achieve the treatment goals), so too may people who come into contact with providers not evaluate provider behavior objectively. For example, it is not uncommon for case management staff or clinical consultants to either favor providers who are very cooperative (always willing to accept an emergency referral, always compliant with administrative requirements) or dislike providers whom they perceive as adversarial or nonresponsive. The former providers may earn a halo and be evaluated positively by case managers on all indicators, clinical and administrative, even if they are weak clinically. In contrast, the latter group of providers may be evaluated negatively on all indicators, even if they are strong in some. Patients may be asked to evaluate the outcome of their treatment or report their level of satisfaction with services. To the extent that they have global positive feelings about their therapist, they may feel obliged to provide a more positive evaluation than is warranted by the clinical situation.

Relevance of Data

The most critical question, of course, is whether the data selected for use in the profile have anything to do with the "quality" of the provider. Since the definition of quality is at least partly values based, within a managed system of care the definition most likely to prevail in the current environment reflects cost-effectiveness, administrative compliance, and patient satisfaction. Whatever the data, they must reflect a range of provider behaviors sufficiently broad to fairly represent a typical provider's repertoire within a system of care.

The quantity of data available for any one individual provider is another systemic problem in assessing the relevance of provider profiles. Unless a single MCO provides a substantial proportion of a provider's clinical referrals, it is likely that there will not be sufficient data to assess performance in a meaningful way. A related issue is the need to track clinical outcomes over a lengthier period of time than is practicable in most clinical and managed care settings.

Moderating Variables—Limiting Factors in Constructing Valid Profiles

There are a number of contextual factors within systems of care that may have a significant impact on a provider's ability to implement an effective treatment plan in particular situations. These factors, which need to be considered in order for profiling data to be meaningful reflections of quality, include characteristics of patients (i.e., patient mix), characteristics of the benefit plan, and characteristics of the geographic area in which a provider practices.

Patient Mix

Since behavioral health professionals are typically trained to treat a fairly broad range of behavioral health problems, the referrals any one provider receives from a managed care company are usually heterogeneous in terms of problem type and severity. As a rule, then, one would expect equal distribution of "difficult" patients across providers. Some providers, however, do become identified by managed care staff as being more capable of dealing with difficult patients and as a consequence they get selected by those staff to deal with more challenging patients. These include practitioners who are consistently responsive to requests for assistance from managed care staff, who are seen as professionals staff members can "count on" in difficult situations.

The kinds of patients classified as challenging may include people whose problems have been refractory to treatment or whose particular diagnoses suggest potential difficulty in developing an effective treatment plan. For patients treated in outpatient care, an example would be someone with a severe coexisting personality disorder; for patients seen in acute care, this category may include long-standing and severe eating disorders and certain disorders of childhood and adolescence. Certainly, profiles for practitioners or facilities that consistently receive more difficult patients should reflect this patient mix.

In managed care systems for publicly funded projects, an additional factor in patient mix is the presence or absence of social supports surrounding a given patient. These include employment, family support, housing, support from other social agencies, and so forth. Describing provider performance and patient response in these situations may require a very different and more complex set of factors than in more traditional "medical" models.

Characteristics of Benefit Plans

A severely limited benefit plan or a plan that does not cover one or more critical treatment modalities, levels of care, or treatment settings may compromise a practitioner or facility's ability to implement an appropriate treatment plan. One example of this is a chemical dependency benefit that includes detoxification services but not rehabilitation. A second example is a mental health benefit that includes no coverage for inpatient or partial hospitalization services, or a plan which reimburses for individual therapy but not for often more appropriate marriage and family treatment. Finally, a benefit with very high copayment requirements might discourage patients from continuing in treatment when continuation would be warranted.

Such benefit plan characteristics, while seeming reasonable to employers or other purchasers of these plans, may severely limit a provider's capacity to maximize his or her effectiveness with particular types of patients. This factor is likely to be particularly significant for a provider who lives in a geographic area that has one very large employer group that is covered by a less than optimal behavioral health benefit plan. A practitioner who is referred a large number of patients with limited benefit plans may not always be able to implement a plan with the most appropriate type, intensity, or level of care. Limitations such as this on the provider's ability to control the selection of treatment (type, level, or intensity) may negatively affect the typical outcome of that provider's patients. Such factors, which might be called "benefit mix," need to be considered in the development of profiles for the affected providers.

Resources Available in the Geographic Area

Metropolitan areas in populous states draw a disproportionately high number of mental health practitioners and often are the sites of a range of highly specialized behavioral health programs and facilities. (Such programs are often found in university-affiliated medical centers.) In these more highly populated areas it may be relatively easy to find an appropriate practitioner, facility, or program, no matter what the treatment needs of a patient. For example, one may find specialized treatment for problems such as Tourette's syndrome, severe eating disorders, and geriatric mental illness. One is also likely to find practitioners and programs specializing in culturally diverse populations or people with a disability (e.g., practitioners fluent in sign language). Rural and other less-populated areas, however, rarely have the luxury of such specialization. Rather, the few practitioners and programs tend, out of necessity, to function as generalists, treating all types of problems and patients, regardless of whether they consider themselves particularly skilled in those areas. One might expect that these providers, who treat whomever with whatever problem that walks through their door, may demonstrate poorer clinical outcomes than providers whose patients are more restricted and more likely to fall within the specialty areas of their providers. This is a patient mix in a different guise from that described above and should be considered in the development of the provider profile. For this, as for all other categorical distinctions among providers, it may be appropriate to compare any given provider to all other providers but also to all providers within a defined group.

USING THE RESULTS OF PROFILING

The subject of provider profiling has been one of the most contentious issues in health services in the last decade, particularly in behavioral health. On the one hand, consumers and payers have demanded access to information about the performance of practitioners and facilities, and certainly health systems have a legitimate need for information to help them improve their performance. On the other hand, practitioners have been suspicious of profiling activities, arguing that profiling models are biased by the values of managed care systems (i.e., they over emphasize efficiency) and are not yet sufficiently sophisticated to reflect the true essence of quality of health services.

Despite the contention, it is generally agreed that payers and purchasers as well as consumers have a right to information about the performance of providers. Furthermore, to the extent that practitioners are evaluated on the basis of profiles, they too have a right to information about their own profiles as well as the profiles of providers to whom they are being compared. Those who create profiling systems, therefore, have a special responsibility to ensure that their models are based on valid data and that the data reflect variables representing the interests of all stakeholder groups (providers themselves, consumers and families, payers, and the managed care company). Further, the data must reflect factors that are meaningful representations of the underlying quality values, and the profiles must be reported in ways that accurately represent what they purport to measure.

Because of the potential for economic harm to a provider whose profile suggests below par performance, the MCO must ensure that the profiling process results in reliable and valid data. In other words, it must be fair. The MCO must, if necessary, be able to defend its profiling model and its results in a court of law. This necessity points to the importance to the MCO of having access to a person with the technical sophistication to create a rigorous model and ensure that it be used appropriately. Such a person would understand issues of reliability, validity, sensitivity of measures, and so on. Interestingly, while industrial–organizational psychologists are the logical choice to have these responsibilities, these professionals are rarely sought out by health systems for this purpose.

As numerous payers and MCOs influence the construction of provider profiles, it may well become problematic for providers to receive different types of profile reports from different payers. In the next several years, national-level efforts may well emerge, both from accrediting bodies and commercial vendors, to provide provider profiles constructed from viewing a provider's total practice and made available to multiple MCOs.

The development of a profiling system must be thought of as an evolutionary process. That is, the original model should be modified over time as the managed care organization evaluates both the model's usefulness to the company and its relevance to the needs of other stakeholders, including providers, consumers, and payers. It is particularly important that providers be involved in this evolutionary process. First and foremost, results of the profiling activity affect providers' standing within the network and most likely the number of referrals they receive. This may be a matter of financial survival for many practitioners. The profile, however, is also intended to be useful to practitioners, to enable them to analyze their strengths and weaknesses and to give them a basis for a professional development program to correct deficiencies or enhance their competence in selected areas. Providers, therefore, must be given ample opportunity to evaluate the profiling model; to critique both its relevance and its usefulness to them. This would most likely take the form of distributing profiles to providers, soliciting feedback from them on questions such clarity and relevance of the indicators, and then modifying the model based on this feedback. A challenge to all participants in the profiling process is to allow profiling to proceed even though all conditions of rigor cannot be met due to the real-life conditions under which profiling must be conducted. The corollary challenge is to continuously enrich the profiling process and its results with new knowledge and statistical techniques as these become known and available.

Reporting Results

If profiling data are to be meaningful and useful to providers, they need to be presented in a way that is easily comprehended, particularly if providers are expected to improve their performance based on the scores on critical indicators. Some profiling models use sophisticated multivariate statistical techniques that combine data and result in global ratings or quality scores. These models that provide complex measures in a summary format will probably not be useful to many providers. (Only clinical psychologists typically receive the training in statistics and research needed to understand multivariate analyses.) Therefore, feedback to providers needs to be in terms of the components (simple variables) that went into the analysis and that appear to be significant discriminators across providers. For example, if a regression model is used, reports to providers need to include their performance on those individual variables determined to be significant predictors in the analysis, rather than in the form of a description of the criterion group.

Results also need to describe each provider's performance relative to scores of a norm group. This norm group may well be the subset of providers determined by the analysis to be of "higher quality" rather than all providers on the network. This will allow each provider to determine where he or she needs to improve, and by how much.

A related issue is the level of reporting about individual provider performance, specifically when that provider is associated with a group, program, or facility. That is, should the performance of individual providers be reported to the administrator of the group or program of which they are a part? And at what level are providers to be held accountable: at the individual level or at the level of an entire group or clinic? This issue will become increasingly important as health care consolidation continues.

Regardless of how profiling results are disseminated, most importantly, they must be useful and must suggest ways in which providers can improve their performance. If the information supplied is not tied to suggested process improvements or technical assistance, the likelihood of performance change is minimal. Continuous feedback is also necessary to encourage sustained performance improvements efforts by providers. This is a substantial difficulty in the current era of rapid consolidation in all areas of the health care system. As payers change, as provider groups merge, and as managed are companies also merge and change, the likelihood of measuring the same items in reliable ways over time is substantially diminished.

DIRECTIONS FOR THE FUTURE

Who Will Do Provider Profiling and Why?

Currently, provider profiling is being carried out primarily by health systems and managed care companies. Each has its own proprietary method and typically does not share its database or its algorithms with other companies or the public. While this approach may allow some organizations to gain market share by demonstrating the superior use of technology and informed decision making, it is unlikely this piecemeal approach will provide overall system improvement. Over the next several years, we may well see the emergence of national-level criteria for profiling of both individual providers and of health care systems as a whole (report card efforts). It will be the responsibility of all parts of the health care system to work together to assure that the results are both reflective and predictive of provider and system performance and not committee-driven descriptions of traditional provider performance. As mentioned earlier, the potential of using population-level data now becoming available promises greater opportunities for understanding what makes health care systems effective.

In the near future, there appear to be three major settings in which profiling may occur. These are MCOs and other payers, independent accrediting bodies, and provider systems themselves. MCOs use of profiling has been discussed extensively earlier. National accrediting bodies may well develop profiling as a way to offer standardized approaches throughout the health care system, much the way the Scholastic Aptitude Tests or other national-level exams purport to measure similar variables across populations. Because accrediting bodies typically do not have access to patient-specific information, their involvement may focus on specifying the elements of profiling and perhaps even the algorithms applied to available data. The development of national-level profiling approaches will take a number of years but again could be one of the lasting valuable contributions of the managed care industry.

As providers begin accepting capitation and working in new relationships with MCOs, they will find themselves in the role of today's MCOs. To enhance their ability to supply high-quality care at a reasonable cost, that is, while allowing them to make a profit, they will need to know which providers are producing the most effective and efficient outcomes. Because none except for the largest and most sophisticated of provider systems could be expected to have the analytic sophistication to perform these tasks, this may be a service purchased from MCOs by provider groups.

Provider Profiling as a Part of a Larger Evaluation System

Systemwide evaluations of health care costs, processes, and outcomes are pressing needs for all stakeholders in the health care system. In behavioral health, where provider behaviors (rather than sophisticated technology or widely accepted standardized techniques) constitute the major item purchased, provider profiling will occupy a disproportionately greater role in the evaluation of larger behavioral health systems. The major categories for evaluating systems are all closely related to the behavior of individual providers and provider groups. The *cost* of care is usually reducible to the number and type of units provided; *satisfaction* is strongly related to the presence or absence of a positive therapeutic relationship; *success* is often measured by provider-supplied ratings (though this is slowly changing with advances in technology); and *ease of access* will be strongly related to factors such as provider responsiveness and availability. It will be interesting to see if the current development of standardized treatment protocols will be enhanced by looking empirically at which providers produce the best results and then determining what were the common factors in successful treatment outcome.

FINAL COMMENT

Provider profiling in behavioral health care is surely in its infancy. This is evidenced by, if nothing else, the great variation in both scope and technical sophistication of the current models. For example, profiling systems currently in use range from very simple models including as few as two data elements—patient satisfaction and utilization—to complex models combining a dozen or more variables using multivariate analytic techniques. Virtually all these systems, however, greatly exceed in sophistication the claims-based utilization profiles most common as recently as 5 years ago.

Within the last decade there have been increasing calls for profiles (reports cards) for health systems, including hospitals, medical groups, and other health systems. Demands have come from governmental agencies, quasi-governmental organizations (such as the National Committee on Quality Assurance), and employer-sponsored groups (business coalitions). In contrast, there has been little organized public demand for profiling systems focused specifically on individual providers.

These latter systems have been developed primarily within the managed health care industry as proprietary products aimed at gaining competitive advantage for the companies that develop them. A uniform, industrywide model of provider profiling and standardized treatment protocols combined with a focus on long-term functional outcomes would provide the basis for defining good systems of care and eliminating the dogma-driven wars about clinical outcomes.

REFERENCES

Eskow, R. H., (1991). Collection, correction, application: The information cycle in managed health care. In P. Boland (Ed.), *Making managed health care work: A practical guide to strategies and solutions* (pp. 445–478). New York: McGraw-Hill.

Hibbard, J. H., & Jewett, J. J. (1997). Will quality report cards help consumers? *Health Affairs, 16*(3), 218–228.

Mayhugh, B. L., & Shueman, S. A. (1994). Development and maintenance of provider networks. In S. A. Shueman, W. G. Troy, & S. L. Mayhugh, (Eds.), *Managed behavioral health care: An industry perspective* (pp. 49–64). Springfield, IL: Charles C. Thomas.

III

QUALITY MANAGEMENT IN PRACTICE

7

The Role of the Managed Care Organization in Ensuring Quality of the Service System

Maintaining the Full Continuum of Services

SUSAN J. PENNER

A preliminary requirement in discussing the role of the managed care organization in maintaining a full continuum of services is to define the target population or populations for a continuum of care in behavioral health. Typically, severely and persistently mentally ill adults have been identified, often referred to as "revolving door" patients, given their frequent acute care readmissions. This is the population for which the community mental health centers program was initiated in the early 1960s, as an alternative to state mental hospitals (Feldman, 1994). By contrast, the largely employed or employee-dependent populations served under managed care plans tend to have relatively low rates of severe chronic mental illness compared to public sector recipients.

However, there are disorders for which a continuum of behavioral health services are indicated in the employed population. Persons with severe substance abuse problems who are prone to relapse may require services ranging from medical detoxification to day treatment, intensive outpatient care, and up to daily contact with a self-help group or sponsor. Children and adolescents, whether suffering from severe psychotic or depressive disorders or from more commonly seen problems such as conduct disorder, may require partial hospitalization, day treatment, and coordination of mental health with school services. The presence of dual or multiple diagnoses, whether a mental illness and concurrent substance abuse or relapse risk, mental illness and a medical co-morbidity, or a combination of mental illness, physical illness, and substance abuse, requires considerable coordination and case management.

Regardless of the nature of the problems presented by the patient in need of a full continuum of behavioral health care, at least two key issues are shared in common, across diagnoses and whether the population is in the public or private sector. One important issues is that the patient's problems are lateral, in other words, require a broad range of behavioral health services and also may require medical social service intervention. In addition, the patient's needs are longitudinal, continuing over a

---

SUSAN J. PENNER • Department of Nursing, Holy Names College, Oakland, California 94619.

Handbook of Quality Management in Behavioral Health, edited by Stricker *et al.* Kluwer Academic / Plenum Publishers, New York, 2000.

substantial time frame, frequently with periods of remission, recovery, and relapse (Penner, 1994). These lateral and longitudinal problems require interorganizational coordination (Hage, 1980) and comprehensive plan coverage if they are to be adequately managed.

One example of multiple diagnoses that managed behavioral health organizations more commonly will need to address is the patient with a mental illness, substance abuse disorder, and human immunodeficiency virus (HIV) infection. The highly interactive dynamics of risk of infection posed by behavioral symptoms such as sexual acting out or injection drug use, risk of depression, and even suicidal gestures or attempts related to HIV diagnoses, neuropsychiatric symptoms that mimic behavioral disorders and the risk of communication of HIV to family, sexual partners, and other drug users presents considerable challenges to managing these cases (Penner, 1994). In many cases, physical and mental disabilities must be managed for years, requiring social support system development as well as a continuum of health, mental health, and substance abuse services. Another example includes the multiple problems presented by the growing elderly population, which increasingly will suffer chronic physical disease or disability and mental disorders such as depression, and who may knowingly or unknowingly abuse prescription or over-the-counter medications.

A failure to aggressively manage the care of these individuals with complex problems is likely to result in patients not utilizing the services they require. Providers may not be aware of all the patient's needs, particularly in cases of dual or multiple diagnoses, and may not be knowledgeable about services that would meet those needs. Benefit limitations may discourage patients from attempting to access services; patients also may be uninformed about services that are available in the community.

ROLES OF MANAGED CARE ORGANIZATIONS

There are several ways in which managed care organizations play important roles in ensuring a full continuum of high-quality patient care services. These approaches set managed care apart from the traditional fee-for-service system and include:

1. Services system planning.
2. Case management.
3. Benefit redesign.
4. Quality management.

Services System Planning

The organizational and financial mechanisms developed by managed care organizations were designed to reduce the fragmentation of services common in mental health systems and to allow "the dollars to follow the patient." Managed care organizations, unlike fee-for-service plans, take a systems view of the patient and of services required to provide a full continuum of care. The patient is seen as potentially moving among various levels of care, from acute to partial hospitalization, day treatment, intensive outpatient, and routine outpatient appointments with a clinician. All levels of care must be developed within the geographic catchment area in order to accommodate these patient needs. The key issue differentiating managed care from fee-for-service approaches is that accountability for continuity of care is assumed by the managed care organization. Hence, managed care organizations develop clinical guidelines for placement in a continuum of treatment programs, may use capitation financing to allow for optimal flexibility in the choice of treatment setting options, and form provider networks that include alternative levels of care.

Guidelines for placement in the most appropriate level of care based on the patient's current medical necessity and severity of risk factors have been developed by a number of managed care organizations (US Behavioral Health, 1994). Other managed care organizations have developed treatment planning guidelines based on diagnostic criteria, rather than criteria based on medical necessity (U.S. Behavioral Systems, 1994). Written guidelines serve several purposes in enabling the managed care organization to ensure an appropriate continuum of care, including:

- Providing guidance to case managers when evaluating or recommending admission, continuing treatment plans, or discharge plans by network providers.
- Educating network providers regarding expectations for treatment and discharge planning, as well as the optimum range of services required in their delivery system.
- Serving as a benchmark for the ideal continuum of services for a population's catchment area, as determined by an expert, interdisciplinary panel of behavioral health professionals. Thus, if these guidelines cannot be followed because alternative levels of care are not available, such gaps are identified and may be remedied via more intensive network development.

Capitation financing is another mechanism that reflects the role of services system planning in managed care. Capitation is of growing interest to funders of public sector plans, because providers are allowed discretion to spend a fixed amount of money on a wide range of services. Providers may select from these services according to the patient's particular needs, thus ensuring individualized treatment, rather than facing perverse incentives that frequently focus care around reimbursable or covered services such as hospitalization. Capitation has become such an integral component of some managed care plans that the two terms are sometimes used interchangeably, although managed care can and does operate without capitation financing.

In the private sector, managed care companies may negotiate capitated rates with payers and pay negotiated fees to providers in the network. The rationale for this strategy is that many providers, whether facilities, groups, or individual therapists, are not prepared to accept the financial risk involved in capitation financing, and thus would be placed at undue jeopardy (Feldman, 1992). In either case, the managed care organization is responsible for monitoring and improving the quality of provider services delivery.

Another important aspect of services system planning in managed care is network development and training. Many managed care organizations guarantee that nearly all their covered members will have timely access (within a given number of miles or minutes of travel) to acute, outpatient, and alternative levels of care. Facilities, clinician groups, and individual clinicians are recruited, credentialed, and contracted on the basis of access, quality, and the provision of specialty services and programs such as for children and adolescents, minority cultures, and special problems (such as eating disorders or dual diagnosis). In addition, providers must agree to offer or coordinate a full continuum of care, with their treatment and discharge plans reviewed and approved by the managed care organization prior to authorization of services.

In some cases, commonly in health maintenance organizations (HMOs), a staff model provider network is developed in which the facilities are owned and the clinicians are employed by the managed care organization. This model permits close oversight and the implementation of practice guidelines throughout the network. However, other managed care organizations develop preferred provider networks (PPOs), in which contracts based on negotiated rates are developed with independent facilities, groups, and clinicians. One rationale for PPO networks is that they allow a "constructive tension" to exist between the managed care organization and the provider, thus facilitating patient advocacy and service quality (Feldman, 1992). The advantages of this constructive tension, however, can only be realized when the proportion of referrals from the managed care organization is small enough that the provider's practice will not be seriously threatened should the provider choose to challenge and possibly leave the managed care network over differences in clinical judgment. Case review, ongoing evaluation of treatment, discharge planning, and contractual requirements for quality management mechanisms enable the managed care organization to monitor quality in a PPO provider network.

Case Management

Elements of case management include case identification, coordination and referral, treatment and discharge planning, and follow-up. In contrast to fee-for-service payment, case managers in managed care organizations authorize services based on the individual patient's specific, current needs. Case management may begin on entry to the managed behavioral care system, when an intake coordinator briefly assesses the patient's presenting problems, identifies whether the situation requires emergency intervention, verifies the benefit coverage, and authorizes a limited number of initial therapy sessions.

If further therapy sessions are requested by the provider, the case manager discusses the patient's status with the clinician or with facility staff, evaluates the provider's recommendations and plan for treatment or discharge, and contacts the provider or patient to ensure the plan is implemented. More intensive oversight is provided by the case manager when the patient is admitted to acute or residential facilities. One role of the case manager is to serve as a qualified peer consultant; it is not uncommon for the case manager to work with the clinician or facility staff to develop an individualized treatment or discharge plan that demonstrates goals based on the presenting problem and diagnosis, interventions to achieve these goals, and realistic time frames for resolution.

Benefit Redesign

One unfortunate characteristic of traditional fee-for-service payment is that it does not subject the provider to review for clinical necessity or clinical quality. As a result, many payers now attempt to reduce unnecessary costs of care by limiting coverage of outpatient care or alternatives to hospitalization such as day treatment programs. As a result, perverse incentives are generated that encourage the use of acute hospital services instead of less expensive and restrictive programs such as partial hospitalization, day treatment, residential care, home visits, and intensive outpatient services. These perverse incentives not only increase care costs and impede quality, but may result in the exhaustion of the patient's or family's benefits. On a case-by-case basis, case managers in a managed care organization must advocate for benefit extensions or substitutions when overly restrictive plans interfere with optimal service delivery.

Managed care organizations also may track cases of benefit extension and exhaustion and report these situations to the payer, not only as they occur, but at the time the managed care organization and the payer renegotiate or renew their contract. In this way, the managed care organization helps reshape the benefit plan to allow for a full continuum of services, such as by allowing the case manager to authorize two units of day treatment in substitution for one unit of hospitalization. Given that managed care organizations contract for the coverage of populations and that an increasing number of Americans receive their health benefits under managed care models, the potential impact of benefit redesign on the development and financing of a full continuum of services is substantial.

Quality Management

Managing quality within managed care service delivery systems is a complex and ongoing task of increasing interest and importance to many players, including payers, accreditors, providers, consumers, and the managed care organization itself. Elements of quality management include credentialing, utilization review, case audits, quality improvement, and mechanisms to ensure accountability.

Credentialing procedures ensure that the pool of providers enrolled or re-enrolled to participate in a managed care network are of adequate quality. At a minimum, health care providers must submit proof of current professional licensure, or in the case of facilities, proof of accreditation from a body such as the Joint Commission for the Accreditation of Healthcare Organizations (JCAHO) or the Commission for the Accreditation of Rehabilitation Facilities (CARF). Proof of current professional liability coverage, hospital privileges and Drug Enforcement Agency (DEA) registration certification (if applicable), professional school graduation, postgraduate training, and specialty board certification must also be submitted, as well as information about legal concerns or infractions, such as pending malpractice claims or violations of narcotics laws. Providers also must report if they are impaired by substance abuse.

In the behavioral health field, credentialing by managed care organizations is more detailed and labor intensive than is required to meet these minimum standards. One reason is that many behavioral health provider networks are made up of an interdisciplinary mix of professionals, including psychiatrists, social workers, psychologists, psychiatric nurses, and counselors, unlike medical–surgical networks that are largely or solely made up of physicians. This multidisciplinary provider network requires designing credentialing forms and procedures that fit these variations in professional discipline. In addition, optimal matching of patients to clinician or treatment setting requires knowledge of numerous subspecialities that the provider may possess, such as the care of children with a history of abuse, ability to speak languages other than English, and skills in treating particular disorders such as bipolar disease or depression. This is not only the case in credentialing clinicians but in facilities as well, where programs rather than overall services may be required. For example, it may not be adequate to know that a hospital has an adult psychiatric service; for appropriate referral the existence and quality of its programs for eating disorders or some other specialty program may frequently be the key factor.

A further concern is access, not only for urgent care (i.e., within 24 hours), but also the ability to schedule weekend or evening appointments on the patient's request. As a result, the development, maintenance, and monitoring of a behavioral health provider network as well as the development of a sophisticated, continually updated provider database pose major challenges for managed care organizations.

Once credentialed, managed care organizations must continually review the quality of care provided by its network and determine which providers should be removed or retained. Providers who are consistently available for referrals and who demonstrate strong skills in treatment and discharge planning that lead to improved outcomes must be differentiated from providers with poor access who provide questionable care. To meet this need, managed care organizations must implement procedures for quality improvement, involving not only monitoring and intervention of individual providers, but developing processes for the overall review and refinement of the provider network.

The reliance on both utilization review and clinical quality case audits is yet another way that managed care differs from fee-for-service. Although substantial overlap exists between utilization review and case auditing in managed care organizations, these functions serve different purposes. Utilization review assures that the managed care company pays claims based on clear evidence of *medical necessity* for the care provided. In contrast, *clinical quality monitoring* by performing case audits not only identifies whether indicators of medical necessity were present, but also evaluates whether treatment was timely, effective, and adequately coordinated (Penner, 1996). Clinical quality monitoring is one issue in the discussion of problems in ensuring a continuum of care.

The managed care organization must have an ethical, appropriate, and logical definition of medical necessity for behavioral health placement and continuation of care. In one managed behavioral health company, medical necessity is based on dimensions that are part of the written guidelines for level of care decisions (US Behavioral Health, 1994). For mental health treatment, the dimensions are functional impairment in affect, behavior, thought processes, or judgment; risk of harm to self or others; and/or serious problems in the patient's social supports. Dimensions determining chemical dependency treatment include risk of toxicity or withdrawal complications, emotional or behavioral conditions or complications, ability to abstain, and the recovery environment. These dimensions may occur separately or in combination, but are usually considered to be interactive.

Accountability to the consumer and payer of services is represented by procedures for grievances and appeals, measures and reports regarding satisfaction and outcomes, and accreditation by entities such as the National Committee for Quality Assurance (NCQA) and the Utilization Review Accreditation Committee (URAC). Managed care organizations must be prepared both to justify decisions about the placement of patients in alternative levels of care and to establish tracking and reporting mechanisms so grievances and appeals are analyzed and reviewed in a timely manner. Methods for measuring consumer and provider satisfaction must be developed and implemented, as well as outcomes measures such as functional improvement.

PROBLEMS IN ENSURING A CONTINUUM OF CARE

Although managed care organizations facilitate improved continuity of behavioral health care, problems remain to be resolved. The following section discusses current problems related to the previous sections of service systems planning, case management, benefits redesign, and quality management. These problems include:

- Insufficient specialty programs and alternative levels of care.
- Utilization of services outside of the managed care network.
- Unsatisfactory treatment and discharge planning.
- Inadequate data collection and utilization to inform and support quality management.

Insufficient Programs and Levels of Care

In many areas of the country, the "infrastructure" for behavioral health specialty programs and a broad range of alternative levels of care to ensure the full continuum of services are missing or inadequate. For example, shortages exist among programs for dual diagnosis (i.e., mental health and substance abuse), children and adolescents, and step-down programs such as intensive outpatient, residential treatment, and day treatment. The issue of dual diagnosis is revisited in the discussion of outcome-based treatment guidelines.

Resolving problems in specialty program development requires attention to resource allocation and incentives. Behavioral health carve-out plans that provide a dedicated, specialty focus for the managing mental health and substance abuse benefits make the development and financing of specialty and alternative programs a priority. There is considerable belief in the managed care industry that integrated systems such as HMOs do not allocate resources to mental health on a parity with medical–surgical services, and resource allocation for treating substance abuse problems is particularly inadequate among HMOs in general. For example, many HMOs spend only about 3–5% of their premium dollars on mental health (up to 6% if required by state mandates), compared to the 8–11% of health care dollars allocated nationally (Bennett, 1994; Freeman, 1993).

HMOs also may allocate inadequate coverage for behavioral health problems in their benefit plan design, in contrast to carve-out organizations, which advocate and negotiate for expanded outpatient access, thereby reducing the need for emergency and acute care. For example, some HMO plans cover detoxification but do not cover chemical dependency rehabilitation, and HMOs frequently limit their standard mental health benefit package to 30 days and 20 visits, compared to the 35–40 days and 35–40 visits typically offered by specialty behavioral health plans (Freeman, 1993; Patterson, 1993). Inadequate financial resources and the lack of coverage for a continuum of care for behavioral health problems hinder the development of alternative programs needed in a high-quality service delivery system.

Some HMOs are addressing these problems by developing "carve-in" entities and by allowing self-referral for behavioral health care. HMOs also may contract with specialized service programs with a reputation of effectiveness and then develop a similar program in-house. For example, one mental health carve-in organization contracted with a local provider who successfully treated Asian populations for depression using acupuncture; after finding that the intervention worked, the organization is testing the usefulness of acupuncture in one of its clinics, as an adjunctive therapy in substance abuse treatment (E. Bonnie, 1995, personal communication).

Accommodation and contracting procedures encourage facilities such as hospitals to devise more flexible alternative arrangements for patients to allow for an improved continuum of appropriate services. For example, an adolescent may be ready for discharge from the 24-hour acute care unit, but may require daily program involvement. The managed care organization negotiates a reduced rate with the hospital to allow the patient to attend the adolescent program during the day for a specified transition time to enhance postdischarge adjustment and reduce the possibility of readmission. Accommodation arrangements with nonnetwork facility programs may lead to credentialing as network facilities given positive patient outcomes. PPO networks offer flexibility in network development and accommodation; integrated managed care organizations such as staff model carve-ins instead must develop a broad range of programs internally.

Technology offers some assistance in resolving the problem of inadequate programs and levels of care. One example is a comprehensive on-line computerized provider database, which includes extensive and continuously updated information regarding programs and services in all of the catchment areas, including nonnetwork providers willing to negotiate accommodation arrangements for patients with needs that cannot be met by the network providers. Another example is the use of telecommunications in patient assessment and treatment, as well as for provider consultation and training (Connecting Urban Doctors and Rural Patients, 1994; Guze, Estep, & Fisher, 1995). Utilization of these technological resources is particularly relevant in addressing the lack of behavioral health programs in rural and other underserved areas.

Nonnetwork Utilization

A major advantage of managed care versus fee-for-service systems is the ongoing review and oversight of the patient's treatment and referral, so patients do not "fall through the cracks," becoming lost to follow-up. However, patients frequently cannot be tracked or their care managed when they choose to utilize nonnetwork clinicians or facilities, or when they avoid clinical contact altogether. This problem may be particularly common in behavioral health care, due to noneconomic factors such as stigma, reliance on the recommendations of friends or relatives for a therapist or treatment program, the proliferation and attraction of nontraditional approaches, and the inclination of some patients or families to maintain control over choice and treatment. Another major reason why patients are lost to the system is relapse to substance abuse.

These difficulties should not preclude the managed care organization from attempting to maintain contact with the individual whenever possible. For example, patients who complete substance abuse treatment may be followed in aftercare contacts scheduled in monthly or quarterly increments for up to a year following discharge. In one managed care organization, intake counselors assess recovering patients for sobriety, risk for relapse, and job/school status, maintaining contact even if the patient is no longer covered by the benefit plan. If a patient has relapsed or indicates a significant risk for relapse, immediate referral to case management for assessment and treatment is arranged. If the patient no longer has benefits, the counselor makes a referral to local community-based programs (US Behavioral Health, 1995).

Another way managed care organizations may reduce the loss of clinical contact is to establish strong ties to the employer's employee assistance program (EAP) or manage EAP services. Although integrated systems such as HMOs argue that behavioral health should be operationally linked to primary care services, the role of the workplace in behavioral health and functioning reinforces the importance of the EAP (Blum & Roman, 1994). If EAP providers are not on the managed care organization's provider network, procedures for effective coordination may be established to ensure a smooth transition from one therapist to the next. Of course, strict protocols ensuring confidentiality must be established and adhered to in cases of management referrals, which involve requirements of employers that dysfunctional employees receive treatment and demonstrate functional improvement before returning to the workplace. Whenever possible, no identification or distinguishing case information should be provided to the patient's employer. In the case of management referrals in which information must be shared, a signed release of information first must be obtained from the patient; even so, only information strictly relevant to the patient's return to the workplace should be shared.

Unsatisfactory Treatment and Discharge Planning

It is essential to ensure not only that the clinician's treatment and discharge planning is adequate, but that the managed care organization adequately monitors and reviews care plans. On the provider side, care plans require close management and review to prevent fragmented services that result in patients falling through the cracks. Contractual requirements for timely documentation and communication of appropriate treatment and discharge plans can help the managed care organization express and achieve its expectations for care planning by the clinician. Documentation also can be structured, to a large extent, via the design of treatment update and patient discharge forms that clearly require specific information relevant to an individualized continuum of care. For example, clinicians should consistently document the patient's medications, risk factors, level of functioning, *Diagnostic and Statistical Manual of Mental Disorders*, 4th edition (DSM-IV) (American Psychiatric Association, 1994) diagnoses across all axes, and time-limited treatment goals linked to the patient's diagnoses, presenting problems, risk factors, physical condition, and social environment.

On the managed care organization's side, staff reviewing the clinician's treatment and discharge plans should possess comparable qualifications as behavioral health professionals. In addition, managed care staff specialty preparation and experience in the care of children and adolescents, the elderly, and in substance abuse treatment allows for better care plan monitoring. Providers should feel that they can request to speak to behavioral health professionals in managed care organizations for which they serve on networks, if the discussion involves a clinical issue (Penner, 1996).

Inadequate Data Collection and Utilization

Data collection and reporting should enable the managed care organization to monitor utilization across levels of care in the service delivery system. It also is necessary to identify problem areas in the transition of patients and close the loop to ensure that problems are resolved, both on a case-by-case basis and at the system level. Most managed care organizations routinely monitor utilization, although specialty behavioral health carve-out organizations are more likely to develop reports breaking down utilization by various levels of service provision than are HMOs. However, automated systems for tracking and reporting quality problems and resolutions at the case and system level are less frequently utilized. One managed behavioral health company developed clinical quality auditing software designed to serve this purpose; the automated system is structured to fit the organization's established procedures for clinical quality reviews. Provider (facility and/or clinician) and case management quality problems, such as the failure to document a comprehensive discharge plan that addresses the patient's special requirements, are recorded, as well as the name of the staff person (such as case management supervisor or provider relations manager) responsible for problem intervention. A brief, proposed action plan is recorded, dated, and tracked until it is resolved by the responsible party, when the selected resolution is entered also into the auditing system. This approach improves accountability and reduces the turnaround time for concurrent clinical quality reviews. In addition, the creation of a coded data base allows system-level reports to be generated so overall quality improvement efforts such as training, education, and monitoring mechanisms can be implemented for the managed care organization's case managers and/or the network providers.

CURRENT AND FUTURE TRENDS

Several trends related to improving the quality of the continuum of care in managed behavioral health systems include:

1. Expansion of managed care models in public sector programs.
2. Increased consumer advocacy and external review mechanisms.
3. The growth of self-help groups for special populations with behavioral health problems.
4. Increasing numbers of the mental health professionals affiliated with programs, facilities, and group practices.

Expansion of Public Sector Managed Care

At least 50 of the more than 70 major health care reform bills debated in 1993 by legislatures in 27 states across the country contained language regarding mental health and substance abuse coverage; most state plans include some form of managed care for their Medicaid recipients. Principles of managed mental health care fit well with the aims of public sector system reform: reducing unnecessary utilization while expanding community-based services; increasing access; monitoring client satisfaction, quality, and outcomes; and planning for current and future needs (Helf, 1994). Current federal budget initiatives proposed by Congress are likely to expand managed care models for Medicare beneficiaries as well. As a result, managed behavioral health organizations may expect to see increasing numbers of patients with complex lateral and longitudinal problems and service needs. In addition, managed care organizations will have to contend with concerns about declining resources from government payers. Nevertheless, these public sector populations will require a comprehensive continuum of care if the managed care organization is to ensure adequate service delivery.

Consumer Advocacy and External Review

Recent years have seen the emergence and expansion of formal external review by payers, accreditation bodies, government regulators, and consumer advocates. Examples include performance standards negotiated by large employers, accreditation standards required by URAC, JCAHO and NCQA, and consumer "report cards" recommended by the Clinton Administration and consumer mental health groups. The managed behavioral health industry may anticipate a proliferation of standards and data sets (such as HEDIS) for rating and comparing the quality of care among behavioral health organizations, and ongoing external monitoring, auditing, and oversight. Managed care organizations also will face increasing demands to develop and implement effective internal monitoring mechanisms and quality improvement systems.

Growth of the Self-Help Movement

Related to a growing and strengthened consumer advocacy movement is the growth of self-help groups serving various special populations with behavioral health problems. Attention to consumer rights already has made a substantial impact on confidentiality laws, restrictiveness of treatment, and, in states such as California, medication administration. Federal provisions require consumer representation in planning for mental health systems (PL 99-660, PL 102-321). Managed care organizations should expect to see growing numbers of their behavioral health patients, both in the public and the private sectors, participating in self-help programs. Increased appreciation of the potential of these voluntary support groups, enhanced procedures for referral and coordination with these programs, and a better understanding of the variety of self-help models (e.g., national vs. locally based, supporting vs. opposing the medical model) are essential.

Mental Health Professional Group Practices

Although mental health professional group practices were virtually unheard of until recently, a growing number of therapists now find tremendous advantages in group affiliations. Group practices enable patients to be more smoothly referred to therapists with specialties that address their presenting problems, diagnosis, or sociodemographic characteristics. Mental health professionals may form groups affiliated with facilities such as psychiatric hospitals, thus strengthening linkages with acute services and discharge planning that may improve the continuum of care. An interdisciplinary team approach is made possible by forming group affiliations, offering several advantages that improve quality. Peer review, whether formal or informal, is more likely when mental health professionals operate in a group versus adhering to solo practice. Patients who might benefit from psychiatric consultation for medication evaluation or medication management may be more smoothly referred when the nonpsychiatrist therapist practices in a group with one more psychiatrists. Group practices have the potential of pooling resources so that they may obtain staff and computer capabilities. As a result, group practices could assign staff to contact patients with complex conditions for more intensive follow-up and can design more comprehensive and sophisticated systems for monitoring and reporting outcomes and quality measures. Managed behavioral health organizations with provider networks are increasingly encouraging the creation of clinician group practices, offering incentives such as referrals and database exchange software systems.

QUESTIONS FOR FURTHER RESEARCH

Considerable work remains to expand the knowledge base required to most effectively and efficiently manage behavioral health services, given the diverse needs and case complexities of patient populations. Several areas for further research include:

1. Outcome-based treatment guidelines for special populations with complex conditions requiring a full continuum of care.
2. Comparative studies of managed care systems in treating patients with complex conditions requiring a full continuum of care.

Outcome-Based Treatment Guidelines

Although in other areas of health care there is increasing reliance on highly structured treatment protocols, the diversity of patient population characteristics and response to treatment in behavioral health care supports a strong role for clinical judgment. However, as empirical research increases that evaluates clinical interventions for specific diagnoses, treatment guidelines can and should be developed that outline the best practices to assist mental health professionals in making decisions about treatment planning. Outcome-based research that would inform the development of treatment guidelines would be particularly useful in the areas of dual diagnosis, addiction programs for women, and axis II disorders.

Dual diagnosis (in this case, comorbid psychiatric disorder and substance abuse) is one of the most pervasive and difficult complications in behavioral health care. Over half of all persons with any drug (other than alcohol) disorder diagnosis have at least one other diagnosis of a mental disorder; of persons with alcohol disorders, over a third have another mental disorder. In addition, 29% of all persons diagnosed with mental disorders have a lifetime diagnosis of a substance abuse disorder (Regier et al., 1990).

Underlying substance abuse is frequently difficult to detect, and the risk of relapse may be missed as patients change therapists or visit various clinics or facilities. Behavioral health professionals must improve their skills in the assessment, treatment, and follow-up care of persons with both a psychiatric and substance use disorder. Moreover, there is a dearth of programs that adequately meets the special needs of these patients. Addiction programs are frequently based on a 12-step model, in which psychiatric patients may be criticized or excluded for using prescribed psychotropic medications. Psychiatric programs frequently overlook issues of substance use and abuse. A better understanding of detection and development of specific interventions effective in dual diagnosis patients would speed recovery, prevent unnecessary acute care admissions, and improve the quality of life for this special population. Recommendations for an appropriate continuum of care services would be a key component of these treatment guidelines.

Women have been long overlooked in the area of addiction treatment, whether the focus is alcohol, other substances, or addictive behaviors such as gambling (American Psychiatric Association, 1994; Harrison & Belille, 1987). Frequently, these women either present a history of physical, emotional, or sexual abuse or are currently in abusive relationships (American Psychiatric Association, 1994; Rohsenow, Corbett, & Devine, 1988; Wallen, 1992). Recent research suggests that women have different issues on entry into a treatment program and may require specific interventions in order for treatment to be effective (Donovan & Mattson, 1994; Miller, 1989). As in the case of dual diagnosis, there are few programs addressing these special needs. Treatment programs and clinical guidelines for women must address their role as family caregivers, thus taking the needs of children and other dependents into account as well as needs of the patient herself.

Axis II disorders, whether primary or comorbid, are difficult to treat effectively (Linehan, Tutek, Heard, & Armstrong, 1994). A cognitive behavioral intervention—dialectical behavior therapy—has been developed that demonstrates efficacy in addressing borderline personality disorder; this approach should undergo further empirical testing and dissemination among clinicians and facilities. Another concern is that some benefit plans do not cover the treatment of axis II disorders as a primary condition; the impact of this restriction on detection, treatment, and patient outcomes should be evaluated.

Comparative Studies of Managed Care Models

The management of service systems in behavioral care is occurring on "shifting sand." Payers, patients, and professionals define managed care in many ways. Some see managed care in terms of utilization review and cost containment; others in terms of capitation, case rate financing, or the use of HMOs. There is a wide variety and range of models represented by managed behavioral care organizations, which may be:

- Part of an HMO—medical staff model.
- Part of a PPO/fee-for-service—network specialty provider model.
- A group practice contracts with HMOs—Independent Practice Associations (IPAs).
- Carve-in and carve-out models—can include EAPs.

The industry is diverse and continually changing, with corporate mergers and acquisitions, as well as trends originating among large purchasers or their consultants. Given the diversity of managed care systems and their potential impact on patient populations, comparative research is needed that examines both costs and outcomes of these different approaches.

SUMMARY AND CONCLUSIONS

From a system-level perspective, mechanisms to develop the provider network, case management oversight of appropriate placement, as well as treatment and discharge planning and quality management mechanisms such as concurrent clinical quality audits, managed care organizations offer substantial advantages in ensuring a high-quality continuum of care services for persons with behavioral health disorders. Problems remain to be resolved, including the loss of some patients to the system and gaps in specialized programs for dual diagnosis and women with addictions. However, current and future trends not only support the expansion of managed behavioral care to the public sector, but also indicate further increases in consumer advocacy, accreditation standards and reviews, self-help interventions, and the formation of mental health professional group practices. These developments are likely to focus attention on problems in continuum of care services. Further research that assists in developing clinical care guidelines for complex disorders and compares the effectiveness of various models of managed care also will contribute to resolving problems in ensuring a high-quality continuum of behavioral health care.

REFERENCES

American Psychiatric Association. (1994). *Diagnostic and statistical manual of mental disorders* (4th ed.). Washington, DC: Author.

Bennett, M. J. (1994). Are competing psychotherapists manageable? *Managed Care Quarterly, 2*(2), 36–42.

Blum, T. C., & Roman, P. M. (1994). *Can EAPs have a prevention effect?* Unpublished review paper.

Connecting urban doctors and rural patients. (1994). *Communication News, 31*(2), 26–29.

Donovan, D. M., & Mattson, M. E. (1994). Alcoholism treatment matching research: Methodological and clinical issues. *Journal of Studies on Alcohol* (Suppl. 12), 5–14.

Feldman, S. (1992). Managed mental health services: Ideas and issues. In S. Feldman (Ed.), *Managed mental health services* (pp. 3–26). Springfield, IL: Charles C. Thomas.

Feldman, S. (1994). Managed mental health—Community mental health revisited? *Managed Care Quarterly, 2*(2), 13–18.

Freeman, M. A. (1993, April). High quality behavioral health benefit programs are possible, but problems must be fixed first. *Managed Healthcare News,* 43.

Guze, B. H., Estep, R., & Fisher, C. (1995). Telemedicine: A review of its use and a proposal for application in psychiatric consultation. *Medical Informatics, 20*(1), 1–18.

Hage, J. (1980). A strategy for creating interdependent delivery systems to meet complex needs. In A.R. Negandhi (Ed.), *Interorganizational theory* (pp. 210–234). Kent, OH: Kent State University Press.

Harrison, P. A., & Belille, C. A. (1987). Women in treatment: Beyond the stereotype. *Journal of Studies on Alcohol, 48,* 574–578.

Helf, C. (1994). *Substance abuse and mental health benefits under state health care reform* (Intergovernmental Health Policy Project State ADM Report). Washington, DC: George Washington University.

Linehan, M. M., Tutek, D. A., Heard, H. L., & Armstrong, H. E. (1994). Interpersonal outcome of cognitive behavioral treatment for chronically suicidal borderline patients. *American Journal of Psychiatry, 151*(12), 1771–1776.

Miller, W. R. (1989). Matching individuals with interventions. In R. K. Hester & W. R. Miller (Eds.), *Handbook of alcoholism treatment approaches: Effective alternatives* (pp. 261–271). Elmsford, NY: Pergamon Press.

Patterson, D. Y. (1993). Dialogue: What percentage of premium should HMOs allocate for behavioral health care? *Behavioral Healthcare Tomorrow, 2*(5), 27–28.

Penner, S. (1994). HIV/AIDS, mental health and community health planning. *Psychosocial Rehabilitation Journal, 17*(4), 125–136.

Penner, S. (1996). Case studies in managed care clinical review. *Journal of Practical Psychiatry and Behavioral Health, 2*(1), 33–38.

PL 99-660. (1986). State Comprehensive Mental Health services Plan Act of 1986. 42 USC 201, *US Statutes at Large*, Vol. 100, 99th congress, 2nd Session, pp. 3794–3797.

PL 102-321. (1992). ADAMHA Reorganization Act. Section 1912. State Plan for Comprehensive Community Mental Health Services for Certain Individuals. 42 USC 300x-1. *US Statutes at Large*, vol. 106, pp. 379–381.

Regier, D. A., Farmer, M. E., Rae, D. S., Locke, B. Z., Kieth, S. J., Judd, L. L., & Goodwin, F. K. (1990). Comorbidity of mental disorders with alcohol and other drug abuse. *Journal of the American Medical Association, 264*(19), 2511–2518.

Rohsenow, D. J., Corbett, R., & Devine, D. (1988). Molested as children: A hidden contribution to substance abuse. *Journal of Substance Abuse Treatment, 5*, 13–18.

US Behavioral Health. (1994). *Guidelines for level of care decisions*. Emeryville, CA: Author.

US Behavioral Health. (1995). *Outcomes manual*. Emeryville, CA: Author.

United Behavioral Systems. (1994). *Manual of preferred clinical practices*. Minneapolis, MN: Author.

Wallen, J. (1992). Comparison of male and female clients in substance abuse treatment. *Journal of Substance Abuse Treatment, 9*, 243–248.

8

Critical Indicators of Quality of a Service System

What Graduate School Never Taught You about Accountability

SHARON A. SHUEMAN AND KATHY ALLEN

This chapter is addressed to behavioral health practitioners who have spent their professional lives in an independent practice setting. More specifically, it targets professionals who have only minimal exposure to the quality management principles and practices familiar to those who have worked in organized care settings such as community mental health centers, specialized treatment programs, and hospitals. The chapter begins with a discussion of the evolving role of accountability within the changing context of behavioral health; it then considers quality-related aspects of behavioral health service delivery under a traditional fee-for-service model. Ways in which expectations for service quality have changed with the advent of managed systems of service delivery and financing and the operational implications of these changes for professionals providing services under managed systems, in turn, round out the picture of quality-driven behavioral health services. The chapter concludes with a brief discussion of the natural advantages of the integrated group practice model in the provision of accountable services.

A FOCUS ON ACCOUNTABILITY

This chapter is essentially about *accountability*—to consumers and purchasers. Accountability to consumers, of course, has always been a primary and explicit concern of independent practitioners. Indeed, much of the dissension expressed by practitioners about current managed systems of service delivery and financing is focused on their perceived inability, under such systems, to discharge their primary responsibilities to their patients, including maintenance of confidentiality and development and implementation of a mutually determined treatment plan.

SHARON A. SHUEMAN • Shueman Troy Associates, Pasadena, California 91106. KATHY ALLEN • Student Health Service, University of California Davis, Davis, California 95616.

Handbook of Quality Management in Behavioral Health, edited by Stricker *et al.* Kluwer Academic / Plenum Publishers, New York, 2000.

Accountability to purchasers, however, has been a most imperfectly developed concept within independent practice, traditionally limited to submission of a claim form with a procedure code and a "nonstigmatizing" diagnosis. The idea that acceptance of third-party funds brought with it a responsibility to the purchaser of care was rarely, if ever, acknowledged. One of the reasons is that the graduate school or residency training provided to most mental health professionals was never intended to instill in trainees any sense of accountability to an external entity. It was (and still is) the rare student, for example, who was ever asked by his or her supervisor to consider the source of the funding for the treatment being provided, even though payment rarely came entirely from the patient. Even within organized care settings, trainees were seldom asked to confront health care financing issues. More often, the trainee was told, explicitly or implicitly, to "work the system" in order to get for the patient that to which he or she was "entitled." This approach was usually rationalized as patient advocacy, and it was rarely balanced against the need of the system to provide for *all* patients. "Independent" (as in independent practitioner) was the operative term. Each practitioner was concerned exclusively with his or her patient and his or her practice. There was no mandate and typically no structure to include consideration of the larger issues related to cost-effective utilization of available resources by the independent practitioner.

Until very recently, providers were not asked to focus on overutilization, nor did they acknowledge that overutilization is potentially a problem. For example, notions such as psychiatric overhospitalization or excessively prolonged or too frequent courses of outpatient therapy were hardly ever considered in the context of the limited contingencies traditionally associated with independent practice.

Beginning with the early and admittedly primitive efforts of the Civilian Health and Medical Program of the Uniformed Services (CHAMPUS) to control costs and evaluate the quality of services provided to its beneficiaries (Bent & Shueman, 1987), and continuing with current (less primitive but still imperfect) efforts by managed care companies to ensure cost-effectiveness, the need for accountability to purchasers has entered the consciousness of providers. For the first time, independent practitioners are being asked to assure employers, governmental entities, unions, and other payers and purchasers that these purchasers' employees, employee dependents, or beneficiaries are in fact receiving services that satisfy specific criteria related to quality and utilization. These criteria, for the most part developed by managed care organizations (MCOs), are in many cases different from those that behavioral health professionals might seek to adopt to evaluate their own performance. In addition, in most cases they are criteria that could not easily be applied under the traditional fee-for-service model of independent practice; rather, they must be implemented within a *system* of care.

The next section provides a context for the presentation of quality monitoring indicators and criteria most commonly used in the current managed systems of care. This context takes the form of a description of "the way things used to be" in the traditional fee-for-service system when services were provided primarily by independent practitioners in solo or nominal* group practices.

*Nominal group in this discussion refers to two or more professionals who share office space and perhaps some types of administrative support, but operate essentially independently of one another.

HOW THINGS USED TO BE

The striking changes that appear to portend the end of independent (solo) practice based on fee-for-service financing have a relatively brief history. As noted above, the first major effort to control costs and monitor quality of care occurred with the CHAMPUS program in the mid- to late 1970s. What follows is a description of the prevailing climate in which independent practitioners operated, then and for the following decade. Six common aspects of care quality are considered, beginning with access to care and concluding with consumer satisfaction issues.

Ensuring Access

Under the traditional fee-for-service model, access was not regarded as a significant quality issue, either by providers or by the purchasers (who were typically insurance companies). No designated entity monitored services to ensure, for example, that a potential patient would have access to a provider or hospital within a certain number of miles or minutes drive from his or her home or place of work.* Further, no entity monitored outpatient provider schedules to ensure that patients would have access to an appointment within a certain number of days or that a patient could get an appointment after work or on a Saturday. Few independent practitioners routinely offered evening or weekend hours and, most often, a person seeking services was obligated to modify his or her work or school schedule to fit the provider's schedule. In addition, there was no external entity monitoring provider access to ensure that a patient in crisis would be able to contact his or her provider in a timely way, day or night.

Determining Necessity for Treatment

Historically, and in principle, third-party payers have reimbursed providers for "medically necessary" services. Typically, this meant that there existed a diagnosable mental or emotional disorder [i.e., as defined in the *Diagnostic and Statistical Manual* (American Psychiatric Association, 1994)] associated with a significant impairment in one or more areas of the person's functioning. Under indemnity programs, however, medical necessity was essentially a meaningless concept since payers had no mechanism for validating necessity. Furthermore, it was the rare provider who ever turned away a potential patient or client (except when his or her schedule was full) because he or she determined that treatment was not necessary. Patients were seen if they wished to be seen rather than if the severity of their functional impairment warranted it. Diagnoses that were submitted to third-party payers to justify continuing care were adjusted to be nonstigmatizing but "reimbursable" (Sharftstein, Towery, & Milowe, 1980). There was never a question of necessity; to the contrary, whether and what type of services were provided was determined by what the patient requested and what the practitioner sought to provide. The same was true for services provided in hospitals and other inpatient or residential programs. Admissions, as with outpatient treat-

*It is doubtful that, prior to managed care, any entity would have had the capability, let alone the mandate, to conduct such monitoring.

ment, were very often "elective" and lengths of stay were frequently determined by the limit of the third-party benefit coverage.

Ensuring Appropriateness of Services

Services delivered were most often determined by what the provider or program typically did. This was done both as a matter of convenience and based on the implicit assumption that one model fit all problems. Most people entering outpatient psychotherapy, for example, were treated in relatively long-term (or at least open-ended), uncovering treatment, and sessions were most often scheduled on a weekly or more frequent basis. Little use was made of flexible scheduling. Homogeneity also prevailed in inpatient and residential programs. For example, patients in chemical dependency treatment programs received the same series of educational sessions and interventions, regardless of their particular problem constellation or previous treatment. (Cynical behavioral health professionals were heard to joke: "Oh, no. Not the liver lecture again!")

Nonmedical professionals were often reluctant to refer a patient to a psychiatrist for a medication evaluation for fear of losing the patient. As a result, many patients who could have benefitted from pharmacotherapy did not receive it.* Many mental health professionals tended to be relatively unskilled with regard to the recognition and treatment of chemical dependency. Others were reluctant to broach this subject with patients, even though the existence of an untreated chemical dependency problem is associated with poorer outcome and higher rates of dropout from treatment.

Little use was made of free or low-cost community-based resources, except in the case where a patient's benefit had been exhausted and he or she was unable to pay for services out-of-pocket. Further, such resources were regarded as inferior to, and a poor substitute for, verbal psychotherapy. Finally, it was the rare provider who routinely offered his or her patients access to alternative types of psychoeducational modalities such as support groups (other than Alcoholics Anonymous) and skills training (e.g., assertiveness, communication, parenting). Such interventions also were often regarded by providers as "second-best" in comparison to weekly individual psychotherapy. In addition, most providers in solo practice or nominal groups did not have the capacity to provide such services (they lacked access to the numbers of patients necessary to support these group modalities). In short, under the traditional fee-for-service system where treatment was provided by independent (mostly solo practice) practitioners, patients generally received what providers and programs were familiar with doing or preferred to do, rather than what their functional impairments necessitated.

Many independent practitioners had neither the expertise nor the interest to serve large numbers of potential patients who did not conform to the image of the desirable patient. Among these patients were persons with serious and persistent mental illness, people with a disability, and ethnic minorities. Such patients were consistently underserved in the private sector and were relegated to public agencies (community mental health systems). Even if they had not been, however, they would

*This reluctance often was also based on uninformed biases among nonmedical professionals about the efficacy of medication.

have been ill-served by a majority of professionals in independent practice who were inadequately prepared and motivated to serve the multiple challenges posed by either disability or human diversity.

Continuity and Coordination of Care

With the exception of proforma discharge planning that occurred when a patient completed inpatient care, little attention was paid to continuity or coordination of care. Patients completing outpatient care (usually when the patient decided he or she was finished) were most typically invited by the provider to call if they ever needed help again. In the relatively rare situation when a patient was under the care of two providers (a psychiatrist for medications and a psychologist or social worker for verbal therapy), effective communication was commonly lacking, particularly that necessary to ensure that the separate treatments were integrated and focused on consistent treatment goals, or that the necessary services could be provided within the compass of the patient's benefit. (For example, seldom would a psychologist reduce the frequency of sessions so that he or she and the psychiatrist could both see the patient within the frequency allowed by the benefit.) Even rarer were instances where the behavioral health provider routinely consulted with the primary care physician when the patient had a coexisting medical problem or where the primary care provider was managing pharmacotherapy. (It must be conceded, however, that such communication inadequacies have invariably existed across the behavioral health disciplinary spectrum, and not only between medical and nonmedical professionals.)

Providers' reluctance to collaborate was often justified by the need to maintain confidentiality. This concern, however, could have been dealt with by an explanation to the patient about the importance of collaboration and a formal request for the patient's consent for the provider to speak with the provider of collateral services. In fact, the reluctance was often due to interprofessional rivalries, at both the individual and the discipline level, and to a lack of understanding among professionals about the importance of effective coordination of care management in the interest of the patient.

Ensuring Patient Improvement

Treatment plans were typically focused on making the patient more comfortable, either by reducing negative thoughts and feelings (e.g., "reduce feelings of stress" and "increase self-esteem") or helping the patient develop insight or understanding. Such goals were typically adopted instead of, rather than in addition to, goals which were specifically targeted at improving the patient's functioning. To focus on functioning (i.e., behaviors) was considered to be ineffective in the longer term. The belief was that if the therapist and patient did not get to the "root" of the problem, this problem would subsequently manifest itself in the guise of "substitute" symptoms. To those (majority of) providers operating under a more analytic or dynamic model, any sense of direction in therapy was considered anathema; indeed, it was the rare practitioner who engaged in collaborative goal setting with the patient, established and adhered to a formal treatment regimen, made suggestions to a patient, or routinely assigned homework.

Patient Complaints and Patient Satisfaction

A very common way for practitioners to construe issues of patient satisfaction was to blame the patient when he or she was unhappy with, or complained about, services. Demonstrable dissatisfaction with treatment was regarded as yet another manifestation of the patient's pathology, and accordingly most providers either did not possess or did not use technology to deal with such matters when they arose. Alternatively, from the consumer's position, a demonstrably failed treatment plan or inappropriate behavior on the part of the provider left patients with little recourse other than to lodge a formal complaint with a state licensing board or an ethics committee of a professional association. For many reasons, however, not the least of which were lack of will and insufficient resources to conduct investigations, these entities were reluctant to follow up on complaints unless there was evidence that the provider's behavior had been manifestly egregious.

HOW THINGS ARE NOW

An overarching goal of an MCO is to create a service system where there previously has been none. Current managed systems are in a relatively early stage of evolution and therefore achieve only a fraction of what they are intended to achieve in the way of utilization management and quality improvement. Such systems usually consist of relatively loosely organized practitioner and facility networks. Managed care organizations develop policies and procedures, relating to matters such as reimbursement and quality management, which are then applied to services provided by the network. These policies and procedures, coupled with the MCO's capacity to monitor service delivery in a very direct way at both the individual provider and the network level combine (presumably) to elicit accountable professional behaviors from practitioners, facilities, and programs and provide a basis for effecting quality improvement.

Ensuring Access

Access has become one of the most critical concerns for purchasers. They typically want to be assured that potential consumers have timely, easy access to appropriate providers and programs. In particular, employers want to be assured of timely access to treatment to minimize the probability that a personal problem will interfere with a person's job performance. This concern is reflected in the types of access criteria almost universally promulgated by MCOs (and, more importantly, almost universally demanded by purchasers). For example:

1. Routine outpatient appointments are offered within 5 business days of the request; urgent appointments occur within 24 hours.
2. An assessment for acute inpatient admission is conducted within 4 hours.
3. Providers are available to patients (through an answering service or pager) 24 hours a day for emergencies.
4. All potential service users have access to a provider or facility within 20 miles or 30 minutes drive time of their home or place of work.

5. Provider offices offer sufficient parking, are near public transportation, and are accessible to the handicapped.

The contracting MCO, then, is responsible for ensuring that the provider and facility network covers the entire geographical area populated by their eligible enrollees. In addition, the organization must ensure that the network is sufficiently large and possesses the range of professional specialties and programs to meet all service needs of the population as well as to ensure timely access to care.

Imperatives for Providers

Policies such as these have significant implications for the individual practitioner. First and foremost, he or she needs to be available to patients for emergencies 24 hours a day, 7 days a week. Typically, this requires immediate access through an answering or paging service. It is not sufficient to have an answering machine that the practitioner regularly checks. The provider also needs to ensure that he or she is able to offer appointments without undue delay. Finally, providers must ensure that their offices satisfy criteria for physical access (e.g., near public transportation, wheelchair accessible).

Determining Necessity

From a quality perspective, a determination of medical necessity is a prerequisite to making an appropriate referral. The concept of medical necessity is perhaps the most problematic aspect of managed care for many providers, since for most of them their training and professional socialization left them with the operational imperative of serving those who ask for service. From the perspective of a managed system, necessity is determined by the patient's past and current level of functioning as well as potential for deterioration if appropriate services are not provided.

As a rule, managed organizations rarely deny patients initial access to services. The decisions MCOs make at the point of access are usually limited to a determination of the need for a specific level, or intensity, of care (e.g., does the patient appear to need acute care). Periodically during treatment, however, the MCO evaluates the condition of the patient to determine whether continued treatment is warranted, and if so, what type, at what level, and with what intensity. As a part of this process, the consistency between diagnosis and the provider's description of the problems and treatment plan is assessed. This is commonly done through the evaluation of written reports, conversations with the provider, or using a second opinion by an independent evaluator. The consistent focus of evaluation is on the functioning of the patient across the spectrum of life's challenges.

Examples of criteria used for determining necessity are as follows:

1. Acute inpatient care is required if the patient is of immediate danger to self (e.g., suicidal attempt, gesture, or serious ideation) or others (e.g., threat to harm another person), or is gravely disabled.*

*The most common example of grave disability is a patient suffering from a psychotic disorder that seriously interferes with his or her ability to attend to his or her self-care needs such as food, clothing, and shelter.

2. Routine outpatient care is required if the patient exhibits functional impairment that significantly interferes with his or her ability to engage in the normal activities of daily living (e.g., interpersonal relationships, job, school, self-care).

Imperatives for Providers

It is incumbent upon the individual provider to understand the concept of necessity, be able to clearly articulate necessity when it exists, and learn to develop solution-focused treatment plans targeting improvement in functioning and the development of coping skills to enable the patient effectively to deal with problems in the future. The overriding premise is that the translation of a treatment plan is designed to *return patient to his or her premorbid level of functioning.*

Ensuring Appropriateness of Services

Since an MCO has access to a wide range of facilities, professionals, and programs, the task of ensuring appropriateness depends on its capacity to assess accurately the patient's needs and to connect the patient to the appropriate services. These services may be provided through the MCO network or by providers and programs that are not part of the contracted network. These external resources might include a range of community-based programs or highly specialized services that are critical but may be infrequently used (e.g., substance abuse treatment program for non-English-speaking pregnant women). Typically, the MCO contracts with these providers on a case-by-case basis.

Network practitioners, facilities, and programs are typically "credentialed" to provide particular types of services, and the MCO maintains written guidelines for selecting services and providers. What this presumes, of course, is that practitioners recognize the boundaries of their competence. Examples of criteria intended to ensure appropriateness of services within managed organizations include:

1. A patient who exhibits signs of a possible substance abuse problem is referred to a specialist (individual or program) for an evaluation to determine whether specialized treatment is required.
2. A patient whose diagnosis, symptoms, or lack of response to treatment suggests that he or she may benefit from psychoactive medications is referred to an MD for a medication evaluation.*
3. Providers refer patients to appropriate community-based resources as adjuncts to their services or for support when active treatment ends.

Imperatives for Providers

The overriding principle is that *the patient should have access to whatever services are necessary whether or not they are directly available from the primary provider.* The primary provider must develop a plan that uses appropriate strategies to deal with the target problems and ensure, where necessary, that the patient has access to other services

*Typically, such guidelines are diagnosis specific. For example, one often-used guideline for depression requires a medication evaluation if the patient has had two or more previous episodes of depression.

and service providers. The primary provider, then, plays a significant role in ensuring appropriateness of care during the course of a patient's treatment. For example, he or she may refer the patient to a chemical dependency program for assessment, to a psychiatrist for a medication evaluation, to some community-based support service (e.g., cancer survivor's group), or to a behavioral health colleague for a psychoeducational or group intervention. Providers must be aware of and understand the utility of the range of alternatives, and they must be willing to make a referral when appropriate.

Ensuring Continuity and Coordination

Unless the individual practitioner is willing to perform a case management function (a function for which few behavioral health professionals have been trained), it is extremely difficult to ensure coordination of care outside of a formal service system. As a consequence, service coordination is one of the most critical responsibilities of an MCO. To facilitate coordination, service systems are typically guided by criteria such as:

1. If multiple behavioral health practitioners are providing services to a patient, the practitioners consult with one another to ensure consistency and integration of treatment plans.
2. If the patient has a medical or physical problem related to the behavioral health disorder being treated, the behavioral health provider consults with the primary care physician or other medical specialist.
3. A patient being discharged from inpatient care has an outpatient visit with a behavioral health provider within (a specified number of) days of discharge.

Imperatives for the Provider

Implications for the individual provider are that he or she must be prepared to consult with other behavioral health professionals who have a role relevant to the behavioral health treatment plan to ensure consistency of treatment goals and implementation strategies and to maximize the value of the benefit. Similarly, the existence of particular types of medical problems (e.g., chronic pain, suspected dementia) will commonly require effective collaboration between the behavioral health provider and a primary care physician or other specialist. In all such cases, patient informed consent is a necessary prerequisite to consultation.

The implication of such criteria for acute care facilities and other programs is that discharge planning policy is sound and procedures are consistently implemented. Facilities and programs must maintain effective mechanisms for ensuring that post-discharge services are scheduled and that the patient is not lost to follow up.

Monitoring Patient Improvement

For the first time in the history of behavioral health services, providers are being asked to achieve demonstrable improvement in patients' functioning. Managed care organizations formally monitor treatment on an aggregate as well as individual basis. To facilitate the evaluation of patient improvement, managed organizations ask providers to use clinical measures, either standardized or "homegrown," to provide an independent estimate of the patient's improvement. Such measures may be used by MCOs as one indicator in the recredentialing process whereby providers are evaluated for continued network membership.

Imperatives for Providers

At the individual level providers are expected to be able to articulate functional goals and demonstrate progress toward those goals. At the aggregate level, providers may be evaluated on the extent to which their patients, as a group, improve. It is therefore incumbent on the provider to learn to work effectively within a goal-focused treatment model, to be able to articulate treatment plans based on goals directly related to the patient's difficulties in functioning, to ensure that the patient understands and concurs with the treatment plan, and to systematically evaluate progress toward goals.

Managing Patient Complaints and Patient Satisfaction

A primary concern of employers and other purchasers of behavioral health services is the level of satisfaction of employees or beneficiaries. Demands from purchasers as well as from external organizations (e.g., National Committee on Quality Assurance, state regulatory agency) compel all MCOs to maintain formal programs for monitoring complaints and evaluating the satisfaction of service users. In addition, states also may require MCOs to submit complaints to state licensing authorities in cases where provider behavior may be in violation of licensing laws or business and professions codes. Under such programs, patient dissatisfaction is manifestly *not* assumed to be a product of the patient's pathology. Criteria commonly guiding the handling of patient complaints are:

1. A complaint must be documented and investigated and a written response must be given to the complainant within 30 days.
2. A provider who is the subject of a patient complaint must respond in writing to the managed care organization within 15 days.

Imperatives for Providers

The implication for the practitioner is that he or she must be prepared to be publicly accountable (to the MCO) for the handling of an episode of care. Ideally, he or she will have internal procedures for dealing directly with patient complaints in order to resolve them prior to their being forwarded to the MCO.

The Value of Organized Group Practices

It should be obvious to the reader reviewing the criteria described above that the quality management responsibilities incumbent on an MCO are much more easily realized if the MCO works with organized group practices rather than individual practitioners. For example, it is relatively easy for a group practice to offer expanded (Saturday and evening) hours and to ensure emergency coverage 24 hours a day, 7 days a week, thereby increasing the probability of timely response to all requests for treatment. Again, integrated, multidisciplinary groups offer providers routine (internal) collateral consultation on clinical management decisions, a process associated with quality improvement.

Multidisciplinary practices also are better able to provide direct access to a range of alternative and adjunctive services such as groups of a therapeutic or psychoeducational nature as well as practitioners in a range of specialties. They also are more likely than individual providers to maintain formalized linkages with community agencies and programs providing services unavailable within the practice.

Because they have operational functional relationships with multiple providers and treatment programs, group practices can better ensure collaboration among providers, coordination of care, and reliable transfer from one level or type of care to another. Because they are "closer" to providers, groups can both mandate such cooperation and follow-up and monitor adherence to these requirements through regular utilization and peer review activities.

Groups can also maintain formal mechanisms to handle and resolve patient complaints. Again, since they are closer to the point of service than is the MCO, they can more immediately and effectively investigate and resolve complaints.

Practice groups are much more able than are solo providers to implement formal programs for monitoring progress and outcomes of treatment. Typically, this is done through regular review of individual episodes of care by utilization management, peer review, or quality management committees. These committees give timely and direct feedback to providers during the treatment episode, feedback that allows providers to modify treatment plans or solicit consultation from colleagues. Group practices also are more likely than solo providers to have computer-based information systems that allow them to monitor treatment at an aggregate level to detect patterns of deficiencies and form the basis for quality improvement activities.

Finally, group practices are the best venue for providing training or continuing education for the practitioners whom they employ. Provider development programs can be tailored to the deficiencies of individual providers or the service system as a whole, as analyzed by the agency's routine utilization and quality monitoring activities. Again, their proximity to the point of service permits groups to better detect skill deficiencies and to develop effective interventions and corrective actions.

CONCLUSION

Perhaps the most significant change required of providers who practice under managed systems is an attitudinal one. A radical shift away from commitment to absolute confidentiality and exclusive accountability to the patient and toward limited sharing of information and accountability to the payer–purchaser or other stakeholders is necessary for practitioners who wish to survive in the era of managed care. Providers who have always held independence and autonomy as the primary source of their professional quality of life (Tryon, 1983) are now being asked to conceptualize a different professional role for themselves: from *independent* provider to *interdependent* member of an integrated system of care. Rather than being all things to all people, providers are asked to evaluate their own competencies and define their potential unique contributions to a system of care.

Accommodation to what is essentially a new set of imperatives is, without question, a difficult challenge for all behavioral health professionals, given the inadequacy of their formal preparation and the disinclination of many to adapt. But adapt they must if they wish to both continue to be reimbursed by the health care dollar and to provide cost-effective services in the public interest. A commitment to the understanding and use of quality assessment and management mechanisms is a nonnegotiable attribute of the accountable behavioral health provider in an age of health reform.

REFERENCES

American Psychiatric Association (1994). *Diagnostic and statistical manual of mental disorders* (4th ed.). Washington, DC: Author.

Bent, R. J., & Shueman, S. A. (1987). History, administrative experiences, and empirical issues: The APA peer review program. *Professional Psychology: Research and Practice, 18,* 102–106.

Sharfstein, S. S., Towery, O. B., & Milowe, I. D. (1980). Accuracy of diagnostic information submitted to an insurance company. *American Journal of Psychiatry, 137,* 70–73.

Tryon, G. S. (1983). Pleasures and displeasures of full-time private practice. *The Clinical Psychologist, 36*(4), 45–48.

9

Challenges to Quality Management in the Public Sector

SUSAN J. PENNER, SHEILA BALER, MARGARET WALKOVER, AND EDWARD COHEN

Founded in 1979 to manage employee assistance programs (EAPs), US Behavioral Health has evolved into a national managed behavioral health care company holding contracts with over 400 large and mid-sized employers, covering an estimated 6 million lives. Public sector contracts include King County and Clark County, both in Washington, and Solano County, California.

Senior executives within US Behavioral Health have a significant amount of experience with public sector mental health programs. The CEO directed the Community Mental Health Center program at the National Institutes of Mental Health when it was initiated in the 1960s. The Senior Vice President for Medical Affairs directed the San Francisco public mental health system and served as a state mental health commissioner. The Vice President of Managed Care, who is responsible for implementing the company's public sector contracts, directed public sector mental health programs in Michigan, Massachusetts, and Colorado. Not surprisingly, then, for its work in both public and private sectors, the company adopts a strong community mental health philosophy and approach with an emphasis on early intervention and a range of community-based outpatient services rather than inpatient and other more restrictive and costly services.

This chapter deals with challenges to quality management in the provision of public program behavioral health services by private sector managed care organizations (MCOs). It is written from the perspective of a particular MCO specializing in carve-out* contracts and programming. Other managed care models, including comprehensive (medical–surgical) health maintenance organizations (HMOs) as well as risk-sharing medical groups or independent practice associations (IPAs), also may be used for the delivery of mental health services. Such programs differ from carve-outs

*A carve-out behavioral health program is one which is financed and managed separately from other health (i.e., medical–surgical) services.

SUSAN J. PENNER • Department of Nursing, Holy Names College, Oakland, California 94619. SHEILA BALER • Menninger Care Systems, Plano, Texas 75093. MARGARET WALKOVER • California Mental Health Directors Association, Sacramento, California 95814. EDWARD COHEN • United Behavioral Health, Oakland, California 94612.

Handbook of Quality Management in Behavioral Health, edited by Stricker *et al.* Kluwer Academic / Plenum Publishers, New York, 2000.

in critical ways, however, and these variations in philosophy and approach would result in challenges different from those faced by a company such as US Behavioral Health (the MCO).* Although focusing on a single company's contractual involvement with the public sector, this chapter is designed to identify and illuminate the variety of obligations and problems MCOs face when entering into public–private arrangements: an exciting nexus for behavioral health systems development and management.

This discussion focuses on the Medicaid and medically indigent public sector populations served through specialized mental health carve-out programs. Typically, Medicaid populations covered through Aid to Families with Dependent Children (AFDC) and Supplemental Security Income (SSI) for the aged and blind receive their health services, including behavioral health, through general medical HMO systems of care. Persons in foster care and disabled persons receiving SSI or Supplemental Security Disability Income (SSDI) often are served through specialized carve-out programs. Medicare beneficiaries and insured public employees represent large and growing markets for managed behavioral health care, but present different challenges, the discussion of which is outside the scope of this chapter.

SERVICES MANAGEMENT ARRANGEMENTS

This section provides a context for the subsequent discussion by describing the general model of triage, assessment, and care management used by the MCO for commercial private sector contracts. These contacts typically cover employed populations.

Triage and Assessment

In managing services under private sector contracts, clinical staff review and preauthorize all initial requests for treatment. Beneficiaries requesting a referral for mental health or substance abuse (sometimes referred to as chemical dependency) services contact the organization's intake counselors via a 24-hour toll-free number. The (masters-level) intake counselor completes a brief assessment of the caller's presenting problem and risk factors, matches the identified needs of the caller to a provider specialty, identifies potential providers by specialty and location, and refers the caller to an appropriate provider in his or her geographic area.

Care managed by the company is provided by a nationwide network of licensed mental health professionals (psychiatrists, psychologists, social workers, and masters-level counselors) and accredited facilities providing a continuum of care, including crisis intervention, acute inpatient, residential, and day treatment. All providers and facilities are credentialed by and formally contracted with the MCO, and services are continuously monitored to ensure appropriate access and quality.

Continual Care Monitoring

Continuing care is reviewed and authorized by care managers. Care managers are licensed mental health professionals with either a master's or a doctoral degree and at least 5 years of prior mental health experience. Some also are credentialed in particular specialties, such as care of children and adolescents or substance abuse

*US Behavioral Health is now United Behavioral Health.

treatment. Care managers supervise the treatment and discharge planning of all children and adolescents, all patients requiring 24-hour care or presenting a dual diagnoses (mental health and substance abuse), patients requiring longer-term care, and other potentially difficult or complex cases. In-house medical directors (board-certified psychiatrists) serve as consultants to care managers and routinely supervise all 24-hour care. A psychopharmacologist is available to care managers on-site for consultation and review of cases involving the use of psychoactive medications.

Quality management at the MCO is supported by programmatic structures, written clinical materials, clinical supervision, ongoing training, and in-service activities. Quality management specifications also are frequently integrated into contracts. The process of developing and maintaining appropriate policies and procedures is considered only one approach to quality management, serving primarily to formalize procedures that are believed to result in increased service quality. These processes are based on a set of fundamental principles. In this chapter, we focus on two issues of critical importance to both private and public sector payers and consumers. These are *access* (i.e., patients must be ensured timely and unrestrained access to appropriate clinical services) and *concurrent quality monitoring* (i.e., services must be appropriate and of adequate quality throughout the course of treatment):

1. *Access*. Quality management of access involves activities such as:
   - Establishing internal decision protocols to help ensure the most appropriate service type and level of care for each person requesting an initial referral or continued care.
   - Ensuring that the provider network offers appropriate specialty and geographic coverage so that all patients are within a reasonable distance of a facility or provider who can offer them appropriate services.
   - Contracting with providers to ensure convenient scheduling of appointments [i.e., requiring them to accommodate requests for evening and weekend appointments and to offer appointments within specific periods of time (within 5 business days)].
   - Privileging providers according to selected subspecialties as well as cultural (ethnic identification, language) and lifestyle (sexual preference, religion) sensitivities.
2. *Concurrent quality monitoring*. The capacity to quickly and efficiently track the performance of network providers and report findings to clinical staff is essential. The effective management of ongoing clinical care involves the following mix of activities:
   - Concurrent case management.
   - Standardized clinical review.
   - Provider quality profiling.
   - Targeted orientation and training of network practitioners.

The obligation of ensuring easy access and quality monitoring of ongoing services constitute the context for this review of quality management challenges specific to the public sector.

PUBLIC SECTOR QUALITY MANAGEMENT CHALLENGES

Beginning in the early 1980s, managed behavioral health carve-out organizations proliferated; they now manage services for an estimated 85 million persons nationwide. These companies typically manage the mental health and substance abuse benefits of employed populations (i.e., employees and their dependents). In the last several years, however, most if not all major managed behavioral health carve-out companies have sought public sector contracts. Local and state governments are increasingly exploring the potential for cost savings and improved service delivery in proprietary managed systems of care. In seeking partnerships with managed care companies, governmental entities endeavor to select companies that are capable of meeting certain critical needs; that is, companies that can provide the technology and administrative expertise that these governments often lack (Bataille, Anderson, & Penner, 1995).

Problems with the Model

Whether private sector managed care models can be directly transferred to public sector systems is a matter of some debate. For example, private sector beneficiaries typically seek treatment for adjustment disorders, anxiety disorders, or depression, conditions most often requiring relatively short-term, usually uncomplicated outpatient therapy and in many cases the management of medication. Inpatient services are rarely required and when they are they are extremely short term with an objective of rapid stabilization and transition to a lower level of care. The systems and processes of private sector MCOs are particularly appropriate for such patients and presenting problems.

By contrast, publicly funded consumers are likely to present with acute episodes of persistent mental illnesses such as schizophrenia or bipolar disorder and are more likely to experience environmental problems (e.g., inadequate housing, the need for income support), which both result directly from their psychiatric disability and complicate treatment. These consumers are known to use significantly more (and more costly) services and have poorer outcomes in comparison to those covered by employment-linked private insurance. They also are more likely than those in employed populations to exhibit cultural or linguistic characteristics that act as barriers to help seeking. To generalize: The problems of public sector consumers of behavioral health services are more likely to be intractable and require long-term, comprehensive, psychosocial approaches characterized by multisectoral involvement.

There also is considerable debate as to the extent to which provider networks typically maintained by private sector companies can or should serve public program consumers. The services public sector consumers use are typically not provided by independent behavioral health practitioners or private facilities and programs. In fact, the modal independent provider has little if any experience with this type of population. The services most often are provided in community-based agencies that can offer a range of psychosocial services and supports. Because of the high cost of treating them, the challenging nature of their service needs, and the fact that they tend to be very different from the "desirable" mental health patient (that is, middle class and socially attractive), public patients generally are not sought out by private sector practitioners and programs: the providers and facilities identified with managed behavioral health care networks. A particular challenge, then, for a managed care company seeking to effectively serve a public contract is its capacity to develop a provider network with the clinical expertise and resources needed to serve chronic and seriously disabled patients.

Problems with Funding

Under traditional publicly funded programs, state and local resource limitations may result in low, noncompetitive provider reimbursement rates, burdensome documentation requirements, and slow payment. Inadequate reimbursement makes it difficult to recruit a highly qualified provider network that will accept public sector referrals, even among providers who have experience with such populations. Although some states, such as New Hampshire, reimburse at competitive rates, those states are not in the majority. Given the often low level of reimbursement rates, paperwork requirements, and the time-consuming appeal process often necessary to obtain payment for Medicaid patients, it is not uncommon for individual providers to deem it more cost-effective to treat a few public patients on a pro bono basis.

The lack of service integration owing to the existence of categorical funding in the public sector also presents quality management challenges to both access and ongoing monitoring. For example, substance abuse treatment may have an entirely separate funding source from mental health services. This separation of funding presents significant challenges to the treatment and management of public sector patients, for whom dual diagnosis of mental illness and substance abuse is common. In addition, in many states, significant funding shortfalls for substance abuse treatment are common.

Other services frequently required by public sector consumers, such as vocational rehabilitation, income support, and housing assistance, also may be poorly integrated with mental health service delivery. This situation compounds the problems of ensuring comprehensive case management and appropriate intervention, and thus jeopardizes the potential for optimal patient outcomes. In some states, such as California, local public mental health funding has split into two systems: patients covered by some public program such as Medi-Cal, California's version of Medicaid, and patients with no entitlement or private coverage. Each funding program is administered separately (Bataille et al., 1995), further complicating the management of care for a vulnerable population of consumers who manifestly need a continuum of mental health services.

Within a state, each governmental authority (state and county) exercises considerable discretion regarding the design, operation, and financing of its mental health system. As a result, procedures, information systems, eligibility criteria, target populations, and other fundamental elements of public mental health systems may vary considerably. The variation across public payers with regard to these factors is much greater than the variation across employers contracting with behavioral health care carve-out organizations (even for employers in diverse industries). Legislative decisions can abruptly alter or terminate programs. In addition, changes in a state's chief executive or the state's philosophy about welfare, mental illness, or health care may affect the scope and adequacy of mental health operations and funding. In those states where counties have a relatively high level of discretion (such as in California), local elections can also result in dramatic shifts in policy and funding (Penner, 1995). Such changes may be difficult to predict and may preclude responsible fiscal planning.

Other Variations Complicating Management of Mental Health Services

States and local government areas differ in their sociodemographic characteristics, philosophy, and political leadership. They further differ with respect to priorities regarding mental health care and services for the most needy in the community and experience in planning for community needs (Blum, 1981). Designing a public sector managed mental health care plan for a multicultural, multilingual population in an economically depressed area with little history of community collaboration or consumer empowerment presents a set of challenges different from those inherent in a largely homogeneous community with a strong tax base and a track record of collaborative achievements in solving social problems and representing needy consumers. Urban versus rural settings and the degree of geographic dispersion of the target population (i.e., with attendant transportation problems) are additional factors that differ across communities. All such differences have implications for consumer access and the management of services quality.

Given the tremendous variation in governments and communities across states and local government areas, it is impossible to design a single template for a public sector managed care system and expect to apply it with minimal adaptation to all public sector customers. In reality, the managed care organization must remain flexible and open to requests for redesign and must be prepared to negotiate and rework elements of the benefit plan throughout the life of the contract. Therefore, the approach taken by the MCO whose policies and procedures inform this chapter is to individually negotiate with each public sector customer to meet the unique design and implementation needs. Although approaches such as specialized case management and technologies such as information systems that track patients and providers may be relatively easily adapted to public sector needs from the MCO's commercial repertoire, it is frequently necessary to develop entirely new strategies and processes for county mental health systems.

What follows is a discussion of our MCO's approximately 2 years' experience with Solano County, California, and 1 year's experience with King County, Washington. Aspects of these public–private contracts exemplify challenges to the quality management of access and clinical services. The discussion focuses on these challenges and the ways in which the company attempted to deal with them.

THE SOLANO COUNTY EXPERIENCE

Solano County, California, is located between the San Francisco Bay Area and the state capital of Sacramento. The county has three cities of over 75,000 residents each and a total population of nearly 362,000. It is in transition from primarily rural and agricultural to mixed urban and suburban rural communities. Approximately 40% of the county population is of ethnic minority origin, largely African American, Hispanic, and Filipino (Bureau of the Census, 1994). In 1994, Solano County was the first local mental health authority in California to move all its fee-for-service Medi-Cal recipients to managed care (Bataille et al., 1995). Approximately 30,000 beneficiaries receive care through the county's mental health carve-out.

The county's lack of staffing and technical resources resulted in their decision to contract with the MCO to provide technical assistance and initially to operate the managed service program in partnership with the county's existing mental health staff. This represented the first public–private collaboration for both the MCO and the Solano County mental health system. The MCO negotiated a technical assistance contract that included independently developing or assisting the county in the development of the following:

- Provider contracting procedures.
- Access protocols for outpatient and inpatient care.
- Protocols to define communication patterns among the MCO, county staff, and facilities in the provider network.
- Training of county mental health staff.
- A 24-hour toll-free telephone access and referral system.
- Medical necessity guidelines.
- Claims payment procedures.
- Eligibility determination procedures.
- Medical economics and forecasting reports.
- Authorization procedures.
- A computerized database integrating all functions.

Access

The first challenge in improving access was developing acceptable medical necessity criteria that met both state and local requirements. As a California field test county in moving to managed mental health, Solano County had few guidelines from which to develop access criteria. Solano County staff followed access criteria established by the state for local mental health programs. These criteria were primarily intended to address care for individuals with long-term mental disabilities, severely and persistently mentally ill adults, and severely emotionally disturbed children. The county also wished, however, to improve access to care for persons who were less severely ill but who still suffered from long-term disorders. In addition, other Medi-Cal-eligible individuals who did not meet California Department of Mental Health target population definitions, such as recipients of the AFDC program and children in foster care, needed access to services.

In order to improve access to all of these underserved groups, medical necessity guidelines had to reflect a full continuum of services, from brief interventions to long-term care. The combined use of the company's level of care guidelines (US Behavioral Health, 1994), designed as general criteria for determining the most appropriate service referral, and medical necessity criteria drafted by the state fulfilled both state and local requirements.

Difficulties arose in ensuring continuity of care because services provided under the county's managed care plan were limited to inpatient and outpatient treatment. Alternative treatment settings, such as day treatment and crisis intervention were, and continue to be, provided separately, out of a general county fund. So, for example, a consumer who required day treatment but who did not meet the county's target population eligibility criteria was unable to qualify for one of the limited number of spaces in day treatment. This limitation continues to present significant obstacles to efforts to ensure appropriateness and continuity of care.

Probably the biggest challenge to consumer access was the low provider reimbursement rate. Before the partnership with the MCO, county staff referred patients to clinicians without providing follow-up to ensure, for example, when and if services were received. These clinicians accepted public sector patients, but frequently placed them on waiting lists, resulting in delays in treatment, and hence inadequate access to care. The MCO staff instituted a policy of intensive follow-up to the referral. They found excessively long provider waiting lists and reported this finding to the Solano

County mental health plan administrators. The staff also intervened with clinicians and emphasized the need to reduce excessive waiting times for scheduled appointments and the importance of the provider's communicating with the MCO if he or she was unable or unwilling to accept additional county referrals. (The information system that the MCO made available for use within the program also helped to improve the referral process. Its centralized, on-line database of providers, with specialty areas and geographic location specified, permitted more effective matching of patients to clinicians. This resulted in improved appropriateness and a reduction of reported transportation problems for patients.)

The low reimbursement rates meant that relatively few clinicians in Solano County accepted Medi-Cal patients. However, after the MCO became involved with the public system, providers expressed more interest in working with public patients, and it was possible to recruit clinicians somewhat more easily. This was particularly true for providers specializing in the treatment of children, which historically was an area of tremendous unmet need (Bataille et al., 1995). The MCO generated waiting list reports—utilization reports that for the first time linked services authorized to claims paid—and used these and other data to justify increasing reimbursement rates in Solano County. The data on access also provided justification for the county to broaden the definition of qualified reimbursable mental health clinicians, formerly limited to psychiatrists and psychologists, to include masters-level social workers and counselors. All these actions further increased the number and quality of clinicians available for the care of public patients.

Clinical Quality

Before entering the public–private relationship, Solano County for the most part utilized the inpatient services of only a single local hospital. Although county staff were not entirely satisfied with the quality of clinical services provided at this facility, they believed that their almost total reliance on this facility left them with little leverage to require changes. The MCO, however, was able to negotiate contracts with other facilities that were somewhat farther away but still accessible to consumers. The company also established communication protocols with these facilities, focusing on treatment planning, discharge planning, and timely communication between the MCO and county staff on treatment and discharge issues. As a result of these interventions, staff reported substantial improvements in the clinical performance and responsiveness of major network acute care facilities. Moreover, there was a reduction in the per member per month costs of services during the first year of the contract, even though patients served were similar in terms of acuity to patients served prior to implementation of the managed care program.

Additional improvements in clinical quality resulted from using the expertise of provider relations staff at the MCO to counsel and, as needed, sanction providers who failed to meet clinical quality standards or contractual obligations. Care managers used an on-line system to rate clinicians and facilities on their assessment, treatment planning, and discharge planning performance. These ratings were automatically aggregated into provider files. An on-line system was also used to report and record complaints about providers and the results of quality assurance committee reviews of clinician and facility clinical performance. The data formed the basis of a provider rating system. These activities and information systems helped shift the provider community (which prior to that time had been largely unaccountable for their public sector practice) in the direction of increased accountability.

After the first year of operation, the MCO and Solano County developed a timeline to transfer all clinical intake, assessment, care management, and member services to the county. The company designed a 60-day training program for county staff, installed information systems at the county, and transferred the toll-free referral to the county in October 1995. The company continues support to the county in the areas of maintenance of provider databases, claims payment, and medical economics reporting. The next step is to transfer the responsibility for financial and utilization report generation.

Solano County has been able to assume responsibility for an increasing number of areas of their managed care system over time, with the transition occurring in a planned and orderly fashion, with technical assistance, training, and backup from the MCO. The county's quality management protocols, policies, and procedures were developed from public and private sources, and are designed to represent the best of both sectors.

THE KING COUNTY EXPERIENCE

King County, Washington, encompasses the Seattle metropolitan area, thus representing a highly urbanized and ethnically diverse community with a total population of over 1.5 million. Approximately 15% of the county population is made up of ethnic groups, largely Asians, African Americans, and Hispanics (Bureau of the Census, 1994). The MCO entered into a public–private partnership with King County to assist in designing and implementing a managed mental health plan for public beneficiaries in 1995, approximately 1 year after the initiation of the Solano County contract. As with the first contract, increasing access and improving the quality of clinical care were two major managed care principles emphasized in the King County Prepaid Health Plan (the plan) program (Jarvis & Mauer, 1995).

The MCO is responsible for a number of areas of management and technical assistance in its partnership with King County, which include:

- Written policies and procedures.
- Billing and reimbursement.
- Management information system project management timelines.
- Member services.
- Provider contracting.
- Provider training and technical assistance.
- Clinical care coordination.

Access

King County has a highly decentralized mental health access system, so patients could request services through any of approximately 40 community agencies or by calling a widely publicized toll-free number. Approximately 9400 persons received services monthly, of whom almost one quarter (2400) are children or adolescents and approximately 80% (7600) are Medi-Cal recipients.

Unlike in many public sector plans, consumers of public services in King County receive a benefits booklet. This booklet, which is translated into many languages, provides information about available services and explains what consumers can expect from the mental health plan. Consumers are ensured choice by a provision allowing them to change their provider agency yearly (or more frequently with cause). When compared to programs in other counties, the plan offers individuals from special populations (e.g., ethnic minority; alternative lifestyles), as well as the agencies serving those populations, more favorable case rates and reimbursement rates, resulting in better access. Specialized agencies also received technical assistance funds. The system was designed to keep services as close as possible to the county's target populations. It appears to have been successful in this regard, since the number of individuals served by the plan increased by 9–20% (depending on the target group) over the course of the first contract year.

Although administrators of the plan wanted to retain the same group of agencies that the mental health system had previously used, the contract established by the MCO included eligibility requirements for agencies. Specifically, the agencies were required to ensure that all appropriate levels of care were accessible to consumers whom they served. For example, a center serving children and families but providing only outpatient services was required to establish and maintain formal linkages with service agencies providing more intensive levels of care to ensure continuity for its consumers. This contractual provision resulted in 16 service agencies being added to the provider network, thus increasing the number of locations through which consumers can access services. The 22 primary agency contracts currently have 56 subcontracts. Benefits have accrued to small "grassroots" organizations previously overlooked by the system, as well as to underserved target populations with special needs such as children and adolescents.

Another improvement was in the handling and disposition of consumer complaints. Prior to the inception of the public–private partnership, county mental health staff referred consumer complaints back to the executive director of the agency against which the complaint was lodged. The MCO appointed a client services staff person, independent of the service agencies, with obligation to respond directly to consumer complaints, questions, and requests for information. This person also worked with consumer-run ombudsman programs, assisted with other consumer-run projects, and developed training programs for county staff based on the information received via consumer complaints and comments. During the first year of implementation, use of the consumer telephone line increased from approximately 50 to over 200 calls per month. In addition, the MCO subscribed to a King County community resource database that facilitated consumers' obtaining information and referrals for housing, educational services, food banks, and other community programs.

Quality of Care

One very simple but effective way in which the MCO began to meet the challenge of managing the quality of clinical care was to pay clinical staff recruited from the community between 5 and 10% more than was typically paid in the local public sector market (as estimated by the plan officials). Since these local staff had had little if any experience in or knowledge of managed care, however, the company also recruited critical project staff who had experience both in managed care and with community and public sector programs. These personnel (some of whom had worked for the MCO) included the project director, office manager, director of contracting, and a child/adolescent clinical supervisor.

The MCO and the county also improved clinical infrastructure by appointing staff medical directors to the Seattle office of the MCO and to the plan. This was a significant change from the county's traditional reliance on psychiatric consultants who had typically only been used on an ad hoc, hourly basis. Under this approach to clinical leadership, the county medical staff focused on clinical policies and community relations and the MCO medical director focused on clinical supervision and consultation.

Under this partnership model, the MCO is responsible for the provider network and contracting, clinical management, client services, and billing and reimbursement. King County staff provide general quality oversight, information systems, and state and local agency liaison.

The MCO clinical staff in Seattle routinely preauthorized services for the most seriously ill individuals who were the highest utilizers within the system. In addition, the staff conducted clinical reviews of a sample of less acute, less complex, and less costly cases from each community agency to ensure monitor quality and continuity of care. Sampling for this case review was initially random, but protocols were subsequently developed to guide review based on clinical risk factors such as the existence of a dual diagnosis, suicidal ideation or intent, and discharge from a higher level of care. Unlike case managers in the typical private sector managed behavioral health care models, the MCO clinical staff working with the plan also spent considerable time making agency visits, which allowed them to perform chart reviews and provide direct case consultation.

The King County Prepaid Health Plan established a quality management section, where system quality indicators and the MCO clinical staff performance were reviewed and evaluated. System quality indicators included measures of access to care by targeted underserved ethnic groups, utilization reports on agencies providing culturally competent services, and findings from consumer satisfaction surveys. A systemwide waiting list was maintained and reviewed regularly and frequently. Reports of outcome measures including reduction of psychiatric symptoms, improved functioning, and improved quality of life were developed for samples of consumers within the target populations.

These reports provided information used to drive significant changes within the service system. For example, monitoring of utilization reports across various benefit plans (used to set case rates based on patient age, risk factors, and other relevant characteristics) revealed apparent overutilization of a benefit plan that allowed weekly outpatient visits. This appeared to be the result of bias on the part of providers toward traditional once-a-week individual treatment as well as providers' inability to conduct the accurate, effective assessments necessary for the development of individualized treatment plans. Closer review of services provided to a sample of these consumers showed significant inadequacies in treatment plans. This finding led to a decision to develop and implement a formal program of provider education, intervention, and monitoring. As a result of these activities, 38% of the consumers formerly assigned to the benefit package in which they were allowed (and were using) weekly outpatient visits were transferred to higher or lower levels of services that more appropriately met their individual needs.

CONCLUSION

The public–private partnership experiences in Solano County and King County exemplify the types of challenges encountered when attempts are made to improve access and quality of services provided to public sector managed mental health care plan beneficiaries. Using sophisticated information system technology, strategies to make reimbursement rates for public sector services competitive, continuum of care approaches that increase the numbers and types of available providers, appropriate eligibility and medical necessity criteria, and intensive follow-up of referrals and waiting list reporting, a behavioral health care carve-out organization helped county mental health systems improve access to care. Importantly, provider clinical quality management improved in these county mental health systems when the behavioral health care carve-out routinely provided review of provider treatment and discharge planning, monitoring of consumer complaints, utilization reports specific to target populations, and contractual requirements for improved agency and facility performance.

Critical Stakeholder Involvement

The managed behavioral health care organization must respond to the input, authority, and requirements of multiple stakeholders in administering any public sector contract. The managed mental health plan staff and administrators, state and local officials, and family and consumer groups must all be included in the planning, design, and formative evaluation of the new system from its inception. In both Solano and King counties, contacts were made and meetings held involving the MCO's staff and stakeholders long before the contract itself had been finalized. This kind of collaboration is particularly vulnerable to inadequacies in the communication process and mastery of the details of the local mental health system.

The consumer of public mental health services is the most central stakeholder. Due in part to legislative requirements, the public sector consumer assumes a far more active role in system design and management than does the consumer of services in the private sector. In 1986, PL 99-660 was enacted into federal law, mandating states to develop plans for the delivery of mental health services to the most needy public recipients; it also included detailed provisions for consumer advocacy and involvement in the planning process (National Institutes of Mental Health, 1987). For innovations such as public–private partnerships to be effective, the vagaries of political considerations require continuous attention. And, critically, consumers and their advocates must be accorded their due as core players in the process of services design and implementation. Quality management principles themselves require nothing less than a proactive, nonpatronizing engagement of consumers and carers by partners: the governmental entity and the managed care organization.

Finally, a successful process of public–private contracting and program development, involving a uniquely demanding set of challenges, depends substantially on a strategic approach to goal setting and resources acquisition and deployment. In this chapter the designated foci of the MCO's quality management endeavor were (1) access and (2) the management of the quality of ongoing services. Rather than attempting to design and apply the same system template to all public sector contracts, these delimited foci enabled the private MCO contractor to incorporate its proven technology within an emerging, dynamic system: public–private collaboration in the public interest.

REFERENCES

Bataille, G., Anderson, K., & Penner, S. (1995). A public–private sector venture in managed mental health: Solano County's experience. *Administration and Policy in Mental Health, 22*(3), 327–344.

Blum, H. L. (1981). *Planning for health: Generics for the eighties* (2nd ed.). New York: Human Sciences Press.

Bureau of the Census. (1994, August). *County and city data book 1994* (12th ed.). Washington, DC: US Department of Commerce, Bureau of the Census.

Jarvis, D., & Mauer, B. (1995, January). *King County prepaid health plan briefing packet.* Unpublished manuscript. Seattle, WA: King County Prepaid Health Plan.

National Institute of Mental Health. (1987). Toward a model plan for a comprehensive, community-based mental health system. Washington, DC: Administrative Document, U.S. Department of Health & Human Services, Public Health Service, Alcohol, Drug Abuse, and Mental Health Administration.

Penner, S. (1995). An evolving managed care system: Public mental health services in San Francisco. *Administration and Policy in Mental Health, 22*(3), 273–288.

US Behavioral Health. (1994). *Guidelines for level of care decisions.* Unpublished manuscript. Emeryville, CA.

10

Quality Management Practice Issues in Behavioral Health Groups

DAVID A. YOUNG AND STEPHEN LONG

INTRODUCTION

Significant changes in the health care industry and in behavioral health care in particular are forcing managers and professionals in the field to reconsider the approaches to "quality." As concepts such as total quality management and continuous quality improvement are increasingly applied to health care delivery (see Gaucher & Coffey, 1993), traditional definitions of quality are being challenged and the term is acquiring new and sometimes widely varying meanings. This is creating considerable confusion, especially for owners, managers, and administrators of start-up behavioral group practices (BGPs) who are increasingly directly responsible for meeting standards of quality that reflect different values and perspectives than they had previously addressed.

As professionals whose training focused mostly, if not solely, on the clinical aspects of care, behavioral health providers have intuitively equated "quality of care" with factors such as the therapist's years of training and practice, internships, post-graduate and continuing education experiences, ethical behavior, the ability to attract and retain patients, and professional reputation. A typical measure of quality has been how well patients like their therapist, as indicated by how long they remain in treatment. Because therapeutic goals of patients being seen in independent practice were often either vague and amorphous or nonexistent, little accountability and few attendant mechanisms were in place to determine whether or not patients' needs and expectations were met.

There is a belief among many therapists that more therapy equals better therapy. This bias, which has dominated the professional community until recently, is in direct conflict with the imperatives of cost-effectiveness and efficient care. Wilson (1992) describes this "maximalist" view as the belief that the highest quality of care is determined by the processes that result in the greatest improvement in health regardless of incremental costs. Managed care and similar arrangements adhere to an "optimalist" view that would exclude interventions whose cost disproportionately exceeded any

---

DAVID A. YOUNG • Pathmakers, Berkeley, California 94705. STEPHEN LONG • Los Angeles, California 90048.

Handbook of Quality Management in Behavioral Health, edited by Stricker *et al.* Kluwer Academic / Plenum Publishers, New York, 2000.

benefit to the patient. In a system (or society) where resources are limited, an optimalist approach is clearly more tenable and offers the best chance to provide the greatest good for the greatest number. However, this approach also forces clinicians to face difficult ethical dilemmas when deciding who should receive care and what type of treatment should be administered. Defining what constitutes an optimum treatment outcome for an individual is also difficult (see Boyle & Callahan, 1995).

Another difficulty many BGPs have in grappling with quality is that the clinicians within the group have been accustomed to viewing cost-benefit decisions in terms of individual patients, rather than in terms of providing a system of care for the health of a given population. Under capitated and other at-risk arrangements, a thorough understanding of population-based orientation is imperative. Shueman and Troy (1994a) argue that such a system of care, as is ideally developed and applied in managed care models, allows the greatest opportunity for effectively monitoring and implementing strategies for improving services. Indeed, for BGPs, a systemic approach is the only way a group can effectively manage all aspects of care, including quality. Indeed, quality management can provide a framework for optimizing all areas of operations within the practice, from clinical to administrative.

WHY SHOULD BEHAVIORAL GROUP PRACTICES CARE ABOUT QUALITY?

Prior to the advent of managed delivery systems, most behavioral health professionals worked independently and gave little thought to formal quality structures and processes. Successful solo practitioners or loosely organized group practices, however, did pay attention to issues that would promote their businesses. Savvy therapists knew they were accountable to their patients and referral sources and would strive to provide good "customer service." Naturally, the amount of time and resources committed to these endeavors depended largely on the practice size, structure, and level of sophistication. Even obvious initiatives such as sending "thank you" cards to referral sources and surveying patient's expectations and responses to their treatment were much easier to undertake and manage when the practice consisted of one therapist or only a few clinicians.

Because these measures were not required or encouraged by any external entity, therapists rarely devoted resources to formally monitoring any aspect of quality routinely or consistently using or reporting this information to anyone. By and large, few outsiders were privy to what happened in the therapist's office, unless a patient filed a grievance with a professional organization or licensing board. Quality of care was assumed as long as complaints were not registered.

Cost-effectiveness was rarely a concern, since fee-for-service reimbursement generally allowed inefficiencies in the provision of care to be passed on to payers (usually patients themselves). As insurance companies have implemented more restrictive limits on mental health benefits, the lack of established reporting structures allowed therapists to revise their billing methods and fee schedules to continue passing all risk for costs to payers. For example, as copayments were increased to reflect a higher percentage of the clinician's fee, some clinicians would increase their fee schedules by a corresponding percentage to allow patients to maintain their current frequency of sessions.

In past years, even formal attempts at comprehensive quality improvement have failed to achieve their goals. Lamb and Lamson (1996) attribute this to a lack of leadership and commitment by senior management and/or to an organizational culture that interferes with the progress toward a quality-driven system. They also cite three specific barriers. In their analysis, outside regulators have historically imposed formidable quality assurance systems that were frequently perceived by clinicians as conflicting, overlapping, and excessive. Gaps in training approaches have not encouraged or required participants at all levels of service to analyze work processes, apply selection criteria, and understand the rationale for a systemic approach for improvement. And, as a third barrier, they point to the current health care environment, which requires rapid adaptation to radical changes in competition, funding, and political climate. The challenge for BGPs is to develop the processes and structures of a true quality-driven organization while struggling to survive as a business.

Driving Forces

In an organized system of care, there are both internal and external forces that compel the BGP to address quality as a central aspect of its organization (see Fig. 1).

Internal Forces

Desire to Improve Services. Behavioral health professionals believe in the benefits of their work and generally desire to continuously improve both their clinical interventions and their systems of care. Increasingly, many are developing programs to evaluate and monitor these factors. Even before the advent of managed care, some conscientious therapists conducted clinical outcome studies and other formal and informal surveys to manage the quality of their clinical services and office staff performance. In addition, as a matter of routine business practice, successful organizations develop financial controls to ensure that the enterprise is operating efficiently and profitably.

Reflection of Organizational Values. The decision to commit limited resources to a bona fide quality management endeavor that may or may not result in short-term financial return is a reflection of an organization's leadership. It says that the owners of the group value quality in the broadest sense, with regard to quality of the system versus having only an interest in the quality of an individual patient's treatment. This also represents a belief in an ethical responsibility to provide services that are truly meeting the needs of "consumers" (patients, referral sources, payers, etc.), as opposed to only considering maximizing financial gain.

Marketing Strategy. Earning a reputation as a "high-quality" practice will not in itself assure the health and success of the enterprise, especially in today's competitive environment. Of course, reputation was and is of paramount importance in traditional fee-for-service practice. However, a quality orientation can be a meaningful long-term strategy that will enable the BGP to position itself as truly committed to organized systems of care. Savvy managers are learning how to capitalize on this reputation to make the practice more competitive in the managed care marketplace.

Organizational Design. In designing or restructuring a BGP, the group leaders must consider how quality is to be managed. Savitz (1992) argues that staff model provider groups may allow for more direct monitoring and supervision of clinicians

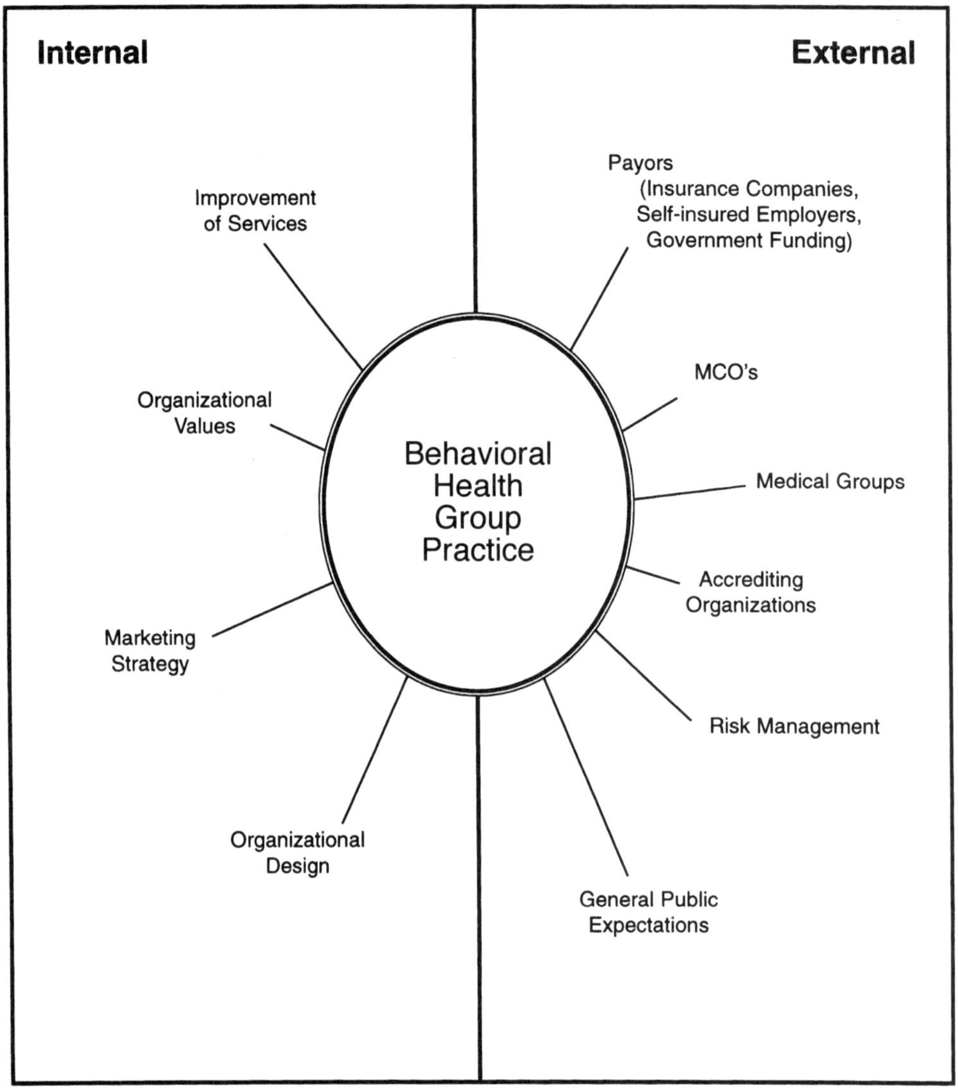

FIGURE 1. Current forces driving quality in behavioral health group practices.

because they are usually smaller and have greater accountability. The clinicians in a staff model also tend to develop more collegial relationships, which allows them to share their common values. Quality under this model may be more easily managed than under an independent practitioners association (IPA) or network model, where clinicians may be located across a wide geographic area and are likely to have more diverse values and less interaction with the group's administration.

External Forces

External forces are increasingly encouraging and even requiring quality-driven systems.

Public Expectations. The personal experiences of patients and the perceptions of the public as a whole have a great impact. The general public's awareness of psychotherapy is greater than in the past. Because of increased media attention, the general population is becoming much more sophisticated about psychological issues. While this is a welcome trend for most practitioners, it may result in some patients having unrealistic expectations about issues such as what their health plan will cover for the treatment of problems that may not be deemed medically necessary. Other patients may have distorted perceptions of how quickly their symptoms should dissipate. Patients need to be educated about the therapeutic process and informed about limitations in their health coverage and benefit structure. With a clearer understanding, their expectations can be managed and guided by the behavioral health professional. A quality management plan should address issues such as how well patients' rights and privileges are shared with them, along with appropriate guidelines for appealing decisions that result in denying the provision or continuation of services.

Accrediting Organizations. Entities such as the National Committee for Quality Assurance (NCQA) and the Joint Commission for the Accreditation of Healthcare Organizations (JCAHO) have strongly influenced quality management structures among health care organizations that need accreditation to maintain their licensure or their place in the health care marketplace (e.g., managed care organizations, medical groups, hospital-based behavioral health care systems). Specific NCQA standards for behavioral health were developed more recently than the standards for general medical care. Nevertheless, they are expected to have a significant impact on how behavioral health care is delivered within both behavioral health and acute medical care systems (see NCQA, 1997). While most BGPs will not need to pursue such accreditation, they can play a crucial role in helping to meet these standards because many of the listed requirements depend on clinician performance. A BGPs understanding of how accrediting organizations view quality and how they go about measuring it can be of great value to managed care organizations (MCOs) and medical groups who depend on their cooperation. Since the responsibility for actually fulfilling some standards can be delegated to provider organizations (e.g., utilization management), there may be an even greater impetus for BGPs to commit the resources to develop a viable quality management plan that can be scrutinized by external parties.

Risk Management. Managing risk is a significant driver in the development of quality management programs. As the number of clinicians in a group grows, it becomes increasingly difficult to track and manage problems as they occur. The key executives of a BGP may never have face-to-face contact with most of their clinicians that practice in remote locations and only see a few contracted patients. If the practice's treatment philosophy is unclear, practice guidelines are nonexistent, and no written quality plan is in place, an errant therapist may continue to perform marginally for an extended period of time without being discovered. Guidelines covering high-risk events (e.g., child abuse, suicidality, danger to others, etc.) can help BGPs avoid adverse outcomes (and litigation) and can assist in resolving disputes when procedures were followed. A formal quality plan not only helps to address problems as soon as they occur, but also can prevent some problems from ever arising. As the community's standards of care evolve, practice guidelines can help providers in a BGP remain current with acceptable and efficacious clinical practices. It is expected that in the near future there will be less variance in the community as these guidelines are adopted widely by large organized systems of care.

Contracting Organizations. In many areas, organized purchasers of health care are increasingly becoming the primary "customers" for BGPs. As such, they are currently the most powerful external driving force for more formalized quality management programs in group practices. Ultimately, BGPs are accountable to the insurance companies, self-insured employers, or federal funding sources that have learned to negotiate not only financial terms but now broad-based quality management issues into their contracts. These might include requirements such as a specific ratio of clinicians to enrollees within a geographic area or a requirement for access to a clinician with a specified period of time.

As more sophisticated BGPs begin to pursue direct contracting (i.e., not through a third-party payer) with employers and other purchasers of behavioral health care, well-developed quality management systems that can demonstrate clinical an administrative accountability will be imperative.

Managed Care Organizations. MCOs also exert significant pressures on BGPs to formalize their systems to manage quality since they act as intermediaries between payers and providers. MCOs themselves must meet regulatory and accreditation requirements for quality assurance and must have their own comprehensive quality management plan. The expectation for a contracting BGP that intends to service the MCO as a "core group" is that it will not only accommodate all the requirements the MCO applies to its network of individual clinicians, but also will present a fairly detailed quality management plan that encompasses all the areas relevant to functioning as a group. Some MCO contracting arrangements even structure the group's compensation based on meeting certain quality and administrative performance standards (Schultz, 1995). For example, bonus payments, or even percentages of baseline compensation may depend on providing services to a minimum proportion of the covered population or for not exceeding a given number of patient complaints.

It is important to consider the philosophy and standards of the contracting MCOs quality plan in developing or amending a BGPs own quality program. Conflicts sometimes arise when a practice contracts with more than one MCO, each with its own program, systems, and requirements. The movement toward national standards may alleviate some of these incongruities, but there will continue to be differences based on varying business imperatives and local regulatory requirements, standards, and customs.

Medical Groups. Depending on how the relationship is structured, a medical group with which a behavioral group practice is affiliated may or may not require rigorous quality management standards by the BGP. As a department or specialist provider for a medical group, a BGP might have its services subsumed under the quality management plan of the larger organization. If there is an independent contractor arrangement, the level of detail and standards themselves may be delineated in the contract. In either case, it is wise to clarify these issues and policies prior to entering into a contractual relationship in order to avoid conflicting expectations and the costs of compliance after the fact. Even a straightforward event, such as a patient filing a complaint, should be addressed with clear policies and procedures. For example, should all complaints be brought to the attention of the medical group administration, even if the patient only complained directly to a therapist? Who is responsible for handling and resolving the complaint? Who is liable if financial consequences result from the complaint (e.g., patient refuses to pay the copayment)?

Since the same NCQA standards apply to behavioral health services offered through the medical group ("carved-in"), as those services that are "carved-out" to a managed care organization, the BGP must clarify which quality activities will be shared and which ones will be delegated to the group. These decisions potentially will have severe financial implications. The implementation of some processes will require extensive systems to monitor and track performance (e.g., utilization management, credentialing, outcome studies) and others can only be accomplished through ongoing training and feedback with clinical staff (e.g., clinical documentation, adherence to clinical guidelines). Since many administrators of medical groups are unfamiliar with NCQAs behavioral health standards, substantial education may be necessary.

With compensation rates continually being driven downward by competitive forces, maintaining a good quality management system may assist a group in arguing for an increase or at least stabilization of these rates. Entities that contract for behavioral health services are beginning to recognize what is known as "value purchasing." This approach involves finding and rewarding organizations that can provide a maximum range of quality services at affordable and sustainable costs. Some payers are using their purchasing power to improve value and outcomes rather than focusing solely on discounts and cost containment (see Keller, 1995). In the face of solid data demonstrating a compromise in the quality of care resulting from further reductions in rates, a responsible payer may see the wisdom in allocating more resources to the BGP. There is a trend among some business coalitions to use their purchasing power to improve value and outcomes instead of focusing only on discounts and cost containment.

In summary, no BGP can afford in any sense to ignore quality issues. The need is established and demands attention. In many if not most cases, a formal, written plan for managing quality is a de facto requirement of practicing in an increasingly competitive and structured environment. Such a plan may be required by payers or other parties and eventually may be needed in order to meet legal and regulatory requirements. In any event, structuring a BGP as a fundamentally quality-driven enterprise has clinical, managerial, and operational benefits and obvious competitive advantages. Providing optimal care and doing so ethically are central to behavioral health care as a healing vocation. Quality management is a route to excellence in fulfilling that mission.

WHAT DO CONTRACTING ORGANIZATIONS EXPECT?

While there is substantial variation in what different MCOs and other contracting parties expect of BGPs with regard to quality management, the industry is moving toward more formalized plans and structures. With the arrival of NCQA guidelines, a minimal set of standards will likely be enforced nationwide. The maturation of the behavioral health industry is resulting in the elimination of provider and payer organizations that are noncompetitive, many because of poor attention to issues that can be said to fall under the general rubric of quality management. As compensation fee schedules and at-risk contracted rates approach a bottom level, competition for contracts will move toward being based more on quality performance and less on price alone. Those BGPs that can demonstrate their commitment to quality and who can follow through on that commitment are better positioned to argue that they can provide behavioral health services effectively and efficiently. While managed behavioral health organizations and other contracting entities (e.g., medical groups, Independent Provider Associations, Preferred Provider Organizations, etc.) will continue to be ultimately accountable for assuring quality standards under industry guidelines, the trend is clearly toward pushing the responsibility for assuring quality (as well as financial risk) down to the providers of health care services.

Some generalizations can be made about the quality requirements of contracting organizations. For our purposes, it is useful to divide these into clinical, administrative, and general requirements.

Clinical Components

Documentation of Clinical Services

This typically includes intake evaluations, treatment plans, clinical progress notes, discharge summaries, and interim reports. All forms should be complete, signed, and dated. There should be a standardized format for reports and clinical notes, if not actual standard forms. Appropriate documentation of case management and utilization management discussions, supervision/collaboration with colleagues, and nonclinical communications (e.g., canceling of appointments) should be present. The purpose of this documentation is to allow the quality of treatment to be compared to norms. An MCO may audit charts for proper evaluation and diagnosis, adequate treatment plans, clear identification of functional impairments that will be the focus of therapeutic interventions, and appropriate care management (e.g., referral for medication evaluation or adjunctive services when indicated under clinical management guidelines). Of course, it behooves the sophisticated BGP to have its own internal monitoring system to assess these same concerns.

Practice Guidelines/Clinical Management Guidelines

These are statements that reflect the group's approach to particular clinical situations. They should reflect some formal, organized process of development that is based on the latest scientific evidence and expert opinion (see Shueman & Troy, 1994b). In larger provider groups these may have been developed for the most frequently seen disorders. Some MCOs have developed their own practice guidelines for every *Diagnostic and Statistical Manual of Mental Disorders*, 4th edition (American Psychiatric Association, 1994) diagnosis. Computerized systems have been developed to support clinical decision making that has clinical pathways or management guidelines integrated into the program. The cost of developing and continually updating theses systems and standards can be enormous. Smaller BCPs are often best served by implementing guidelines that are now available from parties with whom they contract and adapting them to their individual circumstances or by focusing their own internal guidelines on high-risk clinical problems (e.g., danger to self or others) and more complex situations such as psychological disorders with medical complications.

Peer Review Process

Written practice guidelines are the most formal method for ensuring minimal standards of care. Even if such guidelines are not developed, a BGP may employ general standards that all clinicians are expected to uphold. Most contracting payers require some variation of a process in which routine chart review is conducted by peers or their supervisors (such as a clinical director) on a periodic basis to assess adherence to internal if not contracted standards. If a clinician's performance is not in accordance with these standards, there should be established procedures to address this situation with stipulated actions to be taken to correct any deviation and resolve any problems.

Outcome Measures

This generally involves an ongoing program of monitoring and tracking clinical treatment outcomes. There currently are no industry standard measures for clinical outcomes and some groups have developed their own assessment instruments. Others have used published questionnaires. Each BGP has to decide on the most meaningful tools, given resource and time constraints. As the industry becomes more sophisticated in this area, assessment tools will become more rigorous, and BGP's own instruments and methods will need to meet acceptable validity and reliability criteria.

Administrative Components

Internal Communications

Excellent communication between BGP office staff and staff of any contracting party is imperative. It is expected that all administrative personnel handle themselves professionally, and that while disagreements may occur between staff and outside parties, the relationship is professional. Basic customer service precepts apply: phones should be answered promptly and inquiries should be responded to in a timely manner.

Organized Record Keeping

Administrative files that include copies of contracts, fee schedules, current provider lists, and other records supporting business functions should be accessible when communicating with contracting entities.

Accounting/Billing Systems

While there are no specified systems required by the industry, the BGP's systems for billing and claims adjudication must be reliable and sufficient to supply the information necessary to process receivables and payables.

Credentialing Process

Many organizations are now requiring BGPs to perform their own credentialing of clinicians as part of a general trend toward pushing such responsibilities down to the practice level. As the size of a group practice grows, considerable resources could be committed to the process of ensuring that each practitioner's educational degrees have been verified, their licenses and professional liability insurance are current, indicated areas of specialty are verified, and all new clinicians have a completed application form and appropriate references. Any history of professional or legal difficulties must be investigated by a committee or someone representing the BGP. Contracts with individual practitioners should clearly delineate their responsibilities to the BGP, the standards to which they are accountable, and means by which they will be held accountable to them. (This may be accomplished by incorporating the practice's policies and procedures manual and quality management plan into the contract by reference.) All practitioners must agree to cooperate with quality management activities and make their records available for peer review and other quality studies.

Utilization Management Structures and Processes

Systems must be in place to track the utilization of services by individual clinician, as well as for the group as a whole. This not only should include monitoring the number of therapeutic sessions provided, but also should incorporate an evaluation of appropriate documentation to ensure that treatment plans are compatible with stated goals and the patient's functional impairments.

General Components

Availability of Care

Utilization indicators should demonstrate that adequate services are being provided to the population served at both inpatient and outpatient levels of care. A major concern of payers when contracting on an at-risk basis is that access to care will be overly restricted. True quality of care includes adequate and appropriate access to treatment for those in need. This would also include accountability at the intake and triage stage where determinations are made as to the most appropriate level of treatment (e.g., crisis intervention, inpatient setting, medication referral, group setting, etc.).

Accessibility

Offices must be easily accessible, close to freeways and/or mass transportation. Buildings should be wheelchair-accessible. Administration must be easy to contact and available, with an "800" number if appropriate; there should be short periods on hold and rapid response to voice mail. Appointments should be available within 5 days of contact by the patient, and emergencies should be addressed immediately. Rapid response to emergency calls and 24-hour emergency coverage are requirements.

A Functioning Quality Program

A written quality management plan that has been implemented demonstrates that the group has at least made a real commitment to quality. Mechanisms to ensure quality should involve individual responsibility, practice-wide measures, a formal committee with regularly scheduled meetings, and feedback mechanisms that actually result in changes being made to improve the system.

Patient Satisfaction Indicators

While the utility of patient satisfaction surveys are limited because most anonymous respondents to these surveys are either strongly positive or strongly negative, they do add an important subjective dimension to the overall quality picture. Qualitative questionnaires and patient comment cards can provide additional information about how well the office is run and the general satisfaction with its clinical staff.

Quality Management Officer/Designee

At least one individual in the organization must act as the ultimate locus of responsibility for quality management, with formal duties and responsibilities and corresponding authority. Ideally, that individual should have appropriate training, background, and skills and should act as a liaison with payers and other outside parties regarding quality issues. Some MCOs require that a BGP have a designated quality management officer.

Customer Service Orientation

A major challenge to the BGP is having to serve many masters. Patients, of course, are customers. But referring primary care physicians, medical groups and their representatives, and even insurance companies are also part of the chain of customers. Customer service policies and standards must serve all these "customers" efficaciously.

Grievance Processes

There must be clearly established procedures that are followed when any party desires to file a complaint. Every aspect of this process should be specified, including individual steps, forms, duties, responsibilities, and outcomes. Fairness and confidentiality are paramount, as is accountability to and communication with the complainant. Finally, grievance procedures should be designed in such a way as to ensure that any legitimate cause for complaint will not reoccur to the extent that the cause can be controlled by the BGP.

Procedures for Adverse Events

As with any imperfect system, there will be times when mistakes or other unanticipated adverse events occur. A key part of any comprehensive quality management program are measures and methods for evaluating, resolving, and reporting these situations. Adverse events also must be tracked over time in order to discover patterns that may emerge involving particular clinicians, protocols, procedures, or other aspects of the system.

The foregoing is only a summary of what contracting organizations such as MCOs typically expect of behavioral group practices with respect to quality. Specific stipulations depend on the parties involved, the type of contract, and other considerations, but it is clear that the scope of these requirements is broad and includes every aspect of operations in the group practice. Meeting this challenge requires sophistication, planning, and resources.

An important trend in formalizing the measurement of performance of an organized system of care is the development of "report cards" (see Hall, 1996). These tools for monitoring quality indices are gaining popularity among purchasers of health care and consumer advocacy groups. Report cards are used to compare different systems of care in specific areas of performance such as access, clinical appropriateness, treatment effectiveness, utilization, and other aspects of quality. Ultimately, it is presumed that this public scrutiny will motivate providers to improve the quality of their systems and their care.

Finally, behavioral group practices must be aware of the significant impact that a contracting organizations' quality management program may have on them. This could influence the group's planning and structures by either supporting them or making them more complicated. Too often, even experienced practice managers do not recognize and plan for the influence of multiple quality management programs and they may find their practices having to create parallel procedures and repetitive information systems to accommodate different contracts. Ideally, when entering into a contract, BGPs would present their own quality management plan, including standards that the contracting party would agree and also adhere to. For example, forms used for clinical records can be developed by the BGP and designed to meet the data needs of all its MCO contracts; credentialing procedures can be developed to meet universal standards that both the BGP and MCO would satisfy; and MCOs could be held accountable for ensuring a rapid authorization for services with accurate insurance and copayment information to support the BGP's responsibility for rapid access and good customer service.

WHAT DOES "QUALITY" MEAN IN THE BEHAVIORAL GROUP PRACTICE?

Management and professional literature is inundated with definitions, concepts, and acronyms relating to "quality." Presenting a cogent discussion without causing more confusion or being misinterpreted is difficult at best. Some terms (e.g., quality assurance, continuous quality improvement) are strongly associated with specific perspectives, theories, or approaches. Others, such as "quality management," as in the chapter title, are used generically. To the BGP, what represents "quality" depends on context and objectives.

To address quality meaningfully, BGPs must first recognize the various stakeholders in a system of care. In a managed care environment, these include patients, clinicians, contracting organizations, payers, and system administrators. What quality means to each reflects specific needs, biases, and values. Patients may value an empathic therapist, interventions focused on solving their problems, and a courteous office staff. Clinicians may define quality of care in terms of the achievement of goals that have been mutually defined between the therapist and patient. Payers may focus on the greatest efficiencies given an established optimal level of care. Administrators may look at an ideal balance between levels of care offered and patient satisfaction indicators and how smoothly administrative functions are performed.

How can BGPs expect to measure, monitor, and improve quality when the meaning of the term remains so obscure? The various perspectives of the stakeholders are all worthy, yet each one alone is incomplete. A major challenge to group practices is to accommodate these varied interests and standards and integrate them into a system of care that is sensitive to them all. While the specific definition and use of the term may vary somewhat between practices, depending on a variety of factors, each BGP must develop a clear organizational definition that is expressed consistently throughout the practice. To be useful, quality should be viewed from the perspective of the entire clinical and administrative system, rather than by examining only one aspect of care or one administrative activity.

How quality is addressed in the BGP arises directly from the values of its members and leadership. It is not inherently imbedded in its organizational design or derived from its compensation structures. In the past, formal quality management has been limited to larger, multilevel, hierarchical organizations such as hospital settings. These entities often operate on an at-risk basis and employ stringent quality management strategies to monitor the quality of the care they provide and ensure their economic viability. The current and foreseeable business realities are a strong incentive to formalize the quality management activities of the group practice, although these alone are rightly not the only driver. Business imperatives always have meant that cost was a real if unacknowledged component of providing quality behavioral health care. In the past, responsibly attending to cost containment issues allowed a practice to survive financially in order to continue in the profession. The rise of institutional payers has brought this issue to the fore. In today's health care environment, any attempt to assure and improve "quality" in the BGP must address two components: effectiveness of care and cost-effectiveness (sometimes referred to in the literature as "efficiency"). A principle task of the leadership of the contemporary group practice is to manage the tensions between these two components. In this chapter, we use the term "quality" in the context of the BGP to refer to the optimal standard that addresses both treatment effectiveness and cost effectiveness, what we refer to as *efficacious care*.

MANAGING QUALITY IN THE BEHAVIORAL HEALTH GROUP PRACTICE

Establishing the overriding quality goals, designing structures and processes to measure and improve quality, and developing methods for enhancing conformity to quality standards are among the core functions of management in a BGP. Managers must assume the task of defining what will constitute "quality" within the organization, weighing the varying perspectives of all parties holding a stake in the enterprise. This can have significant implications on prior relationships between the practice and outside entities, as well as serious repercussions among the relationships within the organization. For example, managing the transition from a predominantly fee-for-service practice to a system of care that assumes at-risk contracts will require clinicians to be much more accountable to the administration for what happens in a therapeutic session and to learn how to document their clinical work appropriately. Contracting entities, which prior to this change may have had only periodic communication with individual providers within the group, may now insist on a regular reporting schedule of key quality indicators encompassing data from the entire group. BGP management participates in devising these processes in the context of other business considerations.

In measuring quality, the BGP must be able to accommodate different levels of analysis from the point of view of individual patients to the broader perspective of managed care companies. At the level of patient care, indicators involve units of measure such as number of sessions, clinical outcome ratings, and patient satisfaction scores. Managed care organizations and other contractors also are interested in indicators measuring the quality of nonclinical aspects of the system, such as relapse/recidivism rate, telephone response time, and billing accuracy.

Resolving or managing conflicts among differing interests is a key goal of the quality management process for BGPs. Managers must recognize when these may arise either because of inherent tensions within the system or as a result of a lack of understanding or inadequate training. Ensuring that the professional staff has the appropriate training and background to work competently in a managed care system is also the responsibility of management. Much of today's mental health workforce has not been formally trained in the key tenets of managed care, allowing for a broad range of quality in clinicians' performance in these systems. While training is a shared responsibility of practitioners and organizations, this endeavor is very expensive and requires more than a few continuing education courses.

One way that some organizations have encouraged providers to seek training has been to create compensation structures based on merit rather than seniority. Professionals who understand how the system works and are able to contribute beyond the minimal standards are rewarded by receiving a higher volume of patients and/or higher fees or profit sharing of some form, such as participation in a risk pool bonus.

A BGP's size will influence how elaborate a quality management plan it is feasible to implement. A wide range of sizes currently exist, from six to eight clinician groups to Independent Provider Associations consisting of over 200 providers. Most BGPs are on the smaller end and are not able to support a full-scale comprehensive quality program. To do so would require too large a commitment of resources, both human and financial. Nonetheless, they must have some form of quality management, and if the commitment is there, a practice of any size, regardless of how organized, can develop and implement an adequate quality program.

As mentioned earlier, how the practice is structured will also influence the nature of the quality management plan. Staff models generally impose more formal integration among clinicians, and thus create ready-made structures for a quality program. Clinicians are more accustomed to being managed by a centralized administration with expectations to meet certain work standards. Quality standards can be incorporated into their performance reviews and reflected in compensation systems. Quality structures can be derived from existing meetings for clinical and business purposes.

Network models (Independent Provider Associations "group without walls," etc.) that bring together many independently practicing professionals under a more loosely formed structure are generally easier to create but more difficult to manage, especially with respect to quality. Most of the clinicians under these models rarely interact with each other and have varying levels of comfort practicing under managed care systems. They also have different degrees of commitment to the larger organization, as some may organize their practices around referrals from the entity, while others will only desire a few referrals per month to fill out sparse schedules. Administrators must attempt to conduct all the day-to-day business and management of the group via paper, telephone, and fax communications to dozens or more clinicians. While more sophisticated on-line information systems are appearing on the market, full integration between clinical and administrative data sets are still rare and the cost of licensing and installing these programs is prohibitive for all but the most well-financed group practices. This makes identifying, monitoring, and enhancing adherence to quality standards difficult and expensive in the network model. Quality process is heavily weighted on case managers who serve as the main connection between administration and practitioners to enforce organizational policies.

The cultural dynamics of the group practice also have a significant influence on managing quality. Group practices that based their previous success on providing services with a high profit margin, bringing together professionals who primarily shared overhead expenses, must face many challenges. Many of their clinicians were accustomed to defining their success and importance to the group by how many patients they could keep in long-term therapy. Staff meetings focused on sharing clinical information to formulate better conceptualizations of a patient's problems. There were few organizational planning decisions to make and little impetus to be concerned with the effectiveness and efficiency of other clinicians' treatment.

Groups working in organized systems of care are accountable for both the quality of clinical care and the quality of their administration of care. This requires greater cooperation from clinicians to ensure that care is more effective and efficient. Many traditionally trained therapists either are not competent at performing brief psychotherapy or have negative attitudes toward it. Most clinicians who have been practicing independently are resistant to the structures, reporting requirements and general accountability to outside agents that good quality management entails. Office staff members as well may be skeptical and mistrustful of the managed care industry, having preconceived notions based on anecdotal accounts of abuse and confusing messages from the media.

Appropriate education and training to understand the purpose of organized systems of care and to clarify the group's values and appreciate the significance of quality management is critical to overcoming resistance to change. Because the industry is evolving rapidly, it is imperative that everyone working for the group continually be apprised of the changing requirements the practice continuously faces.

A QUALITY MANAGEMENT PROGRAM: THE BASICS

At a minimum, a quality management (QM) program consists of the following elements:

1. A QM officer or designee to plan and coordinate QM activities and act as a "point person" for relevant issues and concerns that may arise. The quality officer may also be responsible for coordinating outcome studies and patient satisfaction surveys. More sophisticated studies should be conducted by professionals with appropriate backgrounds in research methodology.
2. A QM committee or team; a group that collectively has the responsibility and authority for QM over all operational areas of the practice. This typically includes representatives from all key operational areas of the practice such as the executive level, senior clinicians, associates, and office administration.

Representation or close, ongoing communication with contracting parties such as MCOs and medical groups is also important, as is feedback from the community in which the practice is located.

3. A written QM plan that explicitly states the goals of the QM program and details the BGP's standards, policies, procedures, and mechanisms for managing quality, how performance will be monitored and assessed, and methods for actively improving, remediating, and correcting for deviation from standards.

Planning to manage quality is much like any sort of strategic planning. The planning cycle has three parts. First, *assessment* of the situation and circumstances and the internal and external requirements of the system, including feedback from throughout the practice on each identified quality measure. Second, *planning*, which involves identifying and articulating objectives and the strategies and resources required to meet them. Finally, *execution* of the plans formulated. The planning cycle is repeated indefinitely as assessment of the results and outcomes of the execution of the plans is fed back into the process, leading to continuing refinements of the strategy, and, in this case, continuous improvements in quality.

A well-crafted program also includes reflective mechanisms designed to improve the QM program and processes themselves (in addition to the quality that results from them). Ideally, it includes means of assessing the impact of the program and evaluates the utility of the measures chosen and that efficiency of the resources allocated to the effort. Finally, simply devising policies and procedures to measure and manage quality is not the same as actually implementing them. Plans are often developed to satisfy a contractual requirement, then filed and forgotten. Execution and commitment are key to an effective quality management program.

THE SUCCESS FACTORS

Recognition of the Importance of Attending to Quality in All Areas of the Practice

True quality is not unidimensional, and all areas of the practice are interrelated. As in any system, changes in one area may effect other areas.

Commitment from Leadership

This must be demonstrated visibly and supported vocally at every opportunity. Sincere commitment is also indicated by the allocation of resources. While a good QM program does not have to be expensive, it will require some resources to develop and maintain. Key persons must be assigned specific tasks, and data need to be gathered, analyzed, and reported.

Accountability Throughout the Organization

This includes individuals from top management, the QM officer, QM committee, all clinicians, and administrative staff. It is a very powerful message when all members of the practice can see that every other member is willing to be accountable for the quality of their work, and that it is not merely an imposition on those with less authority.

Effective Planning

The plan must be formalized, drafted, and distributed, and it should involve all stakeholders and provide meaningful feedback loops. It should address identified problem areas, as well as potential difficulties, and should be flexible enough to accommodate change as the practice evolves. Remember that while a good QM plan is comprehensive, it should only attempt to address those aspects of quality that can be meaningfully measured and controlled.

Competent Execution and Follow Through

The best laid plan is useless if it is not implemented well. As with any supervisory management, authority to take action when required must be delegated along with the responsibility for doing so, and mechanisms for mutual accountability must be in place. It is important to avoid micromanaging the details of practice operations while not appearing disinterested in them.

Management Information Systems to Support the Program

In a system of care, it is very difficult to manage quality without adequate information systems. Existing mechanisms may be supplemented to address quality issues (e.g., progress note forms, patient registration sheets, etc.), and specific forms or data-gathering tools can be developed (e.g., patient satisfaction questionnaires). An adequate and appropriate computer system to manage quality management data and to generate reports is required.

Compatibility with QM Mechanisms of Contracted Payers

If the BGP's quality program conflicts with key components of a contracted entity, the overall degree of quality will be compromised. For example, if a group's goal is to schedule appointments for patients within 5 days of their first contact but it routinely takes 2 weeks to get an authorization from the MCO, the internal standard will be impossible to meet. Sophisticated and proactive BGPs find that their own quality management policies and procedures can be more rigorous and applicable than those required by slower-moving contracting entities. Also, tailoring a QM plan to the requirements of one contract can cause conflicts with the requirements of others, and at the very least require substantial revisions.

Strong Commitment to Training of Administrative Staff and Clinical Professionals

Much cooperation is required from persons working on the "front lines." If negative attitudes about quality processes exist within the practice, monitoring systems become compromised and measures may be incomplete or inaccurate. Thorough training in both the importance of QM and the BGP's own policies and procedures is essential.

THE QUALITY MANAGEMENT PLAN

The written plan codifies the specific processes and policies that govern QM for the practice. In order to be useful, it must satisfy five key criteria. The plan must be:

- *Simple and easily understood.* It need not and must not be too complex to understand or execute.
- *Powerful, compact, concise but thorough.* If it is too difficult to implement, it will be ignored. All aspects should be well designed, meeting all necessary and significant conditions as well as stated goals.
- *Flexible.* Virtually by definition, a good QM plan must be adaptable to a variety of situations and contract requirements.
- *Neutral.* As discussed, the plan will need to serve the many stakeholders in the practice's quality, including patients, clinicians, office staff, administrators, contractors, and payers. The language and stated goals should reflect the interests of all these parties, without unduly reflecting those of any individual or group.
- *Specific.* It must spell out policies and procedures in detail. Goals must be quantifiable and the indicators operationalized in a manner that is achievable. A good, useful plan will list its objectives, identify assignment of responsibility, state reporting requirements, give measures, describe steps for execution, and offer a time frame for each stage of the program.

Functionally, the plan must also define terms, assign responsibility to promote accountability and clarify expectations, demonstrate commitment from the top of the organization, and allocate appropriate resources. Planning without allocating sufficient resources is the most predictable downfall of the otherwise well-crafted QM plan.

Effective planning in developing the QM document is important to a successful outcome. A number of questions should be answered at the outset. First, the plan must be delimited: How much detail is needed? Given the BGP's current and future contracts, what external requirements will have to be met or can be reasonably anticipated? Will contracting parties play a role in developing the plan?

Who is the audience for the QM document? As with any business communication, this will dictate content, form, and style. Is it principally an internal document? Will it and the performance measures it incorporates be open to public scrutiny? What resources are available for developing the plan and what resources will be budgeted for implementing it? What money, time, and personnel will be available?

Who within the practice will be accountable for the quality plan and its implementation? What segments of the practice should be represented on the committee? Is there commitment from the highest level of the practice? Who will author the plan? Can the practice generate the commitment required? Is there cooperation among clinical and office staff to engage in quality improvement processes? These and other questions must be identified and answered at the outset. Obviously, drafting a useful and viable QM plan is a major initiative in itself.

Once the scope of the project is outlined, the QM objectives of the practice need to be established and clarified. These should reflect the organization's values and be consistent with its mission. The practice needs to decide if quality standards will attempt to meet or exceed customer expectations. Is the goal to create organizational "excellence," or is "beating the competition" the primary objective? Who are the actual "customers" with regard to quality? Have both internal and external customers been considered? What philosophy will the practice take toward setting standards and applying measures to its systems?

The typical goal of QM plans in product-oriented industries is to reduce the variance in processes that produce specific products or results (see Walton, 1986). The assumption is that this will reduce costs because of the inefficiencies implicit in varying from identified standards. Also, presuming the standards set indeed reflect the optimum outcome, improving adherence to them should maximize the "quality" of the results. Is this the approach to standards the BGP will employ? Is it appropriate to behavioral healthcare services? This approach actually can be applied to some aspects of the typical BGP's operations, but human service-oriented enterprises clearly must develop other measures that are more appropriate to their field to manage significant aspects of their practices.

The objectives for a QM program in behavioral health care might include meeting or exceeding quality of care standards, increasing the ability to serve larger patient populations without sacrificing the quality of care, reducing overhead and variable costs with the current volume of patients, or sharing the successful implementation of a plan to demonstrate accountability for quality to a contracting entity. It is important to establish the objectives of the program first, then the goals of the QM plan in order to have a meaningful basis for developing quality standards and measures.

THE ELEMENTS OF THE QUALITY MANAGEMENT PLAN

Quality is expressed in virtually every aspect of operations in the BGP. The QM plan identifies the most significant of those expressions and codifies the means of measuring them, comparing those measurements to established standards, and provides mechanisms and means for improving them as needed. The mechanisms typically involve four parts: accountability, response, feedback, and documentation.

Expressions of Quality

Quality in the BGP is not monolithic. It is expressed in many different ways in different areas of the practice, and so there are necessarily different types of measures that can be applied. Arguably, a QM plan is only as good as its measures that are derived from an understanding of exactly how quality is being expressed in a given area. It is useful to develop at least an informal conceptual model of the operations of the practice to facilitate identifying which expressions of quality are indeed most significant. (In many instances, contracting organizations may have specific requirements in this respect, if not actually specifying which measure, standards, and mechanisms a practice must employ.)

There is a natural division between clinical and nonclinical operations. The nonclinical areas can be further broken into managerial, administrative, financial, information (MIS) and communications, and customer service functions. These groupings are collectively meant to be inclusive of all functions, but some of the distinctions may be arbitrary. This sort of typology is useful in organizing a QM plan and also helps to focus attention on specific areas that might otherwise receive inadequate attention and to disperse accountability by job function.

MEASURES

Measures are the specific criteria used to assess the quality of a given dimensions of the practice. There are a variety of useful measures. The best allow for easy comparison both within the practice over time and with other BGPs when possible. Some measures are direct; others, because of the nature of behavioral health, are less so. Preferably, it is most desirable to measure *outcomes* directly. This is because outcomes (e.g., clinical improvement, patient satisfaction) ultimately reflect the quality of the services provided, and they are the results of appropriate quality processes and structures. In lieu of direct outcome, a specific *process* within the practice may be measured (e.g., adherence to practice guidelines). Where that is unfeasible, measures may be developed that apply to structures (e.g., existence of a QM committee that meets regularly, MIS capability). As a last resort, when none of these approaches is possible but some form of measurement is still necessary, establishing minimum criteria may suffice. An example of the latter, although used in conjunction with others measures, is the practice of credentialing to ensure competency of clinicians. Credentialing does not ensure a practitioner will obtain good clinical results; it merely sets a minimum standard for clinicians who will be allowed to treat patients. Because of the realities of behavioral health care, any quality management plan necessarily uses all of these types of measures.

The quality of some aspects of the practice are by their nature easily quantified, such as days in an inpatient setting. Other dimensions, such as customer service, are harder to quantify and require some creativity. A well-designed MIS can automate the tracking of many measures. In practices above a nominal size an automated computerized MIS is essential.

STANDARDS

Briefly, standards are the benchmarks to which measures are compared in order to assess a given expression of quality. As noted, some standards are supplied by payers as contractual conditions. Others may be developed empirically or by comparison with industry norms.

ACCOUNTABILITY

As with any organization or initiative, accountability on the part of those executing is a requirement of success. Wherever possible, specific individuals should be assigned (by title if not by name) with specific QM duties. The QM officer or designee is an obvious example, but in most BGPs that are quality driven and have a full quality program in place, every employee will have some QM duties. Clinicians and staff are held accountable to the QM officer and the QM committee for executing the plan, maintaining standards, tracking measures where appropriate, and responding and documenting as applicable. It is of the utmost importance to specify who is responsible for responding when measures indicate poor performance relative to standards and bringing measures back into line.

In general, the compliance and accountability of clinicians are greatly enhanced if they are part of the planning process from the outset, rather than simply handed the QM plan. Also, QM should be part of the job description of each employee and be factored into performance reviews.

Response

Setting standards is of no benefit unless policies and procedures are in place to respond when they are not met. This is at the heart of every QM plan. Responses vary widely, of course, depending on what functional area is being addressed and what specific measures and standards are employed.

Feedback

This takes two forms. In the simplest, the information gathered by comparing measures to standards, when responded to effectively, will have a positive effect on the quality of the practice's performance. This is the very reason for implementing a QM plan. In the second, by monitoring the plan and its effectiveness over time, the plan itself can be refined and improve. This reflectivity is the hallmark of a truly well-run QM program.

Documentation

The QM plan itself is a means of documenting the importance the practice gives to quality. There are also specific instances in which documentation is required both internally and externally, such as in the case of adverse clinical outcomes. In another area, patient satisfaction polling might reveal a problem with the manner of a clinician and the procedure for responding to that situation may involve recording the instances, identifying a pattern, bringing it to the clinician's attention, establishing an appropriate intervention, and documenting it in the individual's personnel record.

EVALUATING THE QM PROGRAM

How do we determine if a given QM program is effective? The answer is not simple. Generally speaking, a well-designed and executed QM plan is self-evaluating, that is, will show both improved (or better than targeted) clinical outcomes and greater efficiency over time. By tracking expenses and efficacy, it is possible to do at least a cursory cost-benefit analysis. These generally show a favorable result, which varies with how well the program is run. (And the most sophisticated programs incorporate a certain reflectivity: the QM program itself is subject to the QM plan.) If the key success factors (see previous section) are incorporated, QM programs are by their nature and purpose not harmful to the BGP and typically prove beneficial. In the increasingly competitive behavioral health care environment, the question is less "how do BGP's determine their effectiveness" than "how they can survive without being quality-driven."

FINAL REMARKS

Managing quality in any organization is a continuous process, as opposed to a single attainable goal. It is just as much a reflection of hundreds of small day-to-day decisions as it is representative of key organizational strategies.

In the final analysis, quality as a strategic driver is perfectly suited to the values of behavioral health care professionals. Behavioral health care is a "caring" profession.

Formal QM is the means of expressing this value in a business enterprise. If BGPs are proactive in QM, they can maintain the highest degree of control over the care they provide, while efficaciously managing the tension between their desire to provide the most effective care with the efficiencies demanded in the current health care environment. Embracing quality as a core value of the practice enables them to truly offer the best possible care to the greatest number of people.

REFERENCES

American Psychiatric Association. (1994). *Diagnostic and statistical manual of mental disorders* (4th ed.). Washington, DC: Author.

Boyle, P. J., & Callahan, D. (Eds.). (1995). *What price mental health? The ethics and politics of setting priorities.* Washington DC: Georgetown University Press.

Donahue, M., & Wrecki, M. T. (1995). Knowing what insurers want. In G. Zieman (Ed.), *The complete capitation handbook.* Tiburon, CA: CentraLink Publications.

Ericson, B. (1995). Implementing total quality management. In G. Zieman (Ed.), *The complete capitation handbook.* Tiburon, CA: CentraLink Publications.

Gaucher, E. J., & Coffey R. J. (1993). *Total quality in healthcare.* San Francisco: Jossey-Bass.

Goodman, M., Brown, J., & Deitz, P. (1992). *Managing managed care: A mental health practitioner's survival guide.* Washington DC: American Psychiatric Association.

Hall, L. L. (1996). Report cards accelerate quality and accountability. *Behavioral Healthcare Tomorrow, 5*(3), 57–61.

Keller, J. (1995, July/August). Business coalition initiatives related to behavioral healthcare purchasing and quality improvement. *Behavioral Healthcare Tomorrow, 4*(4), 49-52.

Lamb, R., & Lamson, G. W. (1996). Overcoming barriers to comprehensive quality improvement. *Behavioral Healthcare Tomorrow, 5*(3), 33–37.

National Committee for Quality Assurance (NCQA). (1997). *Accreditation standards for managed behavioral healthcare organizations.* Washington, DC: Author.

Savitz, S. A. (1992). Measuring quality of care and quality maintenance. In J. L. Feldman & R. J. Fitzpatrick (Eds.), *Managed mental health care.* Washington, DC: American Psychiatric Press.

Schultz, T. (1995). Negotiating the contract. In G. Zieman (Ed.), *The complete capitation handbook.* Tiburon, CA: CentraLink Publications.

Shueman, S. A., & Troy W. G. (1994a). Quality assurance in managed systems. In S. A. Shueman, W. G. Troy, & S. L. Mayhugh (Eds.), *Managed behavioral health care: An industry perspective* (pp. 131–148). Springfield, IL: Charles Thomas Publisher.

Shueman, S. A. & Troy W. G. (1994b). The use of practice guidelines in managed behavioral health programs. In S. A. Shueman, W. G. Troy, & S. L. Mayhugh (Eds.), *Managed behavioral health care: An industry perspective* (pp. 149–164). Springfield, IL: Charles Thomas Publisher.

Walton, M. (1986). *The Deming management method.* New York: Dodd Mead & Co.

Wilson, G. F. (1992). Defining and measuring quality. In M. R. Mattson (Ed.), *Manual of psychiatric quality assurance: A report of the American Psychiatric Association Committee on Quality Assurance.* Washington, DC: American Psychiatric Association.

11

Ensuring Quality in the Treatment of Chemical Dependency

DAVID A. ZANIS AND A. THOMAS MCLELLAN

INTRODUCTION

The field of chemical dependency treatment has evolved rapidly over the past ten years as managed care principles have influenced the delivery of behavioral health services. There have been substantial shifts in the utilization of treatment modalities for persons with drug and alcohol dependence; for example, the use of intensive outpatient and partial hospitalization treatment services have increased, while the use of hospital-based inpatient rehabilitative care has decreased. Two factors have driven this service utilization shift: (1) our ability to measure treatment effectiveness, and (2) our ability to measure cost-effectiveness.

While there have been shifts in the types of treatments that are utilized, there has been slow progress toward developing new and more effective treatments over the past 20 years. Although some treatments (i.e., naltrexone combined with psychosocial services for the treatment of alcoholism) have resulted in improved outcomes, there remains no single therapeutic protocol that can be deemed the "best" treatment approach. However, this should not be considered unusual, since drug and/or alcohol dependence like other chronic diseases (diabetes, hypertension, asthma), often require multiple treatment experiences, combined with regular monitoring of the conditions and symptoms associated with the disease following treatment discharge.

Therefore, improving the quality of treatment not only involves continuing the search for new and more effective treatments, but involves reshaping and monitoring the process of how treatment is delivered. Clearly, enhancing the quality of treatment requires substantial effort among many arenas: the scientific community, society, public officials, treatment programs, counselors, and the patients themselves.

This chapter is divided in two general sections: (1) an overview of knowledge and research on addiction and addiction treatment and several issues that affect the quality of treatment; and (2) a discussion of changes toward improving the quality of substance abuse treatment.

DAVID A. ZANIS AND A. THOMAS MCLELLAN • Department of Psychiatry, University of Pennsylvania, Philadelphia, Pennsylvania 19104.

Handbook of Quality Management in Behavioral Health, edited by Stricker *et al.* Kluwer Academic / Plenum Publishers, New York, 2000.

OVERVIEW OF ADDICTION

Incidence and Prevalence of Substance Use

The National Drug and Alcoholism Treatment Unit Survey (SAMHSA, 1995) reported that 944,208 patients were enrolled in both public and private abuse treatment programs in the United States during its 1994 1-day annual survey. In the 1991 National Household Survey on Drug Abuse (NIDA, 1992) it was estimated that over 37% (75 million) of the US population over the age of 12 had used an illicit drug at least once in their lifetime, while 12.7% (26 million) had used an illicit drug in the past year. As reported in Table 1, an estimated 19 million individuals used marijuana and 6 million used cocaine during the 1-year period between 1990 and 1991. Among persons consuming legalized substances, 138 million Americans drank alcohol and 65 million smoked cigarettes during 1991 (Table 2).

It should be noted that these estimates of substance use are considered underrepresentative since they do not include data form hidden and heavily affected populations (i.e., incarcerated, homeless). A more recent report issued by the Office of National Drug Control Policy (1995) indicates the incidence of cocaine use has slightly declined over the past few years, while the incidence of heroin and marijuana use have increased in most regions of the country. Of particular concern has been the reported steady increase in marijuana, cocaine, hallucinogen, stimulant, and inhalant use among adolescents.

Public Health and Social Costs Associated with Substance Use

Substance abuse represents a major public health concern throughout the world and costs the United States economy approximately $150 billion annually in both

TABLE 1. 1991 Population Estimates of Illicit Drug Use in the United States by Age and Gender[a,b]

Age group	Sample size	Any illicit drug		Marijuana		Cocaine		Sedatives		Heroin[c]
		Year	Month	Year	Month	Year	Month	Year	Month	Year
12 to 17	20145	2987	1362	2027	874	302	83	267	95	39
Males	10307	1636	728	1182	514	158	51	109	37	
Females	9838	1351	635	846	360	144	31	158	58	
18 to 25	28496	8305	4390	6994	3714	2186	582	547	191	87
Males	13943	4379	2452	3851	2191	1317	392	286	88	
Females	14553	3926	1938	3144	1522	870	190	260	103	
26 to 34	38737	7125	3467	5590	2705	1959	703	464	141	114
Males	19078	4231	2162	3515	1821	1314	493	245	88	
Females	19659	2893	1306	2074	884	645	211	219	53	
35 or more	115480	7367	3593	4624	2428	1618	523	852	358	142
Males	53913	4059	2031	2967	1609	1157	330	333	81	
Females	61567	3308	1562	1657	820	460	193	520	277	
Total	202859	25783	12813	19235	9721	6065	1892	2130	785	381
Males	97242	14306	7372	11514	6135	3946	1266	973	293	
Females	105617	11478	5441	7721	3586	2120	626	1157	492	

[a]SOURCE: Substance Abuse and Mental Health Services Administration (1991).
[b]In thousands.
[c]Data for heroin use, past month and gender breakdown, unavailable.

TABLE 2. 1991 Population Estimates of Licit Substance Use in the United States by Age and Gender[a,b]

Age group	Sample size	Alcohol		Cigarettes		Smokeless tobacco	
		Year	Month	Year	Month	Year	Month
12 to 17	20145	8122	4092	4053	2183	1223	607
Males	10307	4384	2298	2214	1220	1118	556
Females	9838	3738	1794	1839	962	105	51
18 to 25	28496	23605	18120	11744	9164	2461	1639
Males	13943	11949	9714	5912	4468	2340	1595
Females	14553	11656	8417	5832	4696	121	44
26 to 34	38737	31320	23886	14743	12753	1957	1388
Males	19078	16118	13509	7731	6640	1912	1348
Females	19659	15202	10377	7012	6113	45	40
35 or more	115480	74996	57123	34595	30725	3983	3251
Males	53913	38215	30972	17892	15547	3437	2818
Females	61567	36781	26151	16703	15178	547	433
Total	202859	138043	103232	65136	54825	9624	6885
Males	97242	70666	56493	33750	27875	8806	6316
Females	105617	67377	46739	31386	26950	818	568

[a]SOURCE: Substance Abuse and Mental Health Services Administration (1991).
[b]In thousands.

direct and indirect costs (Rice, Kelman, & Miller, 1991; Harwood, Hubbard, Collins, & Rachal, 1988). Moreover, substance abuse causes a substantial emotional impact, affecting the substance user, the substance users' social network, employers, and victims of substance abuse-related crime.

The United States corrections system has been dramatically affected by inmates convicted of drug-related crimes. By 1993, more than 186,000 persons across the nation were incarcerated in state prisons for drug offenses, compared to fewer than 19,000 in 1980 (US Department of Justice, 1994, 1995). In 1994, a total of 1.1 million inmates (excluding those in local jails) were housed in the state and federal system, of whom 60% are estimated to have a serious substance abuse disorder. The increased arrest, conviction, and incarceration of drug abusers has overcrowded the prison system by nearly 250,000 inmates and has prompted massive prison construction throughout the country. Beyond the $30,000 per year estimate for housing inmates in prisons and jails, correctional institutions have considerable financial outlays to provide intensive supervision, treatment, and rehabilitative services for drug- and alcohol-dependent individuals who have been sentenced to nonjail and prison alternatives.

Substance use also has had a major impact on the United States health care system. Substance-dependent persons consume as much as ten times the health care services as nonaddicted persons, and their families use as much as five times the health care services as families of persons without a substance use disorder. The practice of sharing needles and participating in risky sexual practices has resulted in drug users becoming the second highest at-risk group to transmit and acquire the human immunodeficiency virus (HIV) (Needle, 1994). Overall, it has been estimated that $13.7 billion is spent on the health care of substance users annually (Rice et al., 1991).

Society's Response to the Problem of Substance Abuse

To address the problem of substance abuse on a national level, the federal government has taken a two-pronged approach: (1) interdiction (reducing the supply of drugs both within and outside of the United States), and (2) treatment and prevention of drug users (reducing the demand for drugs). During fiscal year 1995, the federal government spent approximately $13.2 billion on drug abuse control, of which $6.5 billion was allocated to the criminal justice system, $2.7 billion for treatment, $1.6 billion for prevention, $1.2 billion for interdiction, and the remainder for research and other activities.

While the economic costs associated with substance use are staggering, several economic studies have found that substance abuse treatment in general offsets future health care costs (Langenbucher, 1994). Spear and Mason (1991) reported that the health care claims of family members were substantially reduced if an individual within the household received substance abuse treatment compared to households in which the substance abusers who did not receive treatment. Moreover, in a recent California study, researchers found that for each dollar allocated to substance abuse treatment services, more than $7 are saved in societal costs (CALDATA, 1994).

Characteristics of Patients Entering Substance Abuse Treatment

Beyond demographic differences, substance abusers present for treatment with a host of biopsychosocial needs that extend beyond problematic consumption of drugs and alcohol. Nearly 70% of opiate users have a concurrent psychiatric diagnosis (Kebler, 1983). Approximately 30% of acquired immunodeficiency syndrome (AIDS) cases in the United States have been associated with injection drug users (Needle, 1994). Nearly one half of all patients enrolled in publicly funded drug treatment programs are unemployed (NORC, 1995). In addition to these problems, patients entering substance abuse treatment report needing additional treatment services for medical, employment, financial, psychological, family, and other related problems (Table 3). Often it is these related problems that compromise the patients' ability to maintain treatment gains following discharge from treatment.

TABLE 3. Percent of Clients Reporting Service Needs by Modality of Treatment[a]

	Methadone		Long-term residential		Outpatient drug-free		Short-term inpatient[b]
Service type	TOPS (*N* = 2185)	DATOS (*N* = 708)	TOPS (*N* = 1040)	DATOS (*N* = 1234)	TOPS (*N* = 763)	DATOS (*N* = 855)	DATOS (*N* = 1415)
Medical	46.1	56.6	74.6	61.4	29.9	48.3	63.1
Psychological	32.7	56.3	65.8	68.4	70.8	65.5	80.1
Family	24.8	54.4	56.3	77.5	48.9	68.9	86.3
Legal	16.8	19.7	38.1	31.2	13.7	37.5	35.0
Vocational	38.7	55.4	56.7	71.4	34.0	57.8	60.0
Financial	39.1	49.1	61.4	44.4	29.4	46.1	57.1

[a]SOURCE: Etheridge et al. (1995).
[b]TOPS data not available.

Infinite Needs versus Finite Resources: Are Treatment Programs Able to Provide Appropriate Treatment Services?

Although patients present with a wide range of needs, there are limited resources available within the current public sector substance abuse treatment system to meet these needs. For example, Medicaid does not reimburse substance abuse treatment programs for providing social services such as vocational counseling. Therefore, there is little incentive for these agencies to provide such adjunctive services (Duggar, 1991). Treatment programs are left in a dilemma: If the treatment program provides specific social services such as housing assistance, with the objective of stabilizing the patient's social environment to allow the individual to fully engage in drug and alcohol treatment that could result in more effective outcomes, they are not reimbursed. On the other hand, if the treatment programs do not offer these additional social services because they are not reimbursed, it is likely that the patient may not be stabilized to receive the full therapeutic effect of drug and alcohol treatment, and therefore treatment is less effective, possibly resulting in more frequent and/or severe relapse episodes.

Etheridge, Craddock, Dunteman, and Hubbard (1995) reviewed data from the Treatment Outcome Prospective Study (TOPS) collected from 1979 to 1981 and the Drug Abuse Treatment Outcome Study (DATOS) collected from 1991 to 1993 and found a general decline in the range and number of treatment services provided to patients enrolled in community-based treatment programs during this 10-year span (Table 4). While most patients received at least some sessions of adjunct counseling during their stay in treatment, the majority of patients indicated that they needed additional services to address other areas of functioning, such as employment counseling, psychiatric counseling, family counseling, and assistance with other social service needs.

What Are the Goals of Substance Abuse Treatments?

The goals of substance abuse treatment are diverse and can be best understood by examining four different perspectives. From the patient perspective the goal of treat-

Table 4. Percent of Clients Receiving Services by Modality of Treatment from 1981–1991[a]

	Methadone		Long-term residential		Outpatient drug-free		Short-term inpatient[b]
Service type	TOPS 1979–81 (N = 2185)	DATOS 1991–93 (N = 908)	TOPS 1979–81 (N = 1040)	DATOS 1991–93 (N = 1234)	TOPS 1979–81 (N = 763)	DATOS 1991–93 (N = 855)	DATOS 1991–93 (N = 1415)
Medical	32.6	27.0	78.1	55.0	25.5	23.1	33.7
Psychological	15.8	2.8	58.5	12.9	67.5	8.8	7.3
Family	8.6	2.0	33.4	20.2	42.8	8.3	37.4
Legal	2.1	1.6	22.3	13.4	6.0	4.1	0.9
Educational	6.8	1.5	41.7	27.8	21.3	9.6	4.0
Vocational	6.5	1.6	14.3	10.5	13.9	4.6	0.3
Financial	4.4	2.2	18.1	23.3	9.4	4.2	1.2

[a]Source: Etheridge et al. (1995).
[b]TOPS data not available.

ment may be to control or limit the quantity of drugs and/or alcohol consumed (i.e., reduce drinking from 12 alcoholic drinks to 3 drinks daily), or abstain from alcohol/drug use (of which the duration varies). In other cases, the goal of treatment may be to reduce the negative consequences associated with drug/alcohol use (e.g., arrests for driving under the influence; arguments with family members; employment problems). Finally, the individual may seek treatment in order to avoid the negative consequences of not enrolling in treatment (e.g., jail vs. court-ordered enrollment in a treatment facility).

From society's perspective the goals of treatment are to reduce the negative social problems associated with substance abuse (e.g., crime associated with drug use, auto fatalities associated with drug/alcohol use) and to reduce public expenditures allocated for interdiction and treatment efforts (e.g., tax dollars spent on treatment, welfare, disability associated with drug/alcohol related work injuries).

From the treatment provider perspective one goal is to provide the most effective and least costly form of treatment options that will achieve both patient and societal expectations, although the balance between these two competing issues can raise ethical debates. From the counselor perspective the goal of treatment may be to help patients recognize and understand the concepts of denial, disease, and motivation. Given the brief overview of these varied perspectives, finding a formula for balancing the cost and effectiveness in treatment has been difficult, since there are no uniformly accepted criteria to define treatment effectiveness and cost-effective treatment.

Substance Abuse Treatment Programs: Are There Differences in Effectiveness?

There is no single modality of treatment that is most effective for all patients. Although there is general consensus on the primary function of treatment (reduction in drug and alcohol use), there is little agreement on the types, duration, and amounts of treatment services that are necessary to improve patient outcome following treatment. Table 5 presents a brief overview of the common modalities of substance abuse treatment. While the modality of treatment can be an important aspect of matching patients to treatment, not all patients have similar needs and not all programs provide a wide diversity of patient services. Table 4 shows the percentage of clients who received services in the TOPS and DATOS studies by modality of treatment. As can be seen, there is great variation in the types of services provided by treatment modality.

One recently developed method designed to standardize the process of selecting the most appropriate modality of treatment is the American Society of Addiction Medicine's "level of care" criteria, which bases its placement decision on the patients' physical symptoms and general psychosocial functioning. While these criteria serve as a general guide, and potentially a good foundation for treatment matching, there is a lack of empirical evidence supporting the use of these procedures as a standard in the field of addictions (McKay, McLellan, & Alterman, 1993).

McLellan et al. (1994) explored the factors that predicted 6-month outcomes of substance use and social functioning among 22 different treatment programs representing public and private agencies, inpatient and outpatient settings, and serving different types of patients (cocaine, alcohol, and heroin). They found that across all programs similar factors predicted positive outcomes. Overall, the patients' severity of problems negatively predicted better social functioning and substance use rates.

TABLE 5. Modalities of Substance Abuse Treatment

Inpatient detoxification	Designed to stabilize the patient under medical supervision. Medications may be prescribed. Treatment can be in either a hospital or nonhospital-based setting. Length of stay varies from a few days to a few weeks. The goal of detoxification is to stabilize the patient so he or she can engage in rehabilitative services.
Outpatient detoxification	Designed to monitor the medical condition of a patient who does not present with acute withdrawal symptoms. Medications may be prescribed. Length of stay is typically less than 1 week.
Inpatient rehabilitation	Recommended for patients with acute psychosocial dysfunction (e.g, homeless, psychiatric disorders, family conflict, or other conditions that necessitate a change in environment) and for those who have failed outpatient approaches. Length of stay typically ranges from 2 to 4 weeks. Treatment often involves individual, group, and family counseling services. The goal of inpatient treatment is to stabilize substance use and associated conditions toward preparing the patient to participate in continued outpatient treatment.
Partial hospitalization	Also described as intensive outpatient counseling. Intensive counseling and rehabilitation services provided in a structured outpatient facility. Services are provided from 3 to 5 days per week, and 2 to 8 hours per day. Length of stay ranges from 2 to 8 weeks. Treatment is a combination of individual and group counseling.
Outpatient counseling	Individual and/or group counseling and psychosocial services provided in the community. Services typically range from several times weekly to once per month. Sessions may average from 1 to 2 hours per day. Many services are provided during evening hours to accommodate employed patients.
Methadone maintenance	Substitution of a legally prescribed medication to assist the patient in curtailing consumption of illicit opiate use. Additionally, psychosocial services may be provided. Medication is often prescribed on a daily basis. Length of stay ranges from 1 month to 20 or more years.
Halfway house	A transitional living program that combined individual and group substance abuse counseling and psychosocial services aimed toward independent living in the community. Many inmates with substance abuse problems are transitioned back into the community from prison settings. Length of stay ranges from 1 to 6 months.
Therapeutic community	A long-term structured inpatient treatment setting providing intensive individual and group counseling services. Patient population is usually under 35 years of age. Length of stay ranges from 3 to 12 months.

Second, the number and type of treatment services received rather than modality of treatment positively predicted better social functioning in all groups.

In a more recent study, McLellan et al. (1997) reported that matching patients to specific treatment programs (i.e., inpatient vs. partial hospitalization) was not a viable option due to practical factors such as insurance coverage and reimbursement, as well as patient refusal to accept random assignment. Therefore, they matched patient problems to specific treatment services. They found that patients who have employment, family, or psychiatric problems and receive a "dose" of counseling focused on the specific problems (at least three sessions of employment, family, or psychiatric services) had better 6-month outcomes in these problem areas that a comparison group of subjects who were not matched to specific services. The authors concluded that outcome is a function of receiving appropriate treatment services that specifically address problems identified by the patient.

Another important issue is the cost-effectiveness of different modalities of treatment. Several studies have examined cost differences among inpatient and outpatient treatment programs (Alterman et al., 1994; Hayashida, Alterman, O'Brien, & McLellan,

1989; McKay, Alterman, McLellan, Snider, & O'Brien, 1995). In general, intensive outpatient-based programs are less costly (approximately 50% less) and as effective as inpatient programs, when outcome is assessed 6 months following treatment entry. However, there are some patients who benefit more from inpatient treatment than outpatient treatment. Unfortunately, matching patients to treatment modalities is often hindered by external factors such as insurance, patient motivation, and patient characteristics (employed, homeless, etc.). Ultimately, the treatment decisions must reflect the individual patient needs and the ability of an agency to meet these needs through appropriate service provision.

The Growth and Impact of Managed Care

In 1985, fewer than 10% of patients enrolled in substance abuse treatment programs were insured through managed care organizations (MCOs). In 1994, 57% of all workers in the United States were enrolled in MCOs, as were 25% of Medicaid recipients. It is anticipated that these rates of participation in MCOs will grow, particularly in public sector populations. According to the Drug Abuse Treatment System Survey (D'Aunno, 1995), approximately 50% of the nonmethadone and 30% of methadone treatment units had some type of managed care arrangements with either public or private manage care entities (i.e., Medicaid, government, and private insurance companies).

Although very few empirical studies are available to compare the efficacy of MCO practices with fee-for-service (FFS) practices, the current shift from FFS reimbursement to capitated reimbursement may have resulted in a decreased utilization of inpatient modalities of treatment. In a recent evaluation of two systems (private MCOs and FFS, financing coordinated by local government) designed to allocate state Medicaid funds for substance abuse treatment in Medicaid recipients, the Human Organization Science Institute (1995) found widespread systematic differences in the patient referral process and the modalities of treatment utilized. Patients enrolled in MCOs were predominately treated in outpatient settings, while patients enrolled in FFS systems were more likely to be treated in inpatient treatment settings. Unfortunately, the weak methodology of the study and insufficient availability of outcome data did not allow for empirically driven conclusions. The point to be taken is that major differences exist, and determining which system works more effectively has been difficult to evaluate.

As reported in the 1995 Drug Abuse Treatment System Survey (D'Aunno, 1995), a randomly stratified survey of outpatient methadone and nonmethadone treatment programs conducted in 1988, 1990, and 1995, fewer employment, mental health counseling, and routine medical services were offered in 1995 than in 1990 and 1988, among outpatient nonmethadone treatment programs. These data may suggest that the increased growth of patients covered through MCOs may be a factor in the reduced amount and type of services provided to patients, since MCOs often reimburse treatment providers on a per capita basis, rather than reimbursement for specific services provided.

Who Monitors Treatment Quality?

Substance abuse treatment programs must be monitored by an outside entity to ensure that they provide quality treatment services. Patients, for the most part, are uniformed consumers and often rely on the treatment staff to:

1. Educate the patient to understand the illness of chemical dependency.
2. Assess the specific biopsychosocial problem of the patient.
3. Develop a treatment plan to address the problems of the patient.
4. Provide treatment services for the identified problems.
5. Monitor the progress of the patient through the treatment process.
6. Recommend the most appropriate course of treatment following discharge from the treatment program.

Needless to say, it is often difficult for the patient to assess the quality of care provided by the treatment program, since the treatment expectations and motivations of patients vary and are often influenced by the treatment program. Therefore, a monitoring system that is sensitive to the most fundamental elements of treatment is required to ensure consumer protection against programs with poor integrity. The federal government has mandated that each state department of health is responsible to oversee the quality of care provided by treatment programs that receive federal assistance to defray treatment costs. For example, the Pennsylvania Department of Health's, Office of Drug and Alcohol Programs (ODAP) is responsible for licensing and monitoring all providers of drug and alcohol treatment services in the Commonwealth of Pennsylvania on all annual basis.

During 1993, the licensing division of the Pennsylvania Office of Drug and Alcohol Programs monitored 779 substance abuse treatment facilities, of which nearly 50% were found to be out of compliance (Pennsylvania Department of Health, 1994). Many agencies were cited for their lack of performance in important and fundamental areas of treatment. For example, 44% were cited for conducting inadequate psychosocial evaluations; 33% did not provide adequate treatment plans and updates; 33% violated procedures of confidentiality; 32% lacked sufficient short- and long-term goal planning; 25% had insufficient case notes; 23% lacked aftercare plans and discharge summaries; and 15% did not provide adequate training to staff members. These rates of noncompliance are quite high, considering that programs were notified weeks in advance of the site reviews. Treatment programs that are cited for a specific violation are provided with a written report identifying the violation and given a timetable to rectify the situation. Programs that are in violation of specific infractions are usually reinspected within 6 months. Repeated infractions may result in revoking the treatment programs license.

These data substantiate the important role that government plays in ensuring quality. Without these and other monitoring visits coordinated at the local level (county departments of health) and outside licensing agencies (Joint Commission on the Accreditation of Hospital Organizations) it is suggested that the quality of care provided by treatment programs would be greatly diminished.

The Utility of Practice Guidelines

Walker, Howard, Walker, Lambert, and Suchinksy (1995) reviewed the current state of practice guidelines in the field of chemical dependency. In general, they found a number of guidelines, manuals, and treatment protocols that were available to the clinician, but these materials were limited in scope and could not be generalized across patient types or modalities of treatment. Moreover, these locally developed guidelines were based on clinical impressions and did not provide or incorporate data from the available scientific literature. Further, and more importantly, they lacked consensus of experts or peer review.

Practice guidelines are generalizations regarding the extent and nature of treatment for a given disorder rather than protocols by which to prescribe a specific treatment plan for an individual. Determining treatment protocols requires an in-depth evaluation of the individual and his or her specific conditions. Clearly, as our abilities to develop new treatment strategies grow and our abilities to evaluate these procedures grow, practice guidelines will also improve. This is an iterative process that only recently has begun in the field of substance abuse treatment.

The practice guidelines developed by the American Psychiatric Association (1995) provide a general framework for guiding chemical dependency treatment for three types of substance use disorders: alcohol, cocaine, and opioids. These guidelines developed by expert consensus and based on empirical evidence are targeted to the psychiatrist's role in providing and managing treatment. To date, the American Psychiatric Association practice guidelines are the most comprehensive available in the field of substance abuse treatment.

The American Psychiatric Association's practice guidelines are a much needed addition to advancing the quality and consistency of treatment for a specific discipline (psychiatry). At the same time, on the programmatic level the Center for Substance Abuse Treatment (CAST), a branch of the Substance Abuse and Mental Health Services Administration (SAMHSA), has published a series of state-of-the-art protocols and guidelines for the treatment of alcohol and drug abuse disorders. These treatment improvement protocols (TIPS) are developed through a multistage, consensus-building process formulated by a panel of experts composed of clinicians, program administrators, and researchers (Table 6).

Additionally, CSAT publishes a number of reports in their technical assistance publications series, which address important practice, administrative, and treatment issues. Examples of these documents include: (1) *Confidentiality of Patient Records for Alcohol and Other Drug Treatment*; (2) *Approval and Monitoring of Narcotic Treatment Programs: A Guide on the Roles of Federal and State Agencies*; and (3) *Treatment for Alcohol and Other Drug Abuse: Opportunities for Coordination*. These documents represent an important step in developing practice guidelines.

TABLE 6. Treatment Improvement Protocols[a]

State methadone treatment guidelines
Pregnant, substance-using women
Guidelines for the treatment of alcohol and other drug abusing adolescents
Assessment and treatment of patients with coexisting mental illness and alcohol and other drug abuse
Screening and assessment of alcohol and other drug-abusing adolescents
Improving treatment for drug-exposed infants
Screening for infectious diseases among substance abusers
Screening and assessment for alcohol and other drug abuse among adults in the criminal justice system
Intensive outpatient treatment for alcohol and other drug abuse
Assessment and treatment of cocaine-abusing, methadone-maintained patients
Simple screening instruments for outreach for alcohol and other drug abuse and infectious diseases
Combining substance abuse treatment with intermediate sanctions for adults in the criminal justice system.

[a]Available from the Center for Substance Abuse Treatment, Rockville, MD, USDHHS.

RECOMMENDATIONS TO ENHANCE THE QUALITY OF SUBSTANCE ABUSE TREATMENT IN THE UNITED STATES

We describe measures that when properly implemented should enhance the quality of substance abuse treatment. Most of the measures listed below are targeted at the programmatic level. Although some require an investment of staff and money, we strongly believe that these suggestions are cost-effective and will improve the quality of treatment. We have divided these measures into either low-cost activities that require little if any additional funding to implement, or investment strategies that typically require some start-up costs (salary, new services, etc.). We also have described some needed enhancement strategies at the macro level.

Low-Cost Enhancement Strategies for Treatment Programs

Become Consumer Oriented

Substance abuse treatment programs should, without hesitation, answer a simple question: "Is this agency an attractive and supportive option for patients who need treatment for a chronic illness?" In answering this question, the agency should consider some points:

1. How easy is it to access treatment services?
2. Are there rapid admission procedures for treatment entry and reentry?
3. Does the agency offer a range of treatment services that patients want and need?
4. Is the clinic open during convenient hours for working patients?
5. Are child services available?
6. Is there an opportunity or forum available for patients to address program issues?
7. Is there a consumer advocacy board to monitor agency services?

Exploring these issues is rather simple and represents a method of assuring quality. To this extent, conducting periodic patient satisfaction surveys regarding the agencies function as a service provider is worthwhile. The following is a simple illustration of how an agency can become consumer oriented. A substance abuse, outpatient treatment program determined that nearly 50% of the patients who had made a telephone appointment for admission to the treatment program failed to show up for their initial appointment. The agency then instituted a telephone callback procedure to remind patients of the appointment they had scheduled. This procedure resulted in a significantly higher show rate for program admissions and allowed the program to utilize its staff more efficiently (Gariti, Alterman, Holub-Beyer, Prentice, & O'Brien, 1995).

Retention of Patients in Treatment

Simpson, Joe, Rowan-Szal, and Greener (1995) found that patients who engaged in the treatment process during the first month following admission (measured by number of counseling sessions attended) were more likely to remain in treatment longer and have better treatment outcomes following the course of treatment. These data suggest that increasing the intensity of treatment during the initial weeks following admission to the program may positively affect treatment retention and outcome. A cost-effective option may be to offer an orientation group facilitated by a counselor that focuses on retention in treatment. Similarly, other research has found that long-term retention in treatment has often been associated with positive outcomes for patients enrolled in both drug-free and methadone treatment modalities (De Leon, 1991; Ball & Ross, 1991).

Make Use of Self-help Groups

A number of studies have demonstrated that participation in self-help groups in addition to regular treatment services results in better outcomes. McKay, Alterman, McLellan, and Snider (1994) reported that patients who completed day hospital substance abuse rehabilitation and then continued to participate in self-help groups were more likely to have lower rates of alcohol and cocaine use after discharge. Self-help programs can be instituted in a program for little cost (space, time) and little staff involvement (coordinating the activity).

Offer Relapse Prevention Services

Relapse prevention services have demonstrated effectiveness in reducing relapse following substance abuse treatment (Hall, Wasserman, & Havassy, 1991). The costs to provide relapse prevention services are low and may be offset if programs integrate relapse prevention techniques into existing substance abuse counseling sessions. Rounsaville (1986) recommended several important functions for agencies adopting relapse prevention services: (1) programs should develop rapid reentry policies for individuals who relapse following treatment; (2) staff should be appropriately trained in relapse prevention techniques; and (3) the program should contact discharged patients on a regular basis following discharge to assess vulnerability to relapse.

Match Patient Needs to Treatment Services

Rather than randomly assigning patients to program staff, treatment programs could match the needs of patients to staff who have expertise in providing specific treatment services. For example, a staff member who has extensive training in dealing with family systems may be the most appropriate counselor to provide services to patients with substance abuse and family-related problems. The advantage of training each staff member to assume the coordination of a different type of adjunctive service (family counseling, employment, housing, criminal justice referrals, etc.) is that the staff member becomes a local expert in that particular area. Local expertise involves not only understanding what community resources are available to assist a client but also knowing how to access those resources through referral development.

Dennis, Karuntzos, McDougal, French, and Hubbard (1993) reported five strategies that could be used by existing staff when professionally trained employment specialists are not available: (1) develop a community resource directory that identifies local community programs that provide job placement services, GED programs, vocational training and so on; (2) include in the admission assessments and subsequent treatment plans information on patient vocational needs, barriers to employment, employment strengths, and patient motivation to gain employment; (3) train other staff to recognize and address vocational issues to refer patients to outside social service agencies, and to better understand what are realistic versus unrealistic patient expectations; and (4) establish the framework of a job-seekers club, or develop a unit of group counseling that is facilitated by staff that focuses on employment activities.

Make Use of Available Expert Resources

There are a number of excellent resources and available publications that contain information on improving the effectiveness of substance abuse treatment. Generally, materials produced by these organizations are free or can be reproduced for a minimal charge. Examples of these resources include the National Institute on Drug Abuse, the National Institute on Alcoholism and Alcohol Abuse, the National Clearinghouse for Alcohol and Drug Information, the National Institute of Justice, and the Center for Substance Abuse Treatment. In addition to free materials, these agencies offer training seminars and workshops conducted by experts throughout the country. Further, collaboration with local universities can offer agencies an opportunity to receive expert opinion or training at low or often no cost.

Adopt a Set of Practice Guidelines

Treatment programs should adopt a set of practice guidelines such as those published by the American Psychiatric Association or those available through CSAT. Guidelines developed by CSAT are available by calling the National Clearinghouse for Alcohol and Drug Information (NCADI) at 1-800-729-6686. Programs should be cautioned, however, that practice guidelines represent a general overview of a set of standard and effective treatment practices; they should not be used to determine the specific care for an individual.

Develop and Encourage Membership in Professional Organizations

Membership in professional organizations that specialize in chemical dependency provide excellent professional growth opportunities for treatment agencies, treatment providers, and staff. These organizations serve a number of important functions: advocate for the substance abuse professionals on a legislative level (national, state, and local); generate important position papers on special topics (i.e., treatment guidelines and practice parameters); provide testimony to governmental bodies; offer certification for completion of sponsored educational courses; provide fellowship with other professionals; provide a forum to share important clinical findings; sponsor national, regional, and local conferences; and, in some cases, offer and finance fellowships for clinician staff.

INVESTMENT STRATEGIES

Many of the strategies listed below have start-up costs associated with their implementation. However, as stated above, if implemented properly the benefits may offset the costs through improvement in clinic effectiveness and patient outcome.

Conduct Follow-Up Assessments on All Patients who Enter Treatment

Posttreatment follow-up serves two important functions:

1. Follow-up data can be used as an internal quality assurance measure of program effectiveness. Not only can treatment programs monitor their effectiveness (e.g., the percent of subjects who have remained abstinent over a 3-month period), but also the clinical staff can use the information to critique

their own counseling skills by monitoring patient outcome (e.g., did patient *X* follow through with attending Alcoholics Anonymous?).

2. Follow-up is also an effective strategy to reenroll patients into treatment who report that they are at risk for relapsing or who have relapsed. Similarly, patients who present with other non-chemical dependency problems can be referred to appropriate treatment services (e.g., psychiatric counseling).

Zanis, McLellan, Alterman, and Cnaan (1996) randomized 41 discharged patients who reported drug use in the past month to receive either a passive referral or an enhanced referral at the patient's 1-year discharge anniversary. In the enhanced referral condition patients received 30 minutes of brief counseling focused on reenrolling the patient in drug treatment. The comparison condition involved only a referral to treatment. Overall, 63% of the enhanced condition patients reentered treatment and 7% of the passive referral patients reenrolled in treatment. Beyond the individual patient outcomes from this study, the treatment program was able to reduce marketing expenditures by accepting these patients into treatment, and thus allowing the agency to operate at full capacity and optimal cost-effectiveness. Furthermore, Kosten, Rounsaville, and Kleber (1986) reported that patients who reentered treatment within 1 year following discharge from treatment had high rates of retention. These data suggest that discharged patients who relapse and are counseled to reenter treatment may have higher rates of motivation to participate and remain in treatment.

Conducting Follow-Up

In order to effectively implement a follow-up protocol, an agency must systematically prepare for the task. Desmond, Maddux, Johnson, and Confer (1995) described procedures that allowed them to obtain a 98% follow-up rate with subjects:

1. Collect complete locator information at the start of treatment, including name(s), addresses, and telephone numbers, as well as the name address and telephone number of family members and others in the patient's social network.
2. Inform patients that a staff member from the treatment program will contact the patient at a specific point after discharge from treatment (i.e., every patient who enrolls in treatment will be recontacted 3 months following discharge). The program should obtain patient written consent to participate in the follow-up interview upon admission to the treatment program. Finally, the program should provide patients with both a verbal and a written overview of the agencies policy on patient confidentiality.
3. Provide adequate incentive to the patients for completing the follow-up assessment. Examples of incentives include nominal cash payment ($10), food voucher, travel reimbursement, opportunity to return to treatment, referral to social services, and so on.
4. Select qualified staff to locate patients and conduct the follow-up assessment.
5. Document all follow-up activities. Each patient should have a follow-up record that notes each effort to locate the patient. It should include the date and time of the follow-up activity, the specific activity (telephone call, mailing, visit), and a brief explanation of the result.
6. Use available public resources to help locate patients. For example, if a patient

was on parole while enrolled in treatment, it may be advisable to contact that person's parole officer or the local, state, and federal correctional facilities to help track the patient.

7. Develop a follow-up assessment that is concise. Ask only questions that you plan to use to assess a specific function of treatment or to learn about the effects of treatment. For example: "Since discharge 1 month ago, how many days have you attended an AA meeting?"
8. Be realistic and justify follow-up resources and procedures. Establish a budget and rules to allocate follow-up resources.

Design and Conduct Outcome Evaluations

Designing an outcome evaluation study can provide many benefits to a treatment program. However, implementing a design that provides useful information to the program requires adherence to a few basic principles. McLellan and Durell (1995) proposed six general steps necessary for outcome evaluation: (1) use an "intent to treat" design, sampling patients at admission and including "dropouts" in the analyses (please note the procedures suggested in conducting follow-up interviews); (2) measure change from admission to follow-up as well as outcome status at follow-up; (3) monitor the integrity of the delivery of the intervention; (4) evaluate multiple outcomes including substance use as well as psychosocial functioning; (5) use a core of standardized measures to increase comparability with other outcome evaluations; and (6) concentrate on collecting follow-up data on at least 70% of the patients who begin the study.

Conduct both short- and long-term outcomes. There have been several studies that have demonstrated delayed effects in outcome. For example, Woody, McLellan, Luborsky, and O'Brien (1995) found similar outcomes between patients randomized to drug counseling (delivered by counselors) and patients randomized to supportive expressive therapy (delivered by licensed psychologists) when these patients were assessed 1 month following treatment. At the 6-month follow-up point, however, significant improvement was observed among patients in the supportive expressive group but not in the drug counseling group. Depending on resources, an agency may want to sample a subset of patients, such as every third or fourth admission to the treatment program. Regarding follow-up points, the evaluation period should be reasonable, based on the type of intervention. Conducting an intervention 5 years following discharge may yield less important data than conducting the intervention 3 months following discharge.

Develop Pharmacotherapy Services

Pharmacotherapy is most effective when it is combined with psychosocial treatments. The most commonly recognized example of pharmacotherapy has been the provision of methadone with counseling. Methadone, a narcotic substitute, eliminates the physiological withdrawal symptoms caused by heroin use through the daily administration of a legally prescribed and rigidly administered drug. Recently, the Food and Drug Administration has approved two new medications for use in the treatment of substance users: Levomethadyl acetate (LAAM) for opiate dependence and naltrexone for alcohol dependence.

Although some programs maintain a "drug-free" policy toward treating patients with substance abuse disorders, these policies do not take advantage of the combined effects of pharmacological interventions and psychosocial treatments. Often programs do not have the available professional staff necessary to prescribe medications for patients with concurrent psychiatric disorders (i.e., major depression), and therefore rely on referral to community mental health centers for the treatment of psychiatric disorders. While such referrals may be effective, they generate multiple treatment protocols for a patient that may hinder treatment progress if poorly coordinated between treatment settings. Programs with drug-free policies are urged to investigate the empirical data and develop treatment protocols that include proven pharmacotherapy interventions as an on-site service.

Pharmacotherapy should only be considered if appropriate procedures are followed: (1) Consult a qualified psychiatrist or physician, one who preferably has extensive experience in the field of addictions; (2) fully inform the patient of the purpose for the medication, as well as potential side effects, and provide unambiguous communication regarding the effectiveness of the medication; (3) consult empirical studies on the limitations of medications; (4) monitor patients closely; and (5) when possible, include family members in treatment, especially when adjunct medications are part of that treatment. It is important to educate family members regarding the prescription of medications for patients who have substance abuse problems, since an educated family member can help ensure patient compliance. As with other chronic disorders such as asthma, hypertension, and diabetes, medication effectiveness is often directly correlated with compliance of the medication protocol and continued psychosocial support.

Hire Adequate and Appropriate Staff

Gustafson (1991) reported that substance abuse treatment programs in New York State had serious retention problems, particularly with drug counselors. Moreover, these programs were unable to recruit qualified staff to fill vacancies. Four reasons were cited in relation to these recruitment difficulties: (1) inadequate salary and fringe benefits; (2) lack of a desire to work with substance abuse and HIV patients; (3) lack of qualified applicants; and (4) little desire to work in less desirable neighborhoods where treatment programs were often located.

In an informal poll conducted with substance abuse treatment counselors and treatment staff directors, Zanis asked the question, "How would you improve substance abuse treatment?" The respondents overwhelming answered "more money." We then asked a follow-up question, "If you had unlimited financial resources, what would you do with this money to improve substance abuse treatment?" The most frequent responses were: increase salary levels of staff (as a method to attract higher skilled staff); hire more staff (to decrease the counselor to patient caseload); and provide more treatment services (to meet the needs of patients).

It was the general consensus of the respondents that salary levels are too low. This, combined with a job role that offers little professional recognition, make it difficult for programs to attract competent staff to fill job vacancies. This was well illustrated by Woody, McLellan, Luborsky, and O'Brien (1990) who reported that a treatment program advertising in a Philadelphia newspaper for a drug/alcohol counselor offered a $12,000 yearly salary for a full-time position, with no experience necessary. Although the ad is somewhat dated, a quick scan of current classified ads in the Philadelphia area found that while salary levels have increased somewhat ($16,000) and education/experience levels upgraded (high school diploma or GED), some drug/alcohol treatment programs hire, for the most part, inexperienced counseling staff. Furthermore, staff are increasingly asked to take on larger caseloads while providing the same level of treatment services. It is no doubt that counselors have a high rate of turnover, and burnout is considered a hazard of the profession. Potentially, reduced caseloads that allow staff to spend additional time with patients and focus on resolving issues may yield improved satisfaction through giving staff a greater sense of accomplishment.

Match Patient Needs to Treatment Services

Do additional treatment services work? McLellan, Arndt, Metzger, Woody, and O'Brien (1993) found that the provision of enhanced treatment services yielded improved outcomes among patients enrolled in methadone treatment. This study examined three levels of treatment services: minimal (medication and one counseling contact per month); standard (medication and four counseling sessions per month); and enhanced (medication, four counseling sessions per month, and availability of employment, family, and psychiatric services). Overall, patients in the enhanced condition had the best outcomes and patients in the minimal condition had the poorest outcomes.

McLellan et al. (1997) also found that patients who received services that were appropriate to their particular problems were more likely to remain in treatment longer and to have improved functioning following treatment discharge. Finally, McLellan et al. (1994) found that outcome was predicted by similar factors, regardless of the primary substance of dependence, treatment modality, treatment philosophy, or funding type. Increased substance use following treatment was predicted by greater baseline severity of alcohol and drug use. Better social adjustment at follow-up was positively predicted by more psychiatric, family, employment, and medical services provided during treatment. Interestingly, this study found little relationship between the provision of drug and alcohol counseling services provided during treatment with substance use or social functioning improvement 6 months following treatment. Given these findings, it would appear that providing ancillary treatment services and matching them to patients' needs are important ingredients in improving the quality and effectiveness of substance abuse treatment programs.

Enhancement Strategies at the Government Level

While the burden of implementing high-quality treatment services is the responsibility of an individual treatment program, the onus for developing a framework to improve the overall quality of treatment across all treatment programs currently rests with the federal government. It is the government that funds the majority of research activity, monitors treatment agencies, and develops minimal standards for operating treatment programs. Therefore, improving the quality of treatment is largely based on government action.

Enhance Licensing and Certification Procedures

Licensing is a process in which an individual attains a defined level of education and training and successfully passes a state-certified examination composed of peers within a given profession (nursing, physician, psychologist, social worker, etc.). In general, licensing serves a necessary function for maintaining and enhancing quality within a given profession.

Within the field of addictions, there are a number of different types of certifications that are offered. On the counselor level there are both state and national certifications. These certifications represent a minimal test of a counselors' knowledge about substance abuse treatment, although no empirical data have demonstrated a difference in the effectiveness of counselors as a function of certification. However, the certification process does serve several important functions in the field of addictions: (1) it demonstrates commitment by the counselor to work in the field of chemical dependency; (2) it represents a minimal level of skill; (3) it requires the need for ongoing training for recertification; and (4) it is one milestone in the career ladder of the counselor that increases professionalism, and in so doing, potentially reduces burnout and turnover among this highly vulnerable group.

Physician Level of Specialty Training. To date there are few well-structured certification programs for training physicians as specialists in chemical dependency treatment. Recently, the American Board of Psychiatry and Neurology developed an added qualifications in addiction psychiatry specialization that enables board-certified psychiatrists to become board-certified specialists in addictions. This specialized program consists of four 3-month rotations within a certified addiction psychiatry program: an inpatient addiction unit, an outpatient clinic, a partial day hospital program, and a narcotic substitution program. Residents are required to participate in clinical case conferences in which each trainee is required to present a patient case to faculty members on a rotating basis. At the end of the 12-month course, trainees are evaluated by the standing faculty to determine qualification for the board certificate.

As the trend toward health care coverage extends itself to greater use of managed care practices, the gatekeeper for health care is often the primary care physician. Given this, it is necessary for physicians to demonstrate basic competency in the identification of substance abuse disorders, referral procedures for substance abuse treatment, and the ability to deliver brief counseling techniques. Moreover, it is important that all primary care physicians receive more training in substance abuse during their residencies.

Develop Addiction Counselor Residencies

Based on the concept of the American Board of Psychiatry and Neurology, it would seem worthwhile if there were a certification process for counselors that offered a certification based on completing a comprehensive training program. To this extent, we propose the formation of an addiction counselors residency training program. Hypothetically, this residency would offer an advanced counseling certificate. Students would be trained in the core counseling functions such as: (1) screening patients for appropriateness to treatment; (2) multidimensional assessment of patient problems; (3) development of treatment plans; (4) understanding of multiple counseling techniques; (5) understanding of case management techniques; (6) knowledge of drug/alcohol use behaviors; (7) crisis intervention; (8) recording keeping; (9) treatment team counseling; (10) community resources; (11) knowledge of self-help organizations; and (12) interpersonal skills. Exposure to varying concepts and techniques through case studies sessions would provide excellent learning experiences. Such a counselor residency program could serve a critical role by increasing the level of counselor skill and legitimizing a core set of professional competencies through a recognizable certification process.

Increase Monitoring Efforts

Who monitors treatment effectiveness? If you were in need of substance abuse treatment, where would you go? Unfortunately, there are no consumer reports available that rank the effectiveness of treatment programs. Moreover, consumers have little choice in selecting a treatment agency, since insurers often establish the referral networks for substance abuse treatment. Further, there is little public information as to how these referral networks are determined and the extent to which programs in them are selected as a function of their quality versus costs.

A rating system could be established using data on some simple criteria: percent of staff with professional licenses or graduate degrees; average years of experience of staff; average patient-to-staff caseloads; average physician/psychiatrist-to-patient ratios; percent of patients who complete treatment, number and extent of monitoring violations, patient satisfaction, and so on. These ratings could then be made publicly available. While difficult to administer and implement, nominal rating systems that are published annually may be an effective mechanism to motivate and assist programs in developing better quality services. More importantly, they could serve as markers for consumers and insurers to choose programs that fit their needs and provide the necessary treatment to adequately address problems. A rating network could provide treatment programs with an incentive to enhance quality of care, it would provide programs the opportunity to develop pride in their performance, and more importantly it would give staff members a sense of accomplishment.

Greater Coordination across Disciplines Such as Primary Medical Care, Social Services, and Other Publicly Funded Agencies

Not all substance abuse treatment programs provide the same level of services, nor do they provide the same level of effective services to meet the needs of patients. For example, patients who present for treatment with both an affective disorder and a substance abuse disorder should receive treatment in a program that is adequately staffed to provide treatment for both disorders. Unfortunately, many treatment programs will falsely and/or naively claim the ability to provide adjunctive treatment services such as employment counseling, family counseling, or psychiatric counseling. In view of this, it would seem appropriate for monitoring bodies to begin to develop criteria to evaluate a program's capacity to effectively provide adjunctive services. For example, employment services should be provided by a vocational specialist who is degreed in the discipline, licensed in the discipline, or has experience in the field of addictions and vocational rehabilitation. Staff should attend ongoing educational trainings within this discipline. When services are not available in a clinic, programs must develop coordinated referrals with specialized programs.

There are many more people who need treatment than there are available treatment slots. Unfortunately, not all people who need treatment are interested in receiving it. Moreover, many people are unsure of how to access treatment and are "turned off" by treatment when it is difficult to access. To this extent, treatment referrals should be a two-way window. Not only should substance abuse treatment programs develop referral networks to refer patients to other professional treatment services, but substance abuse programs should become aggressive in developing treatment access opportunities with existing human service agencies. Expansion of substance abuse treatment services through referral networks and services located in homeless shelters, welfare programs, Women, Infants and Children (WIC) clinics, HIV clinics and testing sites, and so on, could reach many patients with a substance abuse illness who have not entered the traditional drug and alcohol service delivery system.

Development of a National Data Collection System

Enhancing the quality of treatment for substance abuse requires an empirical basis on which to make decisions. While many local governments and some states have developed systemwide data collection approaches, these systems vary tremendously and often yield insufficient information from which to generate policy. Furthermore, even among the state and local systems that collect similar data, different data collection methods are often used that do not allow for cross-system comparisons. A national data collection system, using a standard methodology across treatment agencies, could produce a representative data bank that could be used as a basis for decisions at the federal, state, local, and even clinic levels. Our current level of computer technology would allow for immediate electronic transfer, collating, and archiving of these data, so that researchers and policymakers can regularly monitor changes and trends in the characteristics of patients entering treatment.

Provide Substance Abuse Treatment Services to Those Incarcerated

Correctional facilities contain a substantial portion of nonviolent offenders incarcerated for problems related to substance dependence. A portion of these "treatable" offenders present no danger to society but cost society up to $30,000 per year for housing. Recently, Inciardi, Lockwood, and Hooper (1994) reported that providing comprehensive rehabilitative services (drug treatment, case management, and employment services) to incarcerated individuals reduced recidivism (return to prison) by 41% and relapse to drug use by 57% compared to standard incarceration services alone. Based on these studies, it would appear that intensive supervision following discharge from prison, in addition to comprehensive treatment services provided during prison, may be a viable course of direction for correction facilities. Unfortunately, not all correctional institutions offer substance abuse treatment services, and there are few data on the quality or effectiveness of those institutions that provide substance abuse treatment services. Treatment programs must work with correctional facilities and parole and probation departments to provide substance abuse services both during and after release from incarceration.

CONCLUSION

Many of the recommendations offered in this chapter require additional financial resources to effectively implement. Therefore, a 1% shift in the allocation of federal dollars from interdiction efforts to drug treatment efforts (approximately $130 million) could potentially prove to be a better utilization of available resources. It is estimated that this level of enhanced funding could create 60,000 new treatment slots for intensive outpatient counseling programs per year or provide substance abuse treatment services to 100,000 inmates per year.

Professionals involved in the field of substance abuse treatment have made great inroads in demonstrating the efficacy of services they provide. At the same time, however, as public funding diminishes and private insurers trim costs, demonstrating better and more effective outcomes require treatment programs to become even more accountable for their services. This requires the active and assertive involvement of treatment programs to demonstrate efficacy in treating a chronic illness and for researchers to further demonstrate the cost-effectiveness of treatment. Although additional funding is not a panacea, it certainly permits expansion of treatment services and can alleviate a number of barriers that restrict the growth of professionalism in the field. If there is to be a shift in the allocation of federal dollars from interdiction to treatment, both the research community and treatment providers must work together to develop an effective strategy that justifies to society and policymakers the benefit of reallocation.

REFERENCES

Alterman, A. I., O'Brien, C. P., McLellan, A. T., August, D. S., Snider, E. C., Droba, M., Cornish, J. W., Hall, C. P. A. H., & Schrade, F. X. (1994). Effectiveness and costs of inpatient versus day hospital cocaine rehabilitation. *The Journal of Nervous and Mental Disorders, 182*, 157–163.

American Psychiatric Association. (1995). *Practice guidelines for treatment of patients with substance use disorders: Alcohol, cocaine, opioids*. Washington, DC: Author.

Ball, J. C., & Ross, A. (1991). *The effectiveness of methadone maintenance treatment*. New York: Springer-Verlag.

CALDATA. (1994). *Evaluating recovery services: The California drug and alcohol treatment assessment*. Sacramento: California Department of Alcohol and Drug Programs Resource Center.

D'Aunno, T. A. (1995). *Treating drug abuse in America: Results from a study of the outpatient substance abuse treatment system 1988–1995*. Ann Arbor: University of Michigan.

De Leon, G. (1991). Retention in drug free therapeutic communities. In R. W. Pickens, C. G. Leukefeld, & C. R. Schuster (Eds.), *Improving drug treatment* (pp. 218–244) (NIDA Monograph #106). Rockville, MD: USDHHS, PHS.

Dennis, M. L., Karuntzos, G. T., McDougal, G. L., French, M. T., & Hubbard, R. L. (1993). Developing training and employment programs to meet the needs of methadone treatment clients. *Evaluation and Program Planning, 16*, 73–86.

Desmond, D. P., Maddox, J. F., Johnson, T. H., & Confer, B. A. (1995). Obtaining follow-up interviews for treatment evaluation. *Journal of Substance Abuse Treatment, 12*, 95–102.

Duggar, B. C. (1991). Community-based drug treatment reimbursement: Progress and barriers. In W. S. Cartwright & J. M. Kaple (Eds.), *Economic costs, cost-effectiveness, financing, and community based drug treatment* (pp. 148–164) (NIDA. Research Monograph Series #113). Rockville, MD: USDHHS.

Etheridge, R. M., Carddock, G. S., Dunteman, G. H., & Hubbard, R. L. (1995). Treatment services in two national studies of community-based drug abuse treatment programs. *Journal of Substance Abuse, 7*, 9–26.

Gariti, P., Alterman, A. I., Holub-Beyer, A., Prentice, N., & O'Brien, C. P. (1995). Effects of an appointment reminder call on patient show rates. *Journal of Substance Abuse Treatment, 12*, 37–45.

Gustafson, J. S. (1991). Do more ... and do it better: Staff-related issues in the drug treatment field that affect the quality and effectiveness of services. In R. W. Pickens, C. G. Leukefeld, & C. R. Schuster (Eds.), *Improving drug treatment* (pp. 52–62) (NIDA Monograph #106). Rockville, MD: USDHHS, PHS.

Hall, S. M., Wasserman, D. A., & Havassy, B. E. (1991). Relapse prevention. In R. W. Pickens, C. G. Leukefeld, & C. R. Schuster (Eds.), *Improving drug treatment* (pp. 279–292) (NIDA Monograph #106). Rockville, MD: USDHHS, PHS.

Harwood, H. J., Hubbard, R. L., Collins, J. J., & Rachal, J. V. (1988). The costs of crime and the benefits of drug abuse treatment: A cost-benefit using TOPS data. In C. G. Leukefeld & F. M. Tims (Eds.), *Compulsory treatment of drug abuse: Research and clinical practice* (pp. 209–235) (Research Monograph Series 86). Rockville, MD: NIDA, USDHHS, PHS.

Hayashida, M., Alterman, A. I., O'Brien, C., & McLellan, A. T. (1989). One-month outcome for inpatient versus outpatient medical alcohol detoxification. *New England Journal of Medicine, 320,* 358–365.

Human Organization Science Institute. (1995). *Evaluation of the implementation of Pennsylvania's Act 152.* Villanova, PA: Villanova University.

Inciardi, J. A., Lockwood, D., & Hooper, R. M. (1994). Through therapy: Delaware treatment programs present promising results. *Corrections Today, 56,* 34–42.

Kleber, H. (1983). Concomitant use of methadone with other psychoactive drugs in the treatment of opiate addicts with other DSM-III diagnoses. In J. R. Cooper, F. Altman, B. S. Brown, & D. Czechowizcz (Eds.), *Research on the treatment of narcotic addiction: State of the art* (pp. 119–148). National Institute on Drug Abuse. Rockville, MD: USDHHS, PHS.

Kosten, T. R., Rounsaville, B. J., & Kleber, H. D. (1986). A 2.5 year follow-up of treatment retention and re-entry among opioid addicts. *Journal of Substance Abuse Treatment, 3,* 181–189.

Langenbucher, J. (1994). Offsets are not add-ons: The place of addictions treatment in American health care reform. *Journal of Substance Abuse, 6,* 117–122.

McKay, J. R., McLellan, A. T., & Alterman, A. I. (1993). An evaluation of the Cleveland criteria for inpatient treatment of substance abuse. *American Journal of Psychiatry, 149,* 1212–1218.

McKay, J. R., Alterman, A. I., McLellan, A. T., & Snider, E. C. (1994). Treatment goals, continuity of care, and outcome in a day hospital substance abuse rehabilitation program. *American Journal of Psychiatry, 151,* 254–259.

McKay, J. R., Alterman, A. I., McLellan, A. T., Snider, E., & O'Brien, C. P. (1995). The effect of random versus nonrandom assignment in a comparison of inpatient and day hospital rehabilitation for male alcoholics. *Journal of Consulting and Clinical Psychology, 63,* 70–78.

McLellan, A. T., & Durell, J. (1995). *Outcome evaluation in psychiatric and substance abuse treatments: Concepts, rationale and methods.* Philadelphia: Treatment Research Institute.

McLellan, A. T., Arndt, I. O., Metzger, D. S., Woody, G. E., & O'Brien, C. P. (1993). The effects of psychosocial services in substance abuse treatment. *Journal of the American Medical Association, 269,* 1953–1959.

McLellan, A. T., Alterman, A. I., Metzger, D. S., Grissom, G. R., Woody, G. E., Luborsky, L., & O'Brien, C. P. (1994). Similarity of outcome predictors across opiate, cocaine, and alcohol treatments: Role of treatment services. *Journal of Consulting and Clinical Psychology, 62,* 1141–1158.

McLellan, A. T., Grissom, G. R., Zanis, D., Randall, M., Brill, P., & O'Brien, C. P. (1997). Patient treatment matching in addiction treatment: A prospective study in four programs. *Archives of General Psychiatry, 54,* 730–735.

National Institute on Drug Abuse (NIDA). (1992). *National household survey on drug abuse: Population estimates 1991.* Rockville, MD: USDHHS, PHS, ADAMHA.

National Opinion Research Center (NORC). (1995). *National Treatment Improvement Evaluation Study.* Chicago, IL: Author.

Needle, R. H. (1994). HIV risk behaviors of heterosexual male drug users. In R. J. Battjex, Z. Sloboda, & W. C. Grace (Eds.), *The context of HIV risk among drug users and their sexual partners* (pp. 11–23) (NIDA Research Monograph Series #143). Rockville, MD: USDHHS, PHS.

Office of National Drug Control Policy. (1995). *Pulse check: National trends in drug abuse.* Washington, DC: Government Printing Office.

Pennsylvania Department of Health. (1994). *Division of drug and alcohol program licensing: Annual report, 1993.* Harrisburg, PA: Pennsylvania Department of Health.

Rice, D. P., Kelman, S., & Miller, L. S. (1991). Economic costs of drug abuse. In W. S. Cartwright & J. M. Kaple (Eds.), *Economic costs, cost-effectiveness, financing, and community based drug treatment* (pp. 10–32) (NIDA Research Monograph Series #113). Rockville, MD: USDHHS.

Rounsaville, B. J. (1986). Clinical implications of relapse research. In F. M. Tims & C. G. Leukefeld (Eds.),

Relapse and recovery in drug abuse (pp. 172–184) (NIDA Research Monograph #72). Rockville, MD: USDHHS, PSH.

Simpson, D. D., Joe, G. W., Rown-Szal, G., & Greener, J. (1995). Client engagement and change during drug abuse treatment. *Journal of Substance Abuse, 7*, 117–134.

Spear, S. F., & Mason, M. (1991). Impact of chemical dependency on family health status. *International Journal of the Addictions, 26*, 179–187.

Substance Abuse and Mental Health Services Administration. (1991). *National Drug and Alcoholism Treatment Unit Survey: 1991 main findings report*. Rockville, MD: USDHHS.

Substance Abuse and Mental Health Services Administration (SAMHSA). (1995). *Overview of the FY94 national drug and alcoholism treatment unit survey (NDATUS): 1995 main findings report*. Rockville, MD: USDHHS.

US Department of Justice. (1995). *Prisoners in 1994*. Washington, DC: National Institutes of Justice.

US Department of Justice. (1994). *Correctional populations in the United States, 1993*. Washington, DC: National Institutes of Justice.

Walker, R. D., Howard, M. O., Walker, P. S., Lambert, M. D., & Suchinsky, R. (1995). Practice guidelines in the addictions: Recent developments. *Journal of Substance Abuse Treatment, 12*, 63–73.

Woody, G. E., McLellan, A. T., Luborsky, L., & O'Brien, C. P. (1990). Psychotherapy and counseling for methadone-maintained opiate addicts: Results of research studies. In L. S. Onken & J. D. Blaine (Eds.), *Psychotherapy and counseling in the treatment of drug abuse* (pp. 9–23) (NIDA Research Monograph #104). Rockville, MD: USDHHS.

Woody, G. E., McLellan, A. T., Luborsky, L., & O'Brien, C. P. (1995). Psychotherapy in community methadone programs: A validation study. *American Journal of Psychiatry, 152*, 1302–1308.

Zanis, D. A., McLellan, A. T., Alterman, A. I., & Cnaan, R. (1996). Efficacy of assertive outreach counseling to re-enroll out-of-treatment, high risk drug users. *American Journal of Psychiatry, 153*, 1095–1096.

12

Quality Management in Practice

Re-visioning Practice Guidelines to Improve Treatment of Anxiety and Traumatic Stress Disorders

DANIEL J. ABRAHAMSON AND KAREN W. SAAKVITNE

- A young woman cannot sleep after a near-miss accident and is troubled by anxiety and persistent fears of driving.
- A veteran cop is irritable and jumpy and experiencing physiological symptoms of anxiety.
- An adolescent boy is compelled to wash his hands repeatedly throughout the day. He is troubled by unidentifiable guilt.
- A survivor of childhood sexual and physical abuse is hypervigilant and unable to be in crowds or in closed spaces. During flashbacks she has chest pain and cannot breathe.
- A child has a specific fear of cats that makes him unable to visit friends' homes.
- A professor is paralyzed with performance anxiety and cannot deliver lectures.

Intolerable anxiety frequently brings clients to seek mental health treatment. Because anxiety is both a cause (symptom) of and a response (defense) to psychological distress, its prevalence is not surprising. Yet many practitioners and clients have experienced frustration and disappointment in treatments that have failed to resolve the anxiety or its precipitants (e.g., traumatic stress, interpersonal conflict). Some clients get stuck in the system and are defined (or come to define themselves) as their symptoms, accepting chronic symptomatology as inevitable.

The authors believe that most current practice guidelines fall short of their goals because of their narrow foundation in symptoms that are isolated from context and the person experiencing them. These guidelines further fail to address the context of treatment, that is, the therapeutic alliance and relationship. Thus guidelines offer disjointed techniques rather than therapeutic strategies.

In this chapter, we offer a critique of current practice guidelines for anxiety disorders and we propose an alternative conception of practice guidelines and describe such a model.

DANIEL J. ABRAHAMSON AND KAREN W. SAAKVITNE • Traumatic Stress Institute, South Windsor, Connecticut 06074-1369.

Handbook of Quality Management in Behavioral Health, edited by Stricker *et al.* Kluwer Academic / Plenum Publishers, New York, 2000.

ARE GUIDELINES USEFUL?

There are good reasons to develop and implement practice guidelines for the treatment of anxiety and posttraumatic stress disorders. Guidelines can benefit clinicians and clients. They steer clinicians toward appropriate treatments. They educate clients about the course of treatment (e.g., Depression Guideline Panel, 1993a). Therapeutic efficacy is improved when both clients and clinicians are informed and can define mutual goals on which to collaborate.

One goal cited for practice guidelines is to reduce arbitrary practice variation and thereby protect clients from inappropriate or ineffective treatments. Often practice variation results from lack of consensus about what constitutes appropriate treatment for a specific condition (Clinton, McCormick, & Bestemen, 1994). Yet guidelines cannot themselves create consensus, which must emerge from academic discussion, research, and theory. Guidelines, however, can be used to identify practices far outside the standard and to flag potentially unethical, ineffective, and unnecessarily costly, prolonged, or restrictive treatments.

In this chapter we argue that the nature of psychological problems and our current state of knowledge are such that guidelines are most appropriately used as a compass and not as a rigid set of directions. A compass can be used to keep one moving in the right direction. It says nothing about the specific course one should take to reach the goal, nor for that matter does it identify the goal.

As questions increase about the cost of health care, there is concern that these trips taken by clinicians and clients are misdirected and too expensive. While the need to reduce unnecessary health care costs is obvious, the implications for psychological treatment are still not clear. Because psychological treatment frequently decreases the necessity of expensive medical procedures, it may prove to be among the most cost-effective treatments currently in use. The physical effects of severe and chronic anxiety and traumatic stress are very expensive. Cost containment is better achieved by developing tools to define the appropriate parameters of ethical, competent approaches to treatment than by investing infinite resources in developing guidelines for specific diagnostic categories.

We need to monitor the purpose and application of therapy guidelines. A political or policy document is not a basis for good clinical work. Working toward cost-effectiveness must occur within the boundaries of our professional clinical training. Treatment guidelines are first and foremost clinical documents, shaped by current knowledge, research, theory, and ethics. While economic and political factors influence guidelines (Abrahamson, 1998), we must not forget that these guidelines are the tools and credibility of our profession. Just as surgeons would not ask a legislative committee to design their scalpels, we must not shirk our responsibilities to develop guidelines based on valid psychological principles.

According to Smith and Hamilton (1994), practice guidelines are being developed in order to counteract the health and economic consequences of inappropriate care. Obviously, it is critical that such guidelines do not compound the problem by forcing people into treatments that may be ineffective or harmful, and as such wasteful and inappropriate. Yet as currently constructed, guidelines can lead to such an outcome.

To summarize, the primary goals of practice guidelines are as follows:

1. To help the clinician select an appropriate treatment modality.
2. To educate clients about psychotherapy and appropriate expectations.

3. To decrease undue practice variation and eliminate unethical, ineffective, or harmful practices.
4. To decrease unnecessary health care costs and increase cost-effective treatments.
5. To decrease the ill consequences of inappropriate care.

Most clinicians, including the authors, support these goals. The obvious question is, "Are we achieving these goals in our current construction of guidelines?" To answer that question, we need to examine the construction of guidelines.

STANDARDS FOR THE DEVELOPMENT OF GUIDELINES

Until recently there has been no systematic framework for the construction of practice guidelines that assures their comprehensiveness and consistency (American Psychological Association, 1995). A first step in developing such a framework is to define the purpose of guidelines.

The Institute of Medicine (IOM) defines practice guidelines as statements systematically developed for the purpose of helping providers and their clients select appropriate health care for specific clinical conditions (Institute of Medicine, 1990). Likewise, Clinton et al. (1994), representing the Agency for Health Care Policy and Research (AHCPR), specify that the purpose of guidelines is to assist in the management of specific clinical conditions. Thus, both the IOM and AHCPR stress the "specific clinical conditions" for which a guideline is intended as inherent to the guideline's purpose. This emphasis underscores a larger problem with most guidelines.

When practice guidelines are defined by specific symptoms or diagnoses (e.g., specific clinical conditions), their generalizability is narrowed and their practical utility is therefore radically reduced. In 1995, the American Psychological Association (APA) published their "Template for Developing Guidelines" based on extensive review of the literature and current guidelines. In this template, generalizability is a key criterion for acceptable and useful guidelines. Specifically, client characteristics such as cultural background, gender, and developmental issues must be included and addressed when developing or using treatment guidelines (American Psychological Association, 1995). Usually, however, such variables are not even mentioned in practice guidelines, most of which identify symptoms as the only variable. It is misleading to assume a symptom is the defining characteristic of a client; symptoms are the focus for change, but change occurs within the context and using the resources of the whole person.

Clearly, the client is only one source of variance in the therapy relationship. When patient variables are combined with individual therapist characteristics and contextual factors, including the therapeutic relationship and its setting, what results is a matrix of almost infinite complexity. Thus, it makes little sense for any particular treatment intervention [e.g., exposure and response prevention for bulimia nervosa (MCC, 1991)] to receive exclusive emphasis, let alone define the entirety of the treatment approach. This principle is taken to its extreme when treatment guidelines define medical necessity as harmful to self or others and actually implicitly encourage clients to remain suicidal or self-harming to justify their need for continued treatment.

A broader approach is more consistent with the criteria identified by the American Psychological Association Task Force on Psychological Intervention Guidelines

(1995).* This report offers a detailed template for the construction of psychological intervention guidelines. It is asserted that such guidelines must show both internal validity, that is efficacy, and external validity, that is clinical utility. To achieve internal validity, the treatment must meet criteria for efficacy based on "both a) the absolute and relative efficacy of the treatment and b) the quality of the studies on which the judgment is made, as well as their replicibility" (p. 30). Eight criteria for efficacy in order of increasing confidence are listed. External validity is measured by confidence in clinical utility on three dimensions: feasibility, generalizability, and costs and benefits. On each of these dimensions, the report identifies specific points for assessment of clinical utility.

Thus, of the three major organizations that have identified and published specific criteria for the development of practice guidelines, two emphasize a focus on specific clinical conditions, while the third emphasizes the need for efficacy, feasibility, generalizability, and balance between costs and benefits. The next section evaluates specific guidelines.

LITERATURE REVIEW

Current Guidelines for Anxiety Disorders

Based on the criteria put forward by the AHCPR (e.g., Clinton et al., 1994), the Institute of Medicine (1992), and the American Psychological Association (1995), there are no well-developed guidelines for the treatment of anxiety and posttraumatic stress disorders. Given the etiological complexity and overdetermined nature of these conditions, the development of extensively validated guidelines is a daunting task.

Generalizability

The extensive literature on anxiety and traumatic stress disorders clearly offers data about general treatment approaches and specific effective treatments. Yet when translated (or abridged) to practice guidelines, the results are inadequate. These guidelines have been summarized by the Task Force on Promotion and Dissemination of Psychological Procedures (1995). This task force worked to establish criteria for and identify a list of empirically validated and "manualized" treatments. Their list includes specific treatments for generalized anxiety disorder, obsessive–compulsive disorder, panic disorder, posttraumatic stress disorder, social phobia, and specific phobias. While this document provides a valuable resource for clinicians who treat anxiety disorders, it in no way represents an established set of guidelines.

One widely cited criterion is the call for practice guidelines to rely on empirically validated treatment techniques. While this standard initially seems sensible, there are several serious flaws in its implementation, including the limits of empirical clinical research. Barron (1995) persuasively articulates the limitations of guidelines and treatment approaches that are based on narrowly defined samples and validated only in highly structured clinical research settings. He questions the generalizability of these findings to real life clinical settings (where exclusion criteria cannot be so

*Daniel J. Abrahamson was a member of this task force.

stringent) and raises concerns about their practicality. On a broader level, he questions the theoretical and philosophical assumptions that underlie treatments that are developed exclusively based on a logical positivist approach to data collection.

Stricker and Trierweiler (1995) also caution about the limited generalizability that results from exclusive reliance on empiricism. The American Psychological Association (1995) echoes this caveat, noting that guidelines are based on assumptions about the meaning of data and reminding us that the prevailing philosophy of science will shape how problems are defined and what data are collected. Seligman (1995) argues that survey data, such as that generated by the *Consumer Reports* study (1995), more clearly reflect actual practice than tightly controlled studies.

Generalizability, then, refers to target population and treatment efficacy. Guidelines must refer to people, including their contexts, and must be applicable to the therapist–client relationship. In addition, the guidelines must be based in theory and techniques that can be implemented in general practice.

Guidelines Generated by Managed Care Companies

Another source of specific treatment recommendations comes from the managed care industry. For this chapter, we contacted several companies known to have specific guidelines for the treatment of anxiety disorders. Only one of these companies, Metropolitan Clinic of Counseling (MCC), was willing to release their guidelines for review. Others did not respond to our request or refused, citing the "proprietary" nature of their guidelines.* The argument they use is that it would make them economically vulnerable to release their specific guidelines. Some companies contend that if clinicians were aware of the treatment guidelines, they would somehow manipulate the system to their advantage. While it is beyond the scope of this chapter to evaluate the managed care industry, it is important to challenge the logic and values represented in these arguments. It seems obvious that all treatment guidelines should be public documents or they are not treatment guidelines but corporate strategies that have no bearing on effective ethical psychological treatment. Honest scientific inquiry requires that guidelines be open to full scientific scrutiny and public policy debate.

While we are extremely appreciative that MCC sent us a copy of their guidelines and references (MCC, 1991, 1992), the documents themselves raise questions about the content and scope of practice guidelines.

In the MCC guidelines on anxiety disorders, the first step is to refer many clients with certain diagnoses (social phobia, panic attacks, generalized anxiety disorder, and posttraumatic stress disorder) for psychiatric evaluation. For other individuals who do not meet the criteria for an initial medication evaluation, a limited number of specific treatment approaches are then recommended. These recommendations, however, are based on an extremely outdated review of the literature (MCC, 1992). This points to an inherent problem with narrowly defined treatment guidelines if they are not updated on a frequent basis. In effect, these guidelines preclude the use of highly effective treatment approaches omitted from the authors' literature review.

When treatment guidelines are developed in such a way that they restrict access to treatment options that have the potential to be beneficial, they compromise the

*Recently, consumer pressure and legislative initiatives have resulted in more managed care companies releasing their treatment guidelines for public scrutiny.

clinician's ethical practice and the client's right to available and effective treatment. The trend for certain managed care companies to arbitrarily rule out certain diagnostic categories or accepted and effective treatment modalities raises serious ethical and legal concerns (de Avila, 1995). Again, guidelines should direct (as a compass) but not prescribe (as a rigid set of directions).

Guidelines for Primary Care Physicians

Another set of guidelines are aimed at a group who are not trained as mental health professionals: primary care physicians. One such guideline for the treatment of anxiety disorders was developed by the Institute for Clinical Systems Integration (1995) to aid primary care physicians working with patients with generalized anxiety disorder and panic disorder. It is a useful diagnostic tool, but does not provide a clinically sophisticated treatment perspective.

In general, efforts to develop mental health treatment guidelines for primary care physicians (e.g., Depression Guideline Panel, 1993) have been found to underemphasize the difficulty of detection, assessment, and treatment (Munoz, Hollon, McGrath, Rehm, & Vanden Bos, 1994). Ideally, such cross-discipline information is invaluable in both directions as we strive to understand the complexities of mind–body influences. Collaborative work between medical and mental health professionals allows appropriate referrals and more accurate differential diagnoses.

An Early Model

An early and successful effort to establish treatment guidelines for anxiety and posttraumatic stress disorders was conducted under the aegis of the Royal Australian and New Zealand College of Psychiatrists (Quality Assurance Project, 1982, 1985a,b). The outcome of this project is what the authors referred to as explicit and detailed treatment outlines. Their model of development was thorough and scholarly. The outlines were developed based on three sources of information: extensive literature review and meta-analysis, a randomized sampling of practicing psychiatrists, and a panel of nominated experts.

The resultant treatment outlines are thorough, specific, and well documented. Because the recommendations are multidetermined, they are sufficiently broad to be of realistic clinical utility. At the same time they are specific enough to provide direction to a less experienced clinician. Additionally, these treatment outlines should be recognized for not overlooking the importance of the therapeutic relationship. For example, under treatment recommendations for posttraumatic stress disorder specific recognition is given to the need for creating a safe framework in which the client can discuss the trauma (Quality Assurance Project, 1985a).

One limit to generalizability in these guidelines stems from the professional sample represented. It appears that only psychiatrists were surveyed to determine customary treatment approaches for this project. Unless guidelines are developed based on the full range of practitioners who treat a given population, the guidelines may be biased in ways that limit treatment options (Rush, 1993).

Another major limitation of this set of specific outlines, based in part on the empirical literature, is that they are more than a decade old. As discussed above, this problem is inherent in any specific treatment guidelines unless there is an unyielding commitment to update them on a regular basis. Unfortunately, this costly and time-consuming process points out the rigors of creating and maintaining specific treatment guidelines.

Specific Populations

Giving primary consideration to client characteristics other than diagnostic category is another way to conceptualize guidelines. Among these guidelines, treatment recommendations stem from awareness of special considerations of the population being treated.

Often the defining characteristic of population is age. For example, the American Academy of Child and Adolescent Psychiatry (AACAP) undertook one such initiative with the development of their "Practice Parameters for the Assessment and Treatment of Anxiety Disorders" (Bernstein & Shaw, 1993). The result is a thorough and concise document that carefully considers the need for a multimodal approach to treatment with children and adolescents.

Although Bernstein and Shaw (1993) utilize a disorder-based classification system, they avoid the oversimplification so common in other diagnosis-specific treatment guidelines. They stay away from a mechanistic approach in which each diagnosis is matched to a specific treatment. Instead, they rely on a much more contextual approach as embodied in this summary paragraph:

> The treatment of anxiety disorders in children and adolescents usually involves a multimodal approach. Comprehensive treatment should include consideration of these components: education of the parents and child about the specific anxiety disorder, consultation with school personnel and primary care physicians, behavioral interventions, psychodynamic psychotherapy, family therapy and pharmacotherapy. (p. 1093)

An additional feature of the AACAP guidelines is the explicit recognition that the course of anxiety disorders in general is exceedingly variable. This naturally leads to the recommendation that for different individuals short-term, intermittent, or long-term treatment and follow-up will be indicated. This is an important distinction from "cookie cutter" or "cookbook" guidelines that presume, based on diagnosis alone, to know the exact treatment needed and the exact length of time it should take without any consideration for the individual being treated.

The flexibility of the AACAP guidelines in no way limits their specificity. The authors include detailed diagnosis-specific treatment recommendations. The only important drawback to the AACAP parameters is the exclusive reliance on physicians for consultation and review throughout the development process. Of the 45 individuals listed as having participated in the development and review of the document, only one was not a physician. Input from psychologists and social workers could only have added to the contextual approach reflected in this document.

Finally, treatment articles about specific groups of clients, although not identified as guidelines, delineate important treatment considerations based on population characteristics and comorbid factors. Smith, Sherrill, and Colenda (1995) consider the unique factors associated with assessing and treating anxiety in an elderly population. Frances and Borg (1993) address the role and treatments of anxiety in clients with alcoholism.

Articles such as these are extremely useful to clinicians who may not regularly work with the specific population or comorbid condition in question. Such articles provide guidance for a clinician who may have general experience treating anxiety-based conditions but limited or no experience with a particular population. These articles, in fact, are potentially far more useful than specific disorder-based treatment guidelines.

Guidelines for Specific Treatment Approaches

Another type of practice guideline that may be more practical than diagnosis-specific guidelines is one that addresses a specific treatment technique. Such guidelines are especially useful for techniques or treatment approaches that are complex or controversial. Such a guideline serves as a resource during treatment selection and implementation and as a safeguard against the inappropriate application of a specific treatment approach or technique.

One such guideline, applicable to assessment and treatment of anxiety and posttraumatic stress disorders, is the guideline for hypnosis published by the American Society of Clinical Hypnosis Press (Hammond et al., 1995). This guideline was written by psychologists, psychiatrists, a nurse, and an attorney. This multidisciplinary perspective is represented throughout the document and adds significantly to its credibility. Again, this is probably a far more useful tool for most clinicians than a directive to provide a specific type of treatment of a specific duration to a client with a particular diagnosis.

An example of a comprehensive treatment approach that has qualities of a useful treatment guideline is the text and workbook on dialectical behavior therapy (Linehan, 1993a, 1993b). These texts describe and detail a treatment protocol for borderline personality disorder (with acknowledged overlap with posttraumatic stress disorder) with specific attention to management of anxiety and other affects. The protocol includes the theory and philosophy of treatment and addresses the therapist's context and need for consultation. Linehan (1995) is emphatic that the consultation group is an essential component of dialectical behavioral therapy. Furthermore, the protocol is so specific, clinicians need extensive training and a community of like-minded clinicians to apply the method. It remains to be seen how effectively the treatment protocol will be implemented in different settings.

Both treatments of technique-specific guidelines are lengthy (books more than guidelines). In order to do justice to the complexity of the work and the individuals involved, guidelines need to be thorough and lengthy. However, such thoroughness potentially changes the purpose and concept of guidelines.

Additional types of guidelines that can be useful regardless of the diagnosis under consideration deal with other features of the assessment or treatment situation. For example, the American Psychological Association (1993) has established record-keeping guidelines as well as guidelines for performing child custody evaluations in divorce proceedings (American Psychological Association, 1994). Saakvitne and Abrahamson (1996) have proposed guidelines for clinicians' contacts with managed care reviewers.

Status of Current Guideline Projects

In light of concerns we have raised about diagnosis-specific treatment guidelines, it is interesting to note that two such guideline development initiatives for anxiety disorders apparently have been recently delayed or canceled. Clinton et al. (1994)

identify treatment of anxiety or panic disorder as one of the proposed AHCPR guidelines. It appears, however, that as of this writing this project has been postponed indefinitely (S. Hollon, personal communication, February 10, 1996). Similarly, the chair of the American Psychiatric Association's Task Force on Treatment Guidelines for Panic Disorder has indicated that that project has been delayed (J. Gorman, personal communication, October 18, 1995).

Is it possible that these delays and postponements in guideline development reflect a growing awareness of the questionable viability of guidelines that focus exclusively on diagnosis and symptoms? Time will tell.

Summary

Therapists who work with people with anxiety and posttraumatic stress disorders need guidance for their work. Such guidance should educate and support the therapist and protect clients from inappropriate treatment. Of the three approaches we examined, those that were organized around specific treatment approaches or population characteristics were more useful than specific diagnostic or symptom categories. When diagnostic categories do serve as the basis for treatment guidelines, the categories and treatments need to be generalizable. It is most useful for the guidelines to identify several options based on a range of contextual factors.

The different guidelines reviewed vary considerably in their usefulness to clinicians. Even the most useful guidelines, however, need to be used in the context of an overarching relational and psychotherapeutic framework if they are to be meaningful in the assessment and treatment of a real person by a real therapist. In the second part of this chapter, such a framework will be presented.

GUIDELINES: A RE-VISION

An Alternative Construction of Practice Guidelines

Let us start with the definition of guideline:

> Guideline: a line by which one is guided as **a**: a cord or rope to aid a passer over a difficult point or to permit retracing a course and **b**: an indication or outline (as by a government) of policy or conduct. (*Websters Ninth New Collegiate Dictionary*, 1986, p. 541)

Both parts of this definition inform our task. The first (a) iterates that guidelines help one stay on a path toward a given goal or destination. They are not the means of transportation but rather the guide to which to refer when one has misstepped or strayed from the path. The second part of the definition (b) identifies the role of guidelines as an expression of standards for a profession or practice. Generic standards must be general enough to allow for individual implementation of particular tasks or specialties within a profession.

We propose that practice guidelines similarly have two purposes and levels. On the one hand, they should reflect overall standards of practice that apply across theoretical orientations, length of treatment, and therapeutic techniques (b). On the other hand, they should provide guidance for treatments that seem lost, misguided, at an impasse, or misdirected (a). We emphasize that the second, more specific, level of guidelines is only useful in the context of the first, more general, guidelines.

This dual model allows the clinician to integrate specific symptom-based techniques or adjunctive treatments into theory-based treatment that is founded on a sturdy therapeutic alliance and designed to address mutually identified therapeutic goals. Thus, a clinician's ability to identify, for example, the need for a psychopharmacology consultation or a behavioral or relaxation technique will be embedded within the framework of the consultation or treatment relationship between the clinician and client.

REDEFINED GUIDELINES

General Guidelines

In therapy outcome research, the most consistent finding is that the relationship with the therapist (including the clients' perception of the therapist's warmth, positive regard, attentiveness, and attunement) is the single most consistent factor in positive outcome (Luborsky, 1994; Strupp, 1960; Strupp, Fox, & Lessler, 1969; Horvath & Symonds, 1991).

*Therapeutic Relationship**

Thus, the first component of any practice guideline should address the development of the therapeutic relationship and alliance. Key elements of the therapeutic relationship must be respect, mutuality, appropriate boundaries, and collaboration. The following components must be addressed.

Frame. All therapeutic relationships develop within the frame of the therapy. The establishment of a clear therapeutic frame creates the context for the work. This process includes setting time frame for sessions, fees and reimbursement, therapist availability, clarifications about roles and responsibilities of each participant, outline of the rules and limits of confidentiality, and establishing mutually agreed upon goals for the work.

Therapist Identity and Role. For therapists, the framework of the therapy must include a definition of role that is both realistic and respectful. Therapists' self-expectations must balance their education, training, and experience (professional knowledge) with humility. Therapists work within the limits of the knowledge of our field, in general, and the limits of their understanding and wisdom about any client, in particular. Therapists must recognize both the extent and the limits of their authority and knowledge and must respect the same in our clients.

Therapeutic Goals. The framework includes the definition of mutual goals and the mutual pursuit of these goals. Thus, there exists a clear definition of each participant's (therapist and client) responsibilities and contributions. The field has too often invited clinicians to believe themselves authorities on the clients rather than consultants to the clients.

*The authors thank Richard Nicastro, PhD, for his helpful contributions to this section.

Person Focused

A second component of our proposed general guidelines is that they are person not symptom focused. A therapeutic relationship is formed with a person, not with that person's symptoms, and one cannot separate a psychological symptom from the person experiencing it.

Yet, how one understands symptoms determines how one treats clients. An adaptation-focused view of psychopathology refocuses the therapist on the person of the client and uses his or her symptoms as sources of information (McCann & Pearlman, 1990; Pearlman & Saakvitne, 1995). Symptoms often motivate someone to seek therapy. They provide information about the client and his or her stress, adaptations, and resources. Often a symptom represents a psychological attempt to cope with an underlying problem, fear, or conflict. The symptom is then viewed as a solution to a problem, and the task of the therapy is to identify the problem and generate alternative solutions. This task defines the client's role as central and collaborative.

A symptom-focused approach tends to define the task of the therapy as eradicating (not understanding) symptoms and define the role of the client as a passive recipient of the therapist's expertise.

Certainly, symptom-focused *techniques* can be useful to clinicians, but they should not be mistaken as treatment guidelines. If we reduce the complexity of the psychotherapeutic process to the practice of techniques, we do a disservice to the complexity of our professions and our work. Further, we underestimate our clients when we let their symptoms define them and our relationship with them. Symptom-focused guidelines too often eradicate individual differences and assume people with certain symptoms are more alike than different.

Person-centered guidelines assume the uniqueness of each client and each treater, and therefore each therapeutic relationship. This approach requires that therapists include each person's particular context (individual, intrapsychic, familial, cultural, biological, social, professional) in the service of treating a given client.

Further, a person-centered approach is consistent with the research on clients' goals and experience of psychotherapy. Henry and Strupp (1994) summarize the literature on therapeutic alliance:

> In discussing therapeutic changes, patients placed relatively minor emphasis on the reduction of symptoms such as anxiety and depression. Rather, they focused on improvements in their interpersonal relationships and self-esteem. In short, patients come to view their symptomatic difficulties in the context of their interpersonal relationships and developed ways to relate and interact more adaptively with others. (p. 53)

Therapist Context and Needs

The third important part of treatment guidelines is a focus on the therapist. The therapist is the key factor in the therapeutic work; he or she is the tool and conduit for information and intervention.

The general guidelines outline necessary components of the therapist's professional practice. The purpose of guidelines is to keep the therapist on track and to support professional standards of practice. To accomplish these goals, we must look farther than the confines of a relationship with a given client. We must set a context that facilitates consistent and appropriate treatment with each client. We identify seven such guidelines below.

Supervision. Our treatment guidelines recommend regular clinical supervision or case consultation for all psychotherapeutic work. By definition, the intricacies of psychotherapy are such that therapists will be limited by their own experiences and constructions. Every clinician's perspective and understanding is bound by his or her perspective and countertransference with each client. Collegial consideration of therapeutic strategies, events, and dilemmas is invaluable to effective therapy. Individual, group, peer, or institutional supervision can provide clinicians with this essential support.

Training. The guidelines recommend clinicians seek appropriate training both for specialty work (e.g., specific techniques, trauma therapy, solution-focused therapy models, couples therapy, family therapy, group therapy, evaluation) and to deepen their understanding of focal details of their work (e.g., countertransference, gender dynamics in therapy, psychotherapy theory). Enrollment in postdoctoral fellowship programs, training institutes, home study programs, and intensive or sequential training workshops can provide access to this type of extensive training.

Continuing Education. The guidelines recommend regular attendance at professional conferences and workshops to maintain standards of excellence, increase awareness of new theory and research, broaden the knowledge base within the field, and maintain participation in the larger professional network. This exposure is necessary in order for practitioners to remain up-to-date on new information, paradigms, and techniques in the field.

Access to Current Research Information. The guidelines recommend clinicians avail themselves of print and computer-generated sources of information about current research and new developments in the field. Journals, computer networks, websites, and bulletin boards, and professional associations provide invaluable information and debates.

Ethical Guidelines. The guidelines recommend that clinicians not only abide by the ethical guidelines of the applicable profession, but review them regularly and implement practice policies to ensure adherence to them. This includes reviewing ethical principles in the face of external pressures and new requirements from reimbursement sources (e.g., make sure disclosure to third-party payers or reviewers are consistent with ethical principles of protected confidentiality) and changes in technology.

Appropriate Limits of Practice. The guidelines recommend clinicians set reasonable limits to their practice, taking into account areas of true talent and expertise, personal stamina, and the demands of the practice. The goal is to ensure the quality and standards of the clinical work by acknowledging the truth of human limitations.

Self-Awareness. The guidelines emphasize the imperative of self-awareness for practicing clinicians. Recognizing the implicit power differential within a therapeutic relationship and the daunting challenge of working toward psychological change and negotiating often complex clinical situations, it is essential that clinicians know themselves. This awareness must be reflected in honest assessment and commitment to attend to areas of need through self-care, professional consultation, and personal psychotherapy.

It should be noted that elements of many of these recommendations are included in the *General Guidelines for Providers of Psychological Services* (American Psychological Association, 1987). These general guidelines address three major areas: therapy relationship, person-centered focus, and therapist context. We believe, if followed, these guidelines set the stage for therapies that are appropriate across clients.

THE SECOND LEVEL: SPECIFIC GUIDELINES FOR CLIENTS WITH A PARTICULAR SYMPTOM CLUSTER

Anxiety Symptoms and Disorders

The literature on guidelines for clients presenting with various symptoms of anxiety has been reviewed earlier in the chapter. Largely, the narrow focus of such guidelines tend to address only the techniques of such therapies, not the therapy as a whole. As such, they fail to address the role or function of such symptoms in the broader context of the person's life and adaptation.

Are All Anxiety Disorders Alike?

One of the misleading implications of many treatment guidelines for anxiety disorders is that of homogeneity. If we entertain the notion that anxiety is a generic defensive response to internal and external stress, we recognize the heterogeneity of clients' experience. This approach allows us to place the symptoms of anxiety in the larger context of the self and belief system of the client.

When a client presents with reports of panic attacks, our treatment approach will be vastly more successful if we assess accurately the precipitants of such attacks. We must determine if these attacks, for example, represent flashback experiences to traumatic events, or dissociative affect flooding, or reflect a focal anxiety response in the context of a current severe stressor.

In addition, anxiety may be masked by defenses against it, and thus emerge as a client makes progress in treatment. In response to the lessening of other symptoms, such as substance abuse or dissociation, which serve to dampen or disconnect feelings, clients often feel more anxious in therapy; thus, the warning that in psychotherapy sometimes one feels worse in the process of feeling better. In fact, reclaiming anxiety as a useful warning sign rather than a paralyzing event is one goal of psychotherapy for anxiety disorders.

As we make these assessments, our treatment plans become more specific. In the frame of the general guidelines discussed above, specific guidelines for anxiety disorders should identify options for intervention and specify particular frame issues.

Techniques as Resources

Clients struggling with debilitating and demoralizing anxiety come to therapy in great distress. They often feel victimized by their physiological reactivity, psychological angst, and emotional torment. Both they and their clinicians want to identify effective sources of relief. For this, techniques that allow the client to reclaim some degree of awareness, understanding, and control over their physiological, psychological (cognitive), and emotional experience are invaluable.

The second level of guidelines can provide information about therapeutic techniques that promote such control. For example, relaxation techniques, guided visualizations, exposure treatments, systematic desensitization, biofeedback, and psychotropic medication are just a few techniques that serve to educate and train an anxiety-ridden client about self-care. Many well-established empirically validated techniques can be found (e.g., Barlow, Craske, Cerny, & Klosko, 1989; Borkovec et al., 1987) in the clinical literature and are now available commercially.

Understanding the Function and Sources of Anxiety

These techniques will be most useful as the therapist and client better understand the function and sources of the client's current anxiety. Anxiety serves an adaptive function; it starts as a warning of some danger or conflict, internal or external. Assessing the threat to the individual or psyche is important and reestablishing security is appropriate. It is, of course, inappropriate to encourage someone who is in real danger not to feel anxious.

Subjective anxiety can reflect the individual's perception of entrapment or helplessness, vulnerability to harm or humiliation, overwhelming fear of annihilation or dissolution, or pervasive mistrust or fears of persecution. These fears often have their roots in interpersonal experiences and internalized object relations. Part of the task of psychotherapy is for the client to develop his or her interpretive skills; that is, to be able to separate past from present, fear from reality, and to use present-day information to evaluate the sources and accuracy of present-day fears.

Affects represented in anxiety vary widely; for example, anxiety can be expressed as incessant worry, crushing shame, shyness, mild apprehension, paralyzing fear, or overwhelming terror. The particular affects direct the exploration of the therapy, both in the understanding of etiology and the prescription for change. Anxiety sometimes staves off other affects, such as grief or anger. Other defenses, such as dissociation or denial, often serve to block anxiety. The client's particular affective style and needs will become clear within the work of therapy.

The client's relationship with both self and others is often both a source of anxiety and the arena in which the anxiety is manifest. As one source of anxiety is conflict, exploration of the way in which beliefs and feelings about self and others are psychologically represented is an important component of this therapeutic work.

Specific Frame Issues

Guidelines for specific symptom clusters also should include relevant frame issues. Are there ways in which the frame of the therapy is modified? For example, many clients with anxiety disorder use psychotropic medication of some sort (e.g., antianxiety medications, certain antidepressants, low-dose neuroleptics). The therapy then must address the negotiation of boundaries and communication with the adjunctive treatment and the relationship with the prescribing physician or nurse. How will communication be handled; what will be communicated and by whom? Similarly, if a client is using any adjunctive treatment, the relationship with the other treaters and a clear framework for communication and information sharing is central.

Within the therapy relationship, if the clinician is using specific techniques such as hypnosis, "homework" assignments, guided visualization, making or giving tapes, or building systematic desensitization hierarchies, both therapist and client need to clarify their roles and the impact of such exercises on their developing relationship. Such treatments are very helpful, but also lend themselves to an authoritarian model of therapy that may work against the larger goals of self-empowerment for the client. The exploration of the client's roles and responsibilities and the limits of the therapist's power and authority can uncover some of the interpersonal components of an anxiety disorder (e.g., the assumed passivity and helplessness experienced by the client in interpersonal contexts).

TRAUMATIC STRESS DISORDERS

A certain percentage of the time, anxiety symptoms occur in the context of posttraumatic disorders (PTSD). PTSD is listed as an anxiety disorder in the *Diagnostic and Statistical Manual of Mental Disorders*, 4th edition (DSM-IV) (American Psychiatric Association, 1994), although symptoms of depression and dissociation are also prevalent in the symptom cluster. Below we present a discussion of treatment guidelines for traumatic stress disorders.

Traumatic stress disorders, unlike other diagnoses, integrate etiology with diagnosis. By doing so, they set the stage for the focus of the work, that is, the understanding of the meaning and context of the traumatic event from the recent or distant past in the client's current psychological, interpersonal, biological, and emotional experience. By understanding the constructions of meaning (McCann & Pearlman, 1990; Pearlman & Saakvitne, 1995; Janoff-Bulman, 1992) and developmental and social contexts (Herman, 1981, 1992; Gelinas, 1993) of traumatic events, the meaning of the client's symptoms and schemas or beliefs become decipherable and thus transformable.

There are several examples of specific treatment approaches for trauma treatment in the literature. Some resemble traditional guidelines, such as the models for short-term intervention for acute adult traumas (Foa, Rothbaum, & Steketee, 1993; Resick & Schnicke, 1992). Others describe longer-term work with specific populations (Pearlman & Saakvitne, 1995; Putnam, 1989; Ross, 1989) or general guidelines for survivors of any trauma (Herman, 1992; Harvey, 1996; McCann & Pearlman, 1990).

We will not present an exhaustive review of these specific treatment approaches here, except to say that these approaches, all published within the last 10 years, represent what we see as a hopeful trend. In general, they are more descriptive. They are more likely to take into account the person of the therapist and the development of the therapeutic relationship. They contextualize symptoms with the person of the client and include the person's particular contexts, that is, present and past psychological, interpersonal, familial, and cultural/social context. For the most part, they tend toward constructivism; that is, they look at the interactive influence of person and event, understanding that the person's perception and construction of the earlier events shape their perception and experience of later events. This premise reframes symptoms as meaningful attempts at adaptation and sets the stage for work within the therapeutic relationship.

Most recently, Pearlman and Saakvitne (1995) identify seven components of relational trauma therapy. They begin the discussion by emphasizing, "Good trauma therapy is first and foremost good theory-based psychotherapy" (p. 19). They then cite the following components:

1. An emphasis on the development of self-capacities (McCann & Pearlman, 1990); that is, development of self-soothing skills, object constancy, and stability of benign self-regard.
2. The need for the therapist to be genuine and present affectively.
3. The primary focus on the development of the therapeutic relationship rather than an exclusive focus on transference.
4. The interpretation of transference should occur earlier in the process and in the context of inviting the client to notice the process of bringing the past into the present.
5. The therapist's comprehension of the role of dissociation in trauma responses.
6. Psychoeducation, particularly information about the normal effects of traumatic events; management of common posttrauma symptoms and adaptations (flashbacks, memory fragments, dissociation); resources for survivors and their loved ones; expectable reactions to the treatment process itself (e.g., people often feel worse before they feel better); and normal child development, that is, typical behavior and psychological abilities at particular developmental stages.
7. Major therapeutic work with trauma survivor clients often takes place in the process of negotiating therapeutic frame and boundaries.

In addition, they emphasize the necessity of supervision for these psychotherapies and specify that the supervision must address theory-based treatment, the dynamics of the therapeutic relationship, countertransference, education about common PTSD symptoms and their management, and vicarious traumatization. Thus, this approach addresses both client and therapist needs.

Harvey (1996) and her colleagues have presented a very useful model of trauma treatment organized around the goals of such treatment, which they define as:

1. Authority over the remembering process.
2. Integration of memory and affect.
3. Affect tolerance.
4. Symptom mastery.
5. Self-esteem and self-cohesion.
6. Safe attachment.
7. Meaning making.

Such approaches represent examples of guidelines, that is, a guide that allows the therapist and client to construct the specific therapy according to the unique person and needs of the client.

CONCLUSIONS AND RECOMMENDATIONS

Our goal has been to broaden and redefine our concept of practice guidelines. Our intent is to improve the efficacy and utility of such instruments. Ideally, improved and re-visioned guidelines will serve as tools to help us achieve the larger goal of "good," respectful, and effective psychological interventions for all people seeking psychological help. And unlike most current guidelines, which are almost never used by practitioners (Abrahamson, in press), it is our hope that these re-visioned guidelines will be experienced as a useful resource by the practice community.

We believe guidelines must serve to protect both clients and therapists. Therapists laboring under false assumptions of their authority or knowledge are at risk for burnout, increased vicarious traumatization (Pearlman & Saakvitne, 1995), and improper or harmful care. Guidelines must be general enough to take into account individual and interpersonal differences among practitioners.

When guidelines are grounded in theory and techniques that highlight individual differences and the whole person rather than symptoms, a model of psychotherapy that emphasizes collaboration, empowerment, and health emerges. The client is an essential component of his or her treatment and cure.

The challenge to practice guidelines reflects the challenge to the DSM-IV (American Psychiatric Association, 1994). It is restricted by its limited goal. Diagnoses are descriptive, emphasizing an individual's symptoms at a given time; they do not create a picture of a person, nor do they capture the essence or complexity of the person's experience. It is a mistake to base treatment guidelines solely on this limited descriptive, categorical tool. Psychotherapy must be tailored to the individual and be responsive to contradictions and complications. Client data that contradict our assumptions are as valuable as those that support our hypotheses.

Ultimately, the value of psychotherapy is not simply symptom reduction or improved worker productivity. Psychotherapy offers us hope for the human condition. Psychotherapy serves to interrupt the cycle of intergenerational transmission of violence or despair and neglect. It serves to offer alternatives to lifetimes (or more) of somatization, substance abuse, depression, shame, and suicide. It returns to society the self of the client previously paralyzed or self-hating. It humanizes our culture.

REFERENCES

Abrahamson, D. J. (in press). Outcomes, guidelines, and manuals: On leading horses to water. *Clinical Psychology: Science and Practice.*

Abrahamson, D. J. (1998). Political issues in practice guidelines implementation. *Behavioral Healthcare Tomorrow, 7,* 32–35.

American Psychiatric Association. (1994). *Diagnostic and statistical manual of mental disorders* (4th ed.). Washington, DC: Author.

American Psychological Association, Board of Professional Affairs, Committee on Professional Standards. (1987). General guidelines for providers of psychological services. *American Psychologist, 42,* 712–723.

American Psychological Association, Committee on Professional Practice and Standards (1993). Record keeping guidelines. *American Psychologist, 48,* 984–986.

American Psychological Association, Committee on Professional Practice and Standards (1994). Guidelines for child custody evaluations in divorce proceedings. *American Psychologist, 49,* 677–680.

American Psychological Association, Task Force on Psychological Intervention guidelines (1995). *Template for developing guidelines: Interventions for mental disorders and psychosocial aspects of physical disorders.* Washington, DC: Author.

Barlow, D. H., Craske, M. G., Cerny, J. A., & Klosko, J. S. (1989). Behavioral treatment of panic disorder. *Behavior Therapy, 20,* 261–282.

Barron, J. (1995). Treatment research: Science, economics and politics. *The Independent Practitioner, 15,* 94–96.

Bernstein, G. A., & Shaw, K. (1993). Practice parameters for the assessment and treatment of anxiety disorders. *American Academy of Child and Adolescent Psychiatry, 32,* 1089–1098.

Borkovec, T. D., Mathews, A. M., Chambers, A., Ebrahimi, S., Lytle, R., & Nelson, R. (1987). The effects of relaxation training with cognitive or nondirective therapy and the role of relaxation-induced anxiety in the treatment of generalized anxiety. *Journal of Consulting and Clinical Psychology, 55*, 883–888.

Clinton, J. J., McCormick, K., & Besteman, J. (1994). Enhancing clinical practice: The role of practice guidelines. *American Psychologist, 49*, 30–33.

Consumer Reports. (1995, November). Mental health: Does therapy help? 734–739.

deAvila, J. (1995) Professional standards by fiat: The undermining of treatment for trauma and dissociative defenses. *Treating Abuse Today, 5*(4/5), 21–28.

Depression Guideline Panel. (1993). Depression in primary care: Vol. 2. *Treatment of major depression* (Clinical Practice Guideline No. 5, AHCPR Publication No. 93-0551). Rockville, MD: Department of Health and Human Services, Public Health Service, Agency for Health Care Policy and Research.

Foa, E. B., Rothbaum, B. O., & Steketee, G. S. (1993). Treatment of rape victims. *Journal of Interpersonal Violence, 8*(2), 256–276.

Frances, R. J., & Borg, L. (1993). The treatment of anxiety in patients with alcoholism. *Journal of Clinical Psychiatry, 54*, 37–43.

Gelinas, D. J. (1993). Relational patterns in incestuous families, malevolent variations, and specific interventions with the adult survivor. In P. L. Paddison (Ed.), *Treatment of adult survivors of incest* (pp. 1–34). Washington, DC: American Psychiatric Press.

Hammond, D. C., Garver, R. B., Mutter, C. B., Crasilneck, H. B., Frischolz, E., Gravitz, M. A., Hibler, N. S., Olson, J., Scheflin, A., Spiegel, H., & Wester, W. (1995). *Clinical hypnosis and memory: Guidelines for clinicians and for forensic hypnosis*. Des Plaines, IL: American Society for Clinical Hypnosis Press.

Harvey, M. R. (1996). An ecological view of psychological trauma and trauma recovery. *Journal of Traumatic Stress, 9*(1), 3–23.

Henry, W. P., & Strupp, H. H. (1994) The therapeutic alliance as interpersonal process. In A.O. Horvath & L. S. Greenberg (Eds.), *The working alliance: Theory, research, and practice* (pp. 51–89). New York: Wiley Interscience.

Herman, J. L. (1981). *Father–daughter incest*. Cambridge, MA: Harvard University Press.

Herman, J. L. (1992). *Trauma and recovery*. New York: Basic Books.

Horvath, A. O., & Symonds, B. D. (1991). Relation between working alliance and outcomes in psychotherapy: A meta-analysis. *Journal of Counseling Psychology, 38*, 139–149.

Institute for Clinical Systems Integration. (1995). *Health care guidelines: Major depression, panic disorder and generalized anxiety disorder in adults in primary care*. Minneapolis, MN: Author.

Institute of Medicine. (1990). *Clinical practice guidelines: Directions for a new program*. M. J. Field & K. N. Lohr (Eds.). Washington, DC: National Academy Press.

Institute of Medicine. (1992). *Guidelines for clinical practice: From development to use*. M. J. Field & K. N. Lohr (Eds.). Washington, DC: National Academy Press.

Janoff-Bulman, R. (1992). *Shattered assumptions: Toward a new psychology of trauma*. New York: Free Press.

Linehan, M. (1993a). *Cognitive behavior therapy for borderline personality disorder*. New York: Guilford Press.

Linehan, M. (1993b). *Workbook: Cognitive behavior therapy for borderline personality disorder*. New York: Guilford Press.

Linehan, M. (1995). Dialectical behavior therapy. American Psychological Association Continuing Education Workshop, August 10, 1995. New York.

Luborsky, L. (1994). Therapeutic alliances as predictors of psychotherapy outcomes: Factors explaining the predictive success. In A. O. Horvath & L. S. Greenberg (Eds.), *The working alliance: Theory, research, and practice* (pp. 38–50). New York: Wiley Interscience.

MCC. (1991). *Preferred practices—Guide*. Eden Prairie, MN: Author.

MCC. (1992). *Preferred practices—References*. Eden Prairie, MN: Author.

McCann, I. L., & Pearlman, L. A. (1990). *Psychological trauma and the adult survivor: Theory, therapy, and transformation*. New York: Brunner/Mazel.

Munoz, R. F., Hollon, S. D., McGrath, E., Rehm, L. P., & Vanden Bos, G. R. (1994). On the AHCPR depression in primary care guidelines: Further considerations for practitioners. *American Psychologist, 49*, 42–61.

Pearlman, L. A., & Saakvitne, K. W. (1995). *Trauma and the therapist: Countertransference and vicarious traumatization in psychotherapy with incest survivors*. New York: Norton.

Putnam, F. (1989). *Diagnosis and treatment of multiple personality disorder*. New York: Guilford.

Quality Assurance Project. (1982). A treatment outline for agoraphobia. *Australian and New Zealand Journal of Psychiatry, 16*, 25–33.

Quality Assurance Project. (1985a). Treatment outlines for the management of anxiety states. *Australian and New Zealand Journal of Psychiatry, 19*, 138–151.

Quality Assurance Project. (1985b). Treatment outlines for the management of obsessive-compulsive disorders. *Australian and New Zealand Journal of Psychiatry, 19,* 240–253.

Resick, P. A., & Schnicke, M. K. (1992). Cognitive processing therapy for sexual assault victims. *Journal of Consulting and Clinical Psychology,* 2(5), 748–756.

Ross, C. (1989). *Multiple personality disorder: Diagnosis, clinical features, and treatment.* New York: Wiley.

Rush, J. A. (1993). Clinical practice guidelines: Good news, bad news, or no news? *Archives of General Psychiatry, 50,* 483–490.

Saakvitne, K. W., & Abrahamson, D. J. (1996). The impact of managed care on the therapeutic relationship. In J. W. Barron & H. Sands (Eds.), *Impact of managed care on psychodynamic treatment* (pp. 27–60). Madison, CT: International Universities Press.

Seligman, M. E. P. (1995). The effectiveness of psychotherapy: The *Consumer Reports* study. *American Psychologists, 50,* 965–974.

Smith, G. R., & Hamilton, G. E. (1994). Dialogue: Treatment guidelines: What are the risks? Provider involvement is critical. *Behavioral Healthcare Tomorrow, 3,* 41–43.

Smith, S. L., Sherrill, K. A., & Colenda, C. C. (1995). Assessing and treating anxiety in elderly persons. *Psychiatric Services, 46,* 36–42.

Stricker, G., & Trierweiler, S. J. (1995). The local clinical scientist: A bridge between science and practice. *American Psychologist, 50,* 995–1002.

Strupp, H. H., Fox, R. E., & Lessler, K. (1969). *Patients view their psychotherapy.* Baltimore, MD: Johns Hopkins Press.

Strupp, H. H. (1960). Nature of psychotherapists' contribution to treatment process. *Archives of General Psychiatry, 3,* 219–231.

Task Force on Promotion and Dissemination of Psychological Procedures. (1995). Training in and dissemination of empirically-validated psychological treatments: Report and recommendations. *The Clinical Psychologist, 48,* 3–23.

Webster's Ninth New Collegiate Dictionary. (1986). Springfield, MA: Merriam-Webster.

13

Practice Guidelines Regarding the Conduct of Psychotherapy with Children and Adolescents

RICHARD J. MORRIS AND YVONNE P. MORRIS

Although we currently find a great deal of interest in the psychotherapeutic treatment of children and adolescents, this is a relatively recent event within the mental health field (Kendall & Morris, 1991; Kazdin, Siegel, & Bass, 1990).* Unlike the adult psychotherapy and related mental health literature, which can be traced back to ancient civilizations, the child therapy literature can only be traced with any clarity to the early 20th century (e.g., Kanner, 1948; Morris & Kratochwill, 1998b). The one notable exception involves those children who have been diagnosed as having a developmental disability. For these children, the treatment literature can be traced to the work of Jean Itard in France and his attempts in the late 1790s to educate the Wild Boy of Aveyron (Itard, 1962; Morris, 1985).

The developments in the early 20th century that contributed substantially to our present-day emphasis on child therapy were: (1) the mental hygiene movement and the work of Clifford Beers in promoting the establishment of improved mental health services for people having emotional problems; (2) the introduction of dynamic psychiatry and Sigmund Freud's 1909 detailed case of "Little Hans," as well as the later play therapy work of Melanie Klein and Freud's daughter, Anna Freud, in the 1920s and 1930s; (3) establishment of child guidance clinics throughout the United States in the first quarter of the 20th century; (4) the intelligence testing movement begun by Alfred Binet in France in the early 1900s; (5) formation of various professional societies in the 1920s that were concerned with the welfare of children (e.g., the Council for Exceptional Children and the American Orthopsychiatry Association), as well as the much earlier established Association of Medical Officers of American Institutions for Idiots and Feebleminded (circa 1876; presently called the American Association on Mental Retardation); and (6) the movement to provide more individualized instruction and special education classes for mentally and emotionally handi-

*Throughout this chapter, "children" or "child" will be used to refer to both children/child and adolescent(s). If discussion necessitates a differentiation, the separate terms will be used.

RICHARD J. MORRIS • School Psychology Program, University of Arizona, Tucson, Arizona 85719.
YVONNE P. MORRIS • Tucson, Arizona 85718.

Handbook of Quality Management in Behavioral Health, edited by Stricker *et al.* Kluwer Academic / Plenum Publishers, New York, 2000.

capped students, with the first teacher-training programs for these children beginning in the early 1910s in Michigan (e.g., Kanner, 1948; Kauffman, 1981; Morris, 1985; Morris & Kratochwill, 1998b).

Other developments affecting our modern-day approach to child therapy included the establishment of psychotherapy methods that were quite different from the psychoanalytic play therapy procedure advocated by Klein and Anna Freud. One of the first new approaches incorporated the psychoanalytic emphasis on the therapeutic relationships, but deemphasized the importance of the Freudian concept of the unconscious in understanding the meaning of children's play activities and verbalizations. For example, such writers as Frederick Allen (1942) and Virginia Axline (1947) emphasized the importance of providing children with a warm, permissive, and accepting environment in which there were few limitations placed on them. The goal of treatment was to help these children achieve there highest level of psychological growth and mental health. In addition, unlike the Freudian approach, these writers emphasized the present reality of the child's life versus past issues. Axline's writings were consistent with the client-centered approach of Carl Rogers (e.g., Rogers, 1942), whereas Allen's therapeutic procedure was more consistent with an ecological perspective and the emerging area of social psychiatry.

The second nonpsychoanalytic approach that developed dates back almost as far as the work of Sigmund Freud and emerged largely out of the experimental psychology laboratory. This therapy approach became known as behavior modification or behavior therapy and was based on psychological theories concerning how people and animals learn to behave; that is, behavior therapy was based on theories of learning and conditioning (e.g., Bandura, 1969; Hull, 1943; Mowrer, 1960; Pavlov, 1927; Skinner, 1938, 1953). Two of the most famous early studies in behavior therapy were conducted by Watson and Raynor (1920), with an 11-month-old child called "Little Albert," and Jones (1924), with a 3-year-old boy named Peter. Like Sigmund Freud's work with "Little Hans," these two latter studies emphasized work on children's fears (Morris & Kratochwill, 1983b).

In this chapter, we present an overview of a prescriptive approach to treating some of the more frequently referred children's behavior disorders. A chapter such as the present one can now be written because of the voluminous scholarly journal articles and books that have been published since the mid-1960s on psychotherapy methods with children and adolescents (see, for example, Kendall, 1991; Kendall & Braswell, 1985; Kratochwill & Morris, 1993; Mash & Barkley, 1989; Matson, 1988; Morris & Kendall, 1991; Morris & Kratochwill, 1983a, 1998; Witt, Elliott, & Gresham, 1988).

THERAPEUTIC APPROACHES AND RELATED ISSUES

Although historically the most prominent form of child psychotherapy involved psychoanalysis, more contemporary views of the development and understanding of children's behavior disorders, as well as the emerging research literature on child therapy, have led to an expansion of the list of the most frequently utilized therapeutic procedures (see, for example, D'Amato & Rothlisberg, 1992; Kratochwill & Morris, 1993; Mash & Barkley, 1989). Specifically, the expanded list now includes, in addition to child psychoanalysis, behavior therapy and cognitive behavior therapy, Adlerian child therapy, family therapy systems, client-centered (humanistic) therapy, reality therapy, ecological and consultation approaches, and pediatric psychopharmacology (Kratochwill & Morris, 1993). Therapy research has also expanded into culturally diverse populations (e.g., Tharp, 1991; Vraniak & Pickett, 1993), medically at-risk children (e.g., Siegel, 1993), developmentally delayed youth (e.g., Cole & Gardner, 1993; Matson & Coe, 1991), the family (e.g., Fauber & Long, 1991), and the prevention of childhood behavior disorders (e.g., Hightower & Braden, 1991; Rhodes, Reyes, & Jason, 1993; Weissberg, Caplan, & Harwood, 1991).

In terms of the most frequently applied psychotherapeutic frameworks with children and adolescents, Kratochwill and Morris (1993) have suggested that behavioral and cognitive–behavioral therapy procedures, child psychoanalysis and related psychodynamic approaches, client-centered therapy, reality therapy, family systems approaches, Adlerian approaches, and ecological interventions are among the most often cited child therapies in the literature. On the other hand, in one of the few data-based studies on the most frequently applied child therapy method(s), Kazdin et al. (1990) found that behavioral, cognitive, eclectic, psychodynamic, and family therapies were rated as "most useful" by the psychologists and psychiatrists that were surveyed. The psychologists in the study, however, rated behavior modification and cognitive approaches as more useful than did the psychiatrists, whereas the psychiatrists rated psychoanalytic approaches as more useful than did the psychologists. In terms of "effectiveness," Kazdin et al. (1990) reported that respondents rated individual psychotherapy and family therapy as "effective most of the time." In addition, they stated, "[t]he majority of either psychologists or psychiatrists, but not both, felt that psychodynamic therapy, play therapy, behavior modification, and cognitive therapy were very effective" (Kazdin et al., 1990, p. 196).

The above findings are consistent with the results of the meta-analysis work conducted by Casey and Berman (1985). They found that children receiving some form of psychotherapy (e.g., client-centered, psychodynamic, cognitive–behavioral, and/or behavioral therapy) improved more at the end of therapy than those not receiving psychotherapy. Casey and Berman also found, however, that for certain types of outcome measures the behavioral therapies were better than were the nonbehavioral therapies, but when the type of measure was controlled for, these differences were no longer found. After reviewing the latter study, as well as others, Kazdin (1991b) concluded that "... meta-analytic reviews have indicated that therapy in general is effective when compared with no treatment" (p. 787). It does not appear, however, that one particular form of child therapy is better than (or more effective than) any other form of therapy procedure that has been studied.

These emerging findings regarding the efficaacy of child therapy procedures have led some writers to conclude what has been discussed for many years in the adult psychotherapy literature, namely, that we can no longer answer the question, "Is child psychotherapy effective?" (see, for example, Goldstein, Heller, & Sechrest, 1966; Kazdin, 1991b, 1993; Kendall & Morris, 1991; Paul, 1967); rather, we have to ask, "Is this *particular therapy method* effective for this *type of child* (e.g., age of child, gender, ethnicity, etc.), having this *presenting problem*, from this *family structure and background*, and implemented by this *type of therapist* (e.g., therapist's expertise and experience, gender, ethnicity, values, etc.), under these *environmental conditions* or constraints?" Unfortunately, our child therapy research literature has not yet reached this level of detail, although some literature exists that does suggest that for certain types of behavior problems particular therapies are more preferred than are others (see, for example, Barkley, 19909; Charlop-Christy, Schreibman, Pierce, & Kurtz, 1998; Kratochwill & Morris, 1991; Mash & Barkley, 1989; Morris & Kratochwill, 1983b).

The effectiveness of treatment also may be influenced by comorbidity factors or those behavior problems that overlap or co-occur with the child's primary diagnosis (e.g., Kendall & Morris, 1991). For example, can a child with a primary diagnosis of attention-deficit hyperactivity disorder (ADHD) be expected to have a better prognosis and improve more quickly than a child who has both ADHD and conduct disorder or ADHD and learning problems? Or, will a child who is both anxious and fearful improve faster than a child who is anxious, fearful, and depressed? Since few data exist that address these types of questions, no definitive answer can be given at this time.

Child therapy outcome is also complicated by the fact that it is not always clear *who is the client* (Kendall & Morris, 1991; Morris & Nicholson, 1993). Unlike psychotherapy with adults, identification of the client is not that easy because oftentimes the child or even the adolescent does not seek out psychotherapy services. In most cases, the child's parent or guardian, school personnel, or the juvenile justice system brings the "client" to the attention of the child therapist. This "adult-oriented" referral process may confuse the therapist and the child as to who is the client, especially if a referral source, such as the school or the juvenile justice system, is expecting an assessment of and progress report on the child, as well as paying for the psychological services that are being provided. A similar level of confusion may occur when parents bring their child to a child therapist. It may be the parents' initial expectation that the child is the client, and learn somewhat later in the therapy process that they, as well a the child's siblings and teachers, also have become integrally tied to the treatment plan.

Therefore, any decision regarding who is part of the therapy process (i.e., who is the client) can only be determined on the basis of a thorough intake assessment, where the child and all other significant persons with whom the child interacts are assessed to determine their relative contribution to the child's emotional and/or behavioral difficulties (e.g., Barkley, 1990; Frame & Matson, 1987; Kendall & Morris, 1991; Morris & Kratochwill, 1983). Once the nature of the child's psychological problems have been assessed, as well as the factors that contribute to their occurrence, then a decision can be made regarding who needs to be involved in the treatment plan. This determination also includes a decision whether parents, teachers, siblings, and significant others will be consultants to the treatment plan versus co-clients and whether the child and/or family needs to be in psychotherapy (Kendall & Morris, 1991). Each person included in the therapy process needs to give their consent to participate in therapy and to permit the therapist to share their respective comments with the other participating clients (Arambula, DeKraai, & Sales, 1993).

DIAGNOSTIC ISSUES

Unlike adults, children are not necessarily viewed as the most reliable and valid sources of information regarding the nature of their particular behavior disorder. Although there are exceptions to this view, particularly with those children and adolescents reporting internalizing disorders, oftentimes it is the socialization agent (i.e., parent, teacher, juvenile justice system, etc.) who brings the child to the attention of a mental health services provider. This is because the child may not construe his or her behavior as problematic, or he or she may view the behavior of the socialization agent as troublesome and maintain that his or her behavior is an appropriate response to a threatening or unkind situation involving the socialization agent (Kendall & Morris, 1991). In addition, some children may assess their behavior difficulties as less intense than their teacher or parent. These circumstances therefore may affect the reliability of any diagnosis made concerning a child's emotional difficulties (e.g., Lachar, 1993).

A related series of factors that may influence the reliability of a child's diagnosis pertain to the developmental and chronological age appropriateness of the assessment instruments that are used (e.g., Edlebrock, Costello, Dulcan, Kalas, & Conover, 1985; Evans & Nelson, 1986; Kazdin, 1991b; Kendall & Morris, 1991; Kendall & Sessa, 1993; Lachar, 1993), the diagnostician's knowledge of cultural issues that impact diagnoses, whether the assessment instruments used were normed on the population to which the child/children in question belongs, and the child's level of acculturalization to and assimilation in the dominant culture (e.g., Gibbs & Huang, 1989; Jacobsen, 1988; Lopez & Hernandez, 1986; Marin, 1992; Mishra, 1980; Tharp, 1991; Westermeyer, 1987).

THERAPEUTIC RELATIONSHIP ISSUES

Systematic research on the contribution of the therapeutic relationship to the outcome of child therapy lags far behind the adult literature on this topic (Kazdin, 1991b; Morris & Nicholson, 1993). This paucity of information has led researchers to speculate about the relative contribution of this variable, in comparison to other treatment components, to therapy outcome. For example, Kendall and Morris (1991), note that although such therapist factors as therapist warmth, therapist empathy, model similarity, ethnicity, and physical contact and verbal encouragement of the child have been discussed or studied, as well as such client variables as presenting problem/pretreatment level of prosocial functioning and level of motivation, no firm conclusions regarding the effects of these factors can be made at this time. In addition, they note that other therapist factors that have ben studied in the adult literature may have relevance to the outcome of child therapy, such as therapist expertise and status, expectancy, values, and self-concept. Kendall and Morris (1991) also indicate that the presence versus absence of confidentiality in child therapy, although not yet studied in a systematic fashion, may further contribute to the outcome and/or to the level self-disclosure during therapy.

Other issues that have emerged that also may affect the therapeutic relationship and the subsequent outcome of child therapy involve psychotherapy work with the following groups: male and female gay adolescents whose psychological difficulties are not construed by them as related to their sexual preference, human immunodeficiency virus (HIV)-positive and other medically at-risk children and adolescents, children living with drug-addicted parents, and physically and/or sexually abused youth who have been placed back into their respective homes by the court (e.g., Morris & Nicholson, 1993; Sobocinski, 1990). The issues that are raised are related to a relatively new parameter in the study of the therapeutic relationship, namely, the therapist's personal beliefs and values regarding the client that he or she is seeing in therapy, as well as the quality of life that the therapist perceives the client to be experiencing.

Since systematic outcome research on the therapeutic relationship in child therapy has not yet been published, few conclusions can be drawn at this time; however, consistent with the theoretical therapeutic frameworks of the major child psychotherapies (i.e., child psychanalysis and psychodynamic therapy, client-centered/humanistic therapy, behavior therapy and cognitive–behavioral therapy, family therapy, and ecological approaches; see, for example, D'Amato & Rothlisberg, 1992; Johnson, Rasbury, & Siegel, 1986; Kazdin et al., 1990; Kratochwill & Morris, 1993), the working assumption in the remainder of this chapter is that the therapy practices discussed are conducted within the framework of the therapist having a sound therapeutic relationship with the child and family.

ASSESSMENT OF CHILDREN'S BEHAVIOR DISORDERS

Consistent with a practice guidelines perspective to child therapy, the clinician must first conduct a psychological assessment of the child and family in order to understand the nature of the child's behavior problem(s). Generally speaking, the following aspects of a child's behavior problem(s) are typically assessed: (1) circumstances and/or settings in which the problem occurs, as well as those conditions under which it does not occur; (2) frequency of occurrence; (3) duration of the problem whenever it occurs and chronicity of the problem over time; (4) intensity or severity level; (5) whether the problem has improved or become worse over time; (6) present developmental appropriateness of the problem, as well as its social and cultural appropriateness; (7) child's/family members' level of personal distress regarding the problem; (8) the child's/family member's/significant others'/teacher's history of previous attempts at remedying the problem; and (9) developmental history relevant to the nature of the problem. This assessment approach not only assists the child therapist in fully understanding the child's behavior difficulties but also permits the therapist to identify the target issues and/or behaviors that need to be addressed in therapy, determine the constraints on the therapy implementation plan, decide who needs to be in therapy and whether significant others and teachers need to be consulted as therapy progresses, and, finally, assign a diagnosis to the behavior problem, especially in those cases involving third-party payment.

The assessment of childhood behavior problems often has followed either a "behavioral" or "traditional" approach to conceptualizing child psychopathology (e.g., Frame & Matson, 1987; Morris & Kratochwill, 1983b). The traditional approach typically focuses on the internal psychological issues, constructs, and/or conflicts that are responsible for the child's difficulties, whereas the behavioral approach focuses on the events and persons in the child's life that are contributing to the maintenance of the child's particular behavioral difficulties (e.g., Morris & Kratochwill, 1983b). The cognitive–behavioral approach adds another dimension to the behavioral approach by assessing what the child says or thinks to her- or himself (including emotions and feelings). This approach also includes an analysis of the duration, intensity, and frequency of the child's cognitive and emotional reactions, as well as her or his motoric behavior. This procedure also stresses obtaining information from significant others in the child's life (e.g., Bernard & Joyce, 1993; Kendall & Sessa, 1993).

Additional approaches that fall somewhere in between the above positions include the Adlerian, ecological, and family systems approaches. For example, assessment within an Adlerian approach is linked to intervention, where the child therapist utilizes the following: observation, the therapist's own feelings about and reactions to the child, the therapist's understanding of the family constellation, assessment of which of the four goals of misbehavior the child uses, genograms, goldmines, private logic, the question, and the two points on a line technique (see, for example, Mosak & Maniacci, 1993). Consistent with the Adlerian approach, the ecological perspective construes assessment as a stage of intervention, since the ecological approach is holistic in its conceptualization of children's behavior disorders. According to Morse (1993), "[a]ssessment requires not only knowledge of the person (the individual pole) and the habitat (the environmental pole), but how these systems *interact*, especially when in discord" (p. 325). Assessment often begins with an examination of the "episodes of conflict" and determines who is involved, what behaviors were manifested, what were the feelings of those involved and how did they perceive the conflict, and what was tried to temper the conflict. Morse also points out that assessment is an ongoing process throughout treatment.

Within a family therapy context, each child within the family, not just the "symptomatic" child, is assessed while also evaluating the mother–father relationship as well as each parent–each child relationship and the respective sibling-to-sibling relationships. According to Everett and Volgy (1993), "... individual features to be assessed include cognitive levels and verbal skills, social and relationship skills, developmental deficits and strengths, expectable level of maturity, coping skills, and current home, school, and peer adjustment" (p. 251).

Whichever assessment approach is utilized, good practice guidelines suggest that the therapist should indicate in any communication regarding the assessment what is her or his level of confidence in the findings and conclusions that are reported. The therapist also should make sure that she or he is knowledgeable of the psychometric properties and other limitations of the assessment instruments that were used.

PRESCRIPTIVE TREATMENT GUIDELINES

Although the child psychotherapy research literature is not as extensive as the equivalent literature on adults, trends have nevertheless emerged from the child therapy literature that permit us to identify certain procedures that appear to be useful in the amelioration of various children's behavioral and emotional problems. Since, in most cases, only limited controlled outcome and/or comparison outcome studies have been published on the various procedures discussed below, the treatment guidelines listed should only be construed as "advisory guidelines" that reflect the current data-based research findings in the field. In this section, we describe treatment guidelines associated with four childhood behavior disorders that are frequently treated by child therapists, namely, childhood fears and phobias and related anxieties, ADHD, childhood depression, and conduct disorder.

Fears and Phobias

Interest in children's fears and phobias has a long tradition of study in the mental health field (see, for example, King, Hamilton, & Ollendick, 1988; Morris & Kratochwill, 1983b). Fears and phobias can have a disruptive influence on a child's learning, development, and socialization, and can set the occasion for the occurrence of mild to severe anxiety and even panic (Morris & Kratochwill, 1983b, 1998a).

Definition and Characteristics

Although distinctions have been made between the terms "fear" and "phobia" in the child therapy and psychopathology literature, these terms have also been used interchangeably in the same literature and with such terms as "anxiety," "stress," and "worry" (e.g., Morris & Kratochwill, 1983b, 1998a). In general, however, *fear* is construed as an intense emotion that is associated with cognitive, motoric, and/or physiological components of anxiety. When a child experiences fear that is not developmentally appropriate and in a setting where there is no obvious danger, the fear is irrational and the child is said to have a *phobia*. When the child begins to avoid the nondangerous situation, even after repeated attempts to encourage him or her to approach the situation, the phobia is commonly referred to as a *phobic reaction* (Morris & Kratochwill, 1983b, 1998a). Marks (1969) has suggested that phobia is actually a subtype of fear that (1) is out of proportion to the demands of the situation, (2) cannot be explained or reasoned away, (3) is beyond voluntary control, and (4) leads to avoidance of the feared situation (p. 3). Miller, Barrett, and Hampe (1974) added that a phobia (1) persists over an extended period of time, (2) is unadaptive, and (3) is not age or stage specific (p. 90). In terms of prevalence information, it is estimated that between 4 and 8% of all clinic referrals are for children's phobias and related severe fears (Morris & Kratochwill, 1983b, 1998a).

Treatment Approaches

Although a fair amount of literature has been published over the past century on the treatment of children's fears and phobias, it has only been within the past 20 years that the research literature has shown that behavior therapy approaches appear to be regularly successful in helping children with this behavior problem (e.g., Kendall et al., 1992; King et al., 1988; Morris & Kratochwill, 1983b, 1998a; Ollendick, King, & Yule, 1994). There are four major behavior therapy methods that have been used on a reliable basis to treat children experiencing fears and phobias: systematic desensitization and its variations, contingency management procedures, modeling methods, and self-instructional/cognitive–behavioral approaches (Morris & Kratochwill, 1983b, 1998a).

Systematic desensitization and its variants—contact desensitization, *in vivo* desensitization, group systematic desensitization—have a substantial amount of outcome data supporting their efficacy (e.g., King et al., 1988; Morris & Kratochwill, 1998a). Some of the behavior problems that have been treated successfully using these desensitization procedures are presented in Table 1.

The basic assumption of the desensitization approach is that the child's fear or phobic response is learned or conditioned and can be counterconditioned by substituting an activity that is antagonistic to this response. Usually, the antagonistic response that is learned by the child is calmness, which is induced by teaching the child how to relax through the use of a relaxation protocol such as the one shown in Table 2; however, the calmness and trust associated with the therapeutic relationship also has ben used in both *in vivo* and contact desensitization procedures (Morris & Kratochwill, 1983b).

TABLE 1. Partial Listing of Child Therapy Procedures Used to Treat Children's Fears, Phobias, and Related Anxieties[a]

Fear/phobia/anxiety	Procedure
Nondangerous animals	Systematic desensitization
	Contact desensitization
	In vivo desensitization
	Modeling
	Positive reinforcement
Driving a/in a car	Systematic desensitization
	Shaping
Physical examination; blood/dental examination; surgical operation	*In vivo* desensitization (with and without modeling)
	Modeling (live or symbolic)
	Self-control
Weight loss	Systematic desensitization
Test anxiety	Systematic desensitization
	Group systematic desensitization
	Modeling
	Self-control desensitization
	Self-control
Water in a swimming pool or bathtub	*In vivo* desensitization
	Contact desensitization
Public speaking/speech anxiety	Systematic desensitization
	Group systematic desensitization
	Self-control desensitization
Social interaction	Positive reinforcement
	Modeling
School phobia	Systematic desensitization
	In vivo desensitization
	Emotive imagery
	Modeling
	Positive reinforcement
	Contingency contracting
	Shaping (with and without positive reinforcement)
	Extinction
Heights	Systematic desensitization
	Contact desensitization
	In vivo desensitization
Fire	Behavioral rehearsal/self-instructional training
Dark/going to sleep at night	*In vivo* desensitization
	Modeling
	Positive reinforcement
	Extinction
	Self-control
Social phobia	Systematic desensitization
	In vivo desensitization
Elective mutism	Stimulus fading
Separation anxiety	*In vivo* desensitization
	Stimulus fading (with and without shaping)
Eating food	Systematic desensitization
	In vivo desensitization
	Positive reinforcement
Academic performance anxiety (reading/math)	Systematic desensitization
	Group systematic desensitization
	Self-control desensitization
	Self-control

[a]Adapted from Morris and Kratochwill (1983b, 1998); Morris, Kratochwill, and Aldridge (1988).

TABLE 2. Program for Teaching Relaxation to Children

Steps in relaxation

1. Take a deep breath and hold it (for about 10 seconds). Hold it. Okay, let it out.
2. Raise both of your hands about half way above the chair or mat, and breathe normally. Now, drop your hands down.
3. Now hold your arms out and make a tight fist. Really tight. Feel the tension in your hands. I am going to count to three and when I say "three" I want you to drop your hands. One ... Two ... Three.
4. Raise your arms again, and bend your fingers back the other way (toward your body). Now drop your hands and relax.
5. Raise your arms. Now drop them and relax.
6. Now raise your arms again, but this time "flap" your hands around. Okay, relax again.
7. Raise your arms again. Now relax.
8. Raise your arms above the couch (chair) again and tense your biceps until they shake. Breathe normally, and keep your hands loose. Relax your hands. (Notice how you have a warm feeling of relaxation.)
9. Now hold your arms out to your side and tense your biceps. Make sure that you breathe normally. Relax your arms.
10. Now arch your shoulders back. Hold it. Make sure that your arms are relaxed. Now relax.
11. Hunch your shoulders forward. Hold it, and make sure that you breathe normally and keep your arms relaxed. Okay, relax. (Notice the feeling of relief from tensing and relaxing your muscles.)
12. Now turn your head to the right and tense your neck. Relax and bring your head back again to its natural position.
13. Turn your head to the left and tense your neck. Relax and bring your head back again to its natural position.
14. Now bend your head back slightly toward the chair. Hold it. Okay, now bring your head back slowly to its natural position.
15. This time bring your head down almost to your chest. Hold it. Now relax and let your head come back to its natural resting position.
16. Now open your mouth as much as possible. A little wider; okay, relax. (Mouth must be partly open at end.)
17. Now tense your lips by closing your mouth. Okay, relax.
18. Put your tongue at the roof of your mouth. Press hard. (Pause) Relax and allow your tongue to come to a comfortable position in your mouth.
19. Now put your tongue at the bottom of your mouth. Press down hard. Relax and let your tongue come to a comfortable position in your mouth.
20. Now just lie (sit) there and relax. Try not to think of anything.
21. To control self-verbalization, I want you to go through the motions of singing a high note—not aloud! Okay, start singing to yourself. Hold that note, and now hard. Relax. (You are becoming more and more relaxed.)
22. Now sing a medium tone and make your vocal cords tense again. Relax.
23. Now sing a low tone and make your vocal cords tense again. Relax. (Your vocal apparatus should be relaxed now. Relax your mouth.)
24. Now close your eyes. Squeeze them tight and breathe naturally. Notice the tension. Now relax. (Notice how the pain goes away when you relax.)
25. Now let your eyes relax and keep your mouth open slightly.
26. Open your eyes as much as possible. Hold it. Now relax your eyes.
27. Now wrinkle your forehead as much as possible. Hold it. Okay, relax.
28. Now take a deep breath and hold it. Relax.
29. Now exhale. Breathe all the air out ... all of it out. Relax. (Notice the wondrous feeling of breathing again.)
30. Imagine that there are weights pulling on all your muscles making them flaccid and relaxed ... pulling your arms and body into the couch.
31. Pull your stomach muscles together. Tighter. Okay, relax.
32. Now extend your muscles as if you were a prize fighter. Make your stomach hard. Relax. (You are becoming more and more relaxed.)
33. Now tense your buttocks. Tighter. Hold it. Now relax.

TABLE 2. *(Continued)*

34. Now search the upper part of your body and relax any part that is tense. First the facial muscles. (Pause 3 to 5 seconds) Then the vocal muscles. (Pause 3 to 5 seconds) The neck region. (Pause 3 to 5 seconds) Your sholder ... relax any part which is tense. (Pause) Now the arms and fingers. Relax these. Becoming very relaxed.
35. Maintaining this relaxation, raise both of your legs (about a 45° angle). Now relax. (Notice that this further relaxes you.)
36. Now bend your feet back so that your toes point toward your face. Relax your mouth. Bend them hard. Relax.
37. Bend your feet the other way ... away from your body. Not far. Notice the tension. Okay, relax.
38. Relax. (Pause) Now curl your toes together as hard as you can. Tighter. Okay, relax. (Quiet ... silence for about 30 seconds.)
39. This completes the formal relaxation procedure. Now explore your body from your feet up. Make sure that every muscle is relaxed. (Say slowly)—first your toes, your feet, your legs, buttocks, stomach, shoulder, neck, eyes, and finally your forehead—all should be relaxed now. (Quiet—silence for about 10 seconds.) Just lie there and feel very relaxed, noticing the warmness of the relaxation. (Pause) I would like you to stay this way for about one more minute, and then I am going to count to five. When I reach five, I want you to open your eyes feeling very calm and refreshed. (Quiet—silence for about one minute.) Okay, when I count to five I want you to open your eyes feeling very calm and refreshed. One ... feeling very calm; two ... very calm, very refreshed; three ... very refreshed; Four ... and Five.

[a]SOURCE: Reprinted from Morris and Kratochwill (1983b).

A second phase of this procedure involves the formation of the child's fear hierarchy/hierarchies. Items on a hierarchy vary from situations or events that are least anxiety or fear provoking to those that produce the highest intensity or level of fear in the child. Hierarchies are highly individualized and oftentimes children experiencing the same type of fear will construct a hierarchy that is substantially different from that of another child. The third phase of this procedure involves the pairing of the calmness that the child experiences with successive items on the fear hierarchy. The pairing can be accomplished through imagery techniques in the child therapist's office or through graded exposure in the very environment that sets the occasion for the fear or phobic reaction. In the case of contact desensitization, as *in vivo* component is also combined with a modeling condition and verbal reinforcement condition where the therapist first models the appropriate response on the hierarchy and then the child is encouraged both verbally and physically to imitate the therapist's behavior.

Although systematic desensitization and its variant procedures have been found to be effective in reducing a variety of children's fears and phobias, such as test anxiety, public speaking anxiety, school phobia, nyctophobia, water in a bathtub or swimming pool, loud noises, gaining weight, nondangerous animals, acrophobia, some of these procedures (e.g., imaginal systematic desensitization) do not appear to be developmentally appropriate for certain age groups. The therapist is encouraged to consult various child therapy textbooks for more specific details on the implementation of these procedures for preschool and primary grade children versus junior high and high school-age children (see, for example, King et al., 1988; Matson, 1988; Morris, 1985; Morris & Kratochwill, 1983b, 1998a; Witt et al., 1988).

Contingency management procedures have a long history of use in the child therapy literature (e.g., Graziano, 1971; Lovaas & Bucher, 1974; Morris & Kratochwill, 1983a,b, 1998; Ollendick & Cerny, 1981). The application of these procedures has its origins in the operant conditioning and learning theory writings of B. F. Skinner (e.g., Skinner, 1938, 1953) and others (e.g., Ayllon & Michaels, 1959; Azrin & Lindsley, 1956; Bijou, 1955; Jones, 1924; Watson & Rayner, 1920). A number of these procedures have been found to be effective in the reduction of directly observable children's fears, phobias, and related anxieties such as those shown in Table 2. For example, positive reinforcement has been used to reduce the frequency and duration of social withdraw and social isolation in children, as well as increase social interaction. When combined with shaping, positive reinforcement also has been used to treat school phobia. Other methods that have been utilized are contingency contracting and stimulus fading techniques.

Modeling consists of an individual called the model (i.e., therapist, teacher, parent, or peer) and a person called the observer (i.e., the child or family member), where the observer watches the model engage in behavior that is fearful to the observer. There are two distinct types of modeling: live modeling and symbolic modeling (Bandura, 1969). In both live and symbolic modeling approaches, the model approaches the feared stimulus situation in a graduated fashion and with caution within a setting where no unsafe consequences are associated with the approach behavior. In symbolic modeling, the modeling activity is performed through videotape, film, or imagination (Morris & Kratochwill, 1983b, 1998a). Like contingency management procedures, these methods have been used more often with clearly identifiable fears and phobias (see Table 2).

Before modeling can take place, the child therapist should be certain that the child can perform the following: (1) attend to the various aspects of the modeling situation, (2) retain what has been learned in the modeling endeavor, (3) motorically reproduce or match what has been observed, and (4) be motivated to perform the observed behavior (Bandura, 1977).

Cognitive–behavioral methods have been used increasingly over the past 15–20 years in child therapy, but only relatively few studies have been published on the use of this procedure with children's fears and phobias (Morris & Kratochwill, 1983b, 1998a). Although appearing to encompass a defined procedure, these methods actually include a number of variations in the application of cognition to the treatment of fears and phobias in children. Each method shares, however, the assumptions that (1) cognitive processes contribute substantially to behavior change and (2) individuals can regulate their own behavior (McReynolds, Morris, & Kratochwill, 1989; Morris & Kratochwill, 1983b, 1998a). These different methods include: self-instructional training, rational–emotive therapy (RET), and self-control. Self-instructional training was initially developed by Meichenbaum and his colleagues (e.g., Meichenbaum & Goodman, 1971) and involves having the therapist model cognitive strategies for the child, with the intent of having the child apply her or his self-talk whenever the child is placed in or approaches situations involving the feared stimulus. Rational–emotive therapy was developed in the early 1960s by Albert Ellis (e.g., Ellis, 1962) and extended to children on a systematic basis by Ellis and his colleagues (see, for example, Bernard & Joyce, 1993). The primary goal of RET is to teach people to identify and change the irrational thoughts or beliefs underlying their fears, phobias, and related anxieties. Children are therefore taught to replace their maladaptive thoughts with more rational thoughts about a feared stimulus.

Self-control and self-regulation procedures have been included in the therapy research literature for many decades (see, for example, Bandura, 1969; Kanfer &

Phillips, 1970; Skinner, 1953). The procedure involves a process through which the person becomes the primary agent in directing those aspects of her or his behavior that lead to preplanned and specific behavioral outcomes and/or consequences (Kanfer & Phillips, 1970). The therapist teaches the child how, when, and where to use various cognitions to facilitate the learning of new behaviors. In the case of fears and phobias, the new behavior learned is nonavoidant behavior whenever the child is exposed to the feared stimulus.

Before applying cognitive–behavioral procedures, the child therapist should first determine whether the child is aware of his or her fear or related anxiety and whether she or he is able to identify the conditions under which she or he becomes fearful or anxious. The therapist should also determine whether the child is motivated to change the maladaptive behavior and whether she or he is willing to accept responsibility for changing the behavior (Kanfer & Schefft, 1988; Morris & Kratochwill, 1983b, 1998a). In addition, the therapist should determine whether the child is developmentally ready to implement the cognitive activity that is required by these methods.

Attention-Deficit Hyperactivity Disorder

ADHD constitutes one of the most frequent reasons for referral to school psychologists and child-based mental health clinics. Prevalence studies indicate that 3 to 5% of school-age children may have ADHD, or approximately one child for every classroom in America, with the disorder occurring more often in boys than girls at a male:female ratio of 3:1 (Barkley, 1990; DuPaul & Barkley, 1998; Morris & Collier, 1987). This behavior problem is also among the most frequently researched childhood behavior disorders in the psychological assessment and child therapy literature.

Definition and Characteristics

ADHD has been defined over the years in various ways, with some of the definitions involving such concepts as brain dysfunction, developmental disorder of social conduct and self-regulation, and as a disorder of rule-governed behavior (e.g., DuPaul, Guevremont, & Barkley, 1991; Morris & Collier, 1987). More recently, the American Psychiatric Association (APA) (1994) has defined ADHD as a disorder consisting of a child manifesting at least six of nine behavioral symptoms, in one or both of the following two categories, for at least 6 months: Inattention and Hyperactivity-Impulsivity.

The behaviors associated with the *inattention* category are: careless mistakes and inattention to details; difficulty sustaining attention in various activities; not listening; not following through on instructions and failing to complete assignments; difficulty in organizing tasks; avoiding tasks requiring sustained mental effort; often losing things; being easily distracted; and often forgetful. The *hyperactivity–impulsivity* category consists of the following frequently occurring behaviors: fidgets; leaves seat; runs around or climbs excessively; difficulty playing or being involved quietly in leisure activities; acts "driven" or "on the go"; talks; blurts out an answer before a question is finished; difficulty awaiting one's turn; interrupts others. In addition, these behaviors must occur before the child turns 7 years of age; cause some impairment in the child's functioning in two or more settings; involve a "clinically significant impairment in social, academic, or occupational functioning"; and, cannot be manifested "exclusively" during pervasive developmental disorder or the presence of schizophrenia or any other psychotic disorder, and cannot be explained by another mental disorder (APAP, 1994, p. 65).

Barkley (e.g., 1990), one of the more active researchers in the field, has revised his earlier conceptual view of ADHD as a disorder of rule-governed behavior and has recently reconceptualized it as an "... impairment in delayed responding to the environment in the development of higher order cognitive skills" (DuPaul & Barkley, 1998, p. 133). This conceptualization, according to DuPaul and Barkley (1998) accounts for the myriad behavioral difficulties that children with ADHD encounter, and in turn it focuses treatment programs on adapting the child's environments in order to accommodate for the impairment.

Treatment Approaches

Given the voluminous research that has been published over the past two decades (see, for example, Barkley, 1981, 1990; DuPaul & Barkley, 1998; Weiss & Hechtman, 1993), there is now sufficient literature available to suggest rather focused treatment guidelines regarding ADHD.

Following a thorough assessment of the child, the family, and the environment(s) in which the behavior difficulties occur, a treatment program should be developed that focuses on the target behavior problems that were identified in the assessment and that contributed to the diagnosis. The treatment program consists of a tripartite approach to this disorder, namely, psychostimulant medication, parent training in behavior management procedures, and classroom behavior management and teacher consultation (e.g., Barkley, 1990; DuPaul & Barkley, 1998; DuPaul et al., 1991). A fourth possible additional component of this treatment regimen involves individual relationship-oriented child therapy that includes self-instructional training; however, it should be pointed out that this component has received appreciably less empirical support in the treatment literature as being a necessary part of treatment. The tripartite treatment regimen places the child therapist in the role of "coordinator of services" and "consultant" where she or he (1) refers parents to a parent training program on behavior management; (2) refers the parents to a medical professional for a medication review of the child and the prescribing of psychostimulant medication; and (3) consults with school personnel on classroom management regarding the child's behavior.

The *parent training* component can be conducted on a group basis, where the parents are referred to an ongoing parent training program, or it can be conducted by the therapist on an individual basis with the parents. The majority of the training follows a behavior modification approach to the management of the child's behavior problems. Barkley (1981, 1990) outlines the specific aspects of an eight-session training program that need to be covered by the child therapist: (1) information about and overview of ADHD, (2) parent–child relations and behavior management principles, (3) establishing and improving parental attention to the child's behavior, (4) paying attention to the child's appropriate behavior, (5) developing a home-based token reinforcement program, (6) application of response cost and time-out programs, (7) managing the child's behavior in public situations, and (8) managing the child's future problem behaviors. This training is followed every 4 to 6 weeks with "booster" sessions where the therapist meets with the parents to review their progress in applying the behavior management procedures and to problem solve any difficulties that they may have.

The *classroom management* component of the treatment program for ADHD follows a consultation approach like that proposed by Bergan (e.g., Bergan, 1977; Bergan & Kratochwill, 1990) and involves problem solving the particular difficulties that the teacher or other school personnel are having with the child and developing a classroom management strategy for resolving the problem. The classroom management strategy that is typically recommended by the therapist is based on behavior modification principles.

The *medication* component of the treatment program is one of the more controversial aspects of the regimen, while also being the component that has an appreciable amount of research supporting its efficacy in enhancing particular cognitive, academic-related, and behavioral processes (DuPaul & Barkley, 1998; DuPaul et al., 1991). The stimulant medications most often prescribed for the treatment of ADHD, as well as the recommended dosage levels by child's weight, are listed in Table 3. The available data suggest that as long as these children remain on the medication—at times, from 2 to 10 years—the gains found in the cognitive, behavioral, and academic domains will be maintained; however, when the medication is discontinued, the observable gains decrease and sometimes revert back to the level that the child demonstrated when the medication was first initiated (DuPaul & Barkley, 1998).

The fourth, less empirically supported component, *relationship-oriented therapy* emphasizing self-instructional training, is applied to assist the child in addressing issues of low self-esteem, discouragement, poor or mediocre social relationships, and a home and classroom environment that often has been associated with negative feedback to the child. Play therapy is used with the child, where the emphasis is on rapport building and social skills training through modeling and behavior rehearsal. Problem-solving and self-instructional training are also often included and are ori-

TABLE 3. Stimulant Medications, Tablet Sizes, and Dose Ranges[a]

Brand name[b]	Tablet sizes	Dosage regimen	Dose range[c]
Ritalin	5 mg		2.5–25 mg
(methylphenidate)	10 mg		
	20 mg	Twice daily	
	SR 20 mg[d]	Once daily	20–40 mg
Dexedrine	5-mg spansule		2.5–25 mg
(dextroamphetamine)	10-mg spansule		
	15-mg spansul	Once daily	
	5-mg tablet		
	5-mg/5-ml (elixir)	Twice daily	2.5–25 mg
Cylert	18.75 mg		18.75–112.5 mg
(pemoline)	37.5 mg		
	75 mg	Once daily	

[a]Reprinted from DuPaul and Barkley (1998).
[b]Generic name in parentheses.
[c]Dose range for each administration is provided.
[d]SR, Slow release.

ented toward problematic situations that the child encounters in various settings (e.g., Kendall & Braswell, 1985; Morris & Morris, 1992).

Considerations

A child therapist's decision to treat a child having ADHD must take into consideration the long-term nature of the treatment and the high probability that the therapist will be associated with the child, family, and child's school for many years. It is therefore important that the therapist feels comfortable working with the child and family and that appropriate resources and services are available to support the therapeutic endeavor. The literature on the parent training component is limited to children between 3 and 11 years of age. For older children, a combination of family therapy following a family systems or Adlerian therapy model and individually oriented cognitive–behavioral therapy emphasizing problem solving and self-instructional training may be helpful. It should be noted, however, that appreciably less research literature is available regarding the treatment of adolescents having ADHD.

The child therapist also should be aware of possible comorbidity issues associated with ADHD. Concurrent behavior problems such as depression, oppositional behavior, and conduct problems, as well as academic underachievement and related learning problems, have been noted in the literature (see, for example, Abikoff & Klein, 1992; Hinshaw, 1992). The presence of these and/or other comorbid behaviors and learning problems should be ruled-out during the initial assessment.

Last, if medication is being considered for a child or adolescent, one must take into account a number of issues, such as: (1) if the child therapist is not the prescribing physician, then the child therapist must make sure that the treating physician is in agreement with the overall treatment program being applied, the child therapist's therapeutic framework and philosophy regarding the child's psychotherapeutic treatment, and with the fact that the physician is part of the treatment team (the others, in the case of an ADHD child, being the child therapist, parents, teacher(s), child, and significant others); (2) the parent's support of the use of medication for their child; (3) the potential side effects of the medication; (4) what objective measures will be used to determine the effectiveness of the medication; (5) the initial dosage level used; (6) the length of time of the trial use of the medication to determine its relative effectiveness; (7) whether the child or adolescent can take the medication safely; (8) whether there is sufficient family monitoring and supervision of the child's or adolescent's use of the medication; and (9) whether the medication will be taken in the prescribed manner and under the conditions imposed by the physician.

Childhood Depression

Although interest in the treatment of childhood depression has increased tremendously over the past decade, the amount of child therapy research published in this area is relatively limited (see, for example, Kaslow & Rehm, 1991; Kazdin, 1989; Reynolds, 1990; Stark, Dempsey, & Christopher, 1993). The major symptom of this behavior disorder is the same as it is with adults, namely, dysphoric mood that is also associated with various physical, behavioral, and cognitive symptom clusters. It is estimated that approximately one out of six children (16.66%) who are seen in a psychiatric setting has a diagnosis of depression (Reynolds, 1990). In addition, among elementary school-age children, there does not appear to be a gender difference in prevalence rates; however, for adolescents, females tend to have more depressive symptoms than males.

Definition and Characteristics

Various definitions of childhood depression have been discussed in the literature (see, for example, Kaslow & Rehm, 1991; Kendall, Cantwell, & Kazdin, 1989; Reynolds, 1990). One of the problems associated with clearly defining the term "depression" is the mixed use of the word as both a descriptor of behavior (i.e., symptom) and a cluster of behaviors (i.e., syndrome or behavior disorder). Although depressive symptoms in children and adults are generally similar, the manner in which particular symptoms are manifested may vary in children according to their respective age grouping; however, Stark et al. (1993) report that "[o]ver 90% of the depressed youths that have participated in our research ... have reported low self-esteem" (p. 115). They further point out that many depressed youth also report feelings of worthlessness.

A review of the childhood depression literature suggests that the most common definition used for this behavior disorder is the one listed in the *Diagnostic and Statistical Manual of Mental Disorders*, 4th edition (DSM-IV) (APA, 1994). This view of depression indicates that a child must manifest at least two continuous weeks of depressed mood or irritable mood, or loss of interest or pleasure in most activities, compared with previous functioning, plus at least four of the following symptoms: (1) significant weight loss not due to dieting, or weight gain, or failure to achieve expected weight gains, or increase or decrease in appetite almost every day; (2) insomnia or hypersomnia almost each day; (3) psychomotor retardation or agitation each day; (4) loss of energy or fatigue almost every day; (5) feelings of worthlessness or excessive or inappropriate guilt; (6) diminished ability to concentrate, or being indecisive, almost every day; (7) recurrent thoughts of death or recurrent suicide ideation, or a suicide attempt or a specific plan for committing suicide (APA, 1994, p. 327).

Treatment Approaches

Compared to other childhood behavior disorders, there are relatively few psychotherapy outcome studies published on childhood depression, although a number of studies have been published on the use of antidepressant medication. The treatment guidelines discussed in this section should therefore be viewed with caution.

Of the psychotherapy approaches discussed in the literature, the ones that have received increasing attention involve cognitive and cognitive–behavior therapy approaches and problem solving/skills training approaches (see, for example, Kaslow & Rehm, 1991; Kazdin, 1989; Stark et al., 1993). The *cognitive therapy* approach follows Beck's model (e.g., Beck, Rush, Shaw, & Emery, 1979) and examines the distorted cognitions and related attributions that a child may have about his or her current life experiences, as well as the cognition associated with the child's low level of self-esteem and feelings of helplessness and rejection. An alternative *cognitive–behavioral* approach follows the self-control model of Rehm (1977). This model assumes that depression results from deficits in such self-control areas as self-evaluation, self-monitoring, self-reinforcement, and attributions. Therapy, therefore, would focus on teaching children adaptive skills with regard to the way in which they self-monitor, self-reinforce, self-evaluate, and attribute the causes of good and bad outcomes. These skills are taught during the therapy session and homework assignments are initiated to assist the children in practicing the self-control procedures in those settings in which they feel depressed (e.g., Kaslow & Rehm, 1991; Stark, Reynolds, & Kaslow, 1987).

Another cognitive–behavioral approach follows the rational–emotive therapy work of Ellis (e.g., Bernard & Joyce, 1993). In this procedure, the child therapist examines the irrational statements that the child makes about himself, such as, "No one is really interested in who I am or what I have to say. Even if someone did become interested, he would soon discover—as I already know—that I am not worth it" (Bernard & Joyce, 1993). The *problem solving/skills training* approach involves the identification of the problematic social skills that a child manifests and teaching him or her to respond in a manner that is more likely to lead on a regular basis to positive reinforcement and feedback from significant others in his or her environment. Modeling, role playing, and social reinforcement are also used in this approach to assist in the education of the children (e.g., Frame, Matson, Sonis, Fialkov, & Kazdin, 1980; Kaslow & Rehm, 1991).

Other treatment approaches, such as psychoanalysis, Adlerian therapy, and client-centered therapy, also have been utilized in the treatment of childhood depression; however, given the paucity of research on the efficacy of these approaches, as well as the lack of comparison outcome studies between these latter procedures and the cognitive, cognitive–behavioral and behavior therapies, no conclusions can be made regarding the relative effectiveness of any one of these procedures over the others.

With respect to *pharmacological treatment*, placebo-controlled findings involving the use of tricyclic antidepressants have failed to demonstrate that tricyclics are effective in reducing the symptoms of depression in prepubertal children having major depression (Pomeroy & Gadow, 1998). On the other hand, according to Pomeroy and Gadow (1998) some promising results have been published using selective serotonin reuptake inhibitors (SSRIs), such as Prozac (fluoxetine) and Zoloft (sertraline). They indicate that results published by several researchers (e.g., Elmslie, Kowatch, Costello, Travis, & Pierce, 1995a; Elmslie et al., 1995b; Tierney, Joshi, Llinas, Rosenberg, & Riddle, 1995) have suggested that both prepubertal children and adolescents show a positive antidepressant response to these medications. Pomeroy and Gadow (1998), however, indicate that the use of SSRIs are not presently approved by the Federal Drug Administration (FDA) for use with children.

With respect to adolescents, according to Pomeroy and Gadow (1998), there is some disagreement in the field regarding the relative effectiveness of tricyclic antidepressants with adolescents, and there is encouraging findings regarding the use of SSRIS, where the side effects of these latter drugs appear to be less serious. Monoamine oxidase inhibitors (MAOIs) are rarely used with adolescents.

Considerations

Before any child therapy method is chosen to treat depression, particular attention should be given to the child's age and developmental level to determine whether the child is developmentally ready to participate in the type of therapy proposed. The parents of the child also need to be seen in therapy, since the cognitive strategies and/or behaviors that the child manifests may be modeled from the parents; therefore, the parents may need to learn alternative strategies for teaching their child how to more effectively deal with various life events. The parents also may need to be taught how to deal more effectively with conflict between one or both of them and their child.

The child therapist also should be aware of possible comorbidity issues associated with childhood depression. For example, concurrent behavior problems such as ADHD, oppositional behavior, phobia, and conduct problems, as well as mild learning problems, have been noted in some cases. The presence of these and/or other comorbid behaviors should be ruled-out during the initial assessment. Last, if medication is recommended or being considered, the same precautions and concerns mentioned in the ADHD section above should be reviewed by the child therapist before proceeding with such treatment.

Conduct Disorder

One of the most frequently occurring childhood behavior disorders is conduct disorder. This disorder accounts for a large percentage of those children who are described by their teachers as being "difficult to teach," described by their parents as being "difficult to control," described by people within the legal system as being "juvenile delinquents," and described by their school peers and others as being "aggressive," "troublesome," and/or "involved in illegal activity" (see, for example, Kazdin, 1991a, 1998; McConaughy & Skiba, 1993; Short & Shapiro, 1993; Webster-Stratton, 1993). The behaviors of these children clearly deviate from those found in the typical classroom or home setting, especially with respect to the frequency, severity, duration, social appropriateness, developmental appropriateness, and/or chronicity of the behaviors.

It is estimated that 3 to 10% (approximately 1.3 to 1.8 million children) of all school-age children in the United States demonstrate a pattern of behaviors that are consistent with the diagnosis of conduct disorder, with the disorder occurring approximately three times more often in boys than in girls under 10 years of age. For adolescents, however, the disorder appears to occur in equal numbers in both males and females. In addition, it is estimated that between 33 and 73% of all clinic referrals involve children who have the diagnosis of conduct disorder (e.g., Kazdin, 1998; Kazdin, Siegel, & Bass, 1992; McConaughy & Skiba, 1993; Short & Shapiro, 1993; Webster-Stratton, 1993). This disorder also appears to be fairly stable over time (e.g., Kazdin, 1998; Kazdin, Siegel, & Bass, 1992; McConaughy & Skiba, 1993; Short & Shapiro, 1993), and that teachers have approximately two children per year in their classrooms that demonstrate behavioral characteristics consistent with conduct disorder (Webster-Stratton, 1993).

Definition and Characteristics

Increasingly, writers have construed conduct disorder as a series of behaviors that are antisocial, chronic, and impair the child's educational performance and social interactions (e.g., Kazdin, 1998; McConaughy & Skiba, 1993; Short & Shapiro, 1993; Webster-Stratton, 1993). The DSM-IV indicates that this disorder involves "[a] repetitive and persistent pattern of behavior in which the basic rights of others or major age-appropriate societal norms or rules are violated ..." (APA, 1994, pp. 90–91). In order to make this diagnosis, according to the DSM-IV, a child must manifest at least three of the following behavioral characteristics over the past 12 months, and at least one of the following characteristics over the past 6 months: (1) often bullies or threatens others, (2) has frequently started physical fights, (3) has used a weapon on or toward another person, (4) being physically cruel to people, (5) being physically cruel to animals, (5) stealing from another person when the person is present, (6) forcing a person into sexual activity, (7) involved in fire setting, (8) has destroyed other's property, (9) has broken into a person's house or car, (10) has lied to obtain goods, (11) has engaged in shoplifting, (12) has stayed out all night prior to 13 years of age without parent's consent, (13) has run away from home at least twice, and (14) has been truant from school starting before 13 years of age (APA, 1994).

With respect to comorbidity, it appears that a fairly large percentage of children with conduct disorder also demonstrate behavioral characteristics consistent with the diagnosis of ADHD or oppositional defiant disorder (e.g., Abikoff & Klein, 1992; McConaughy & Skiba, 1993; Webster-Stratton, 1993).

Treatment Approaches

Psychotherapy with a child diagnosed as having a conduct disorder is long term, multimodal, multidomain and costly; therefore, any treatment planning and/or guidelines must take into consideration the fact that short-term treatments have generally not been found to be effective over time (see, for example, Abikoff & Klein, 1992; Short & Shapiro, 1993; Webster-Stratton, 1993). Although numerous forms of child therapy have been applied to the treatment of conduct disorder, relatively few have an empirical basis to them with respect to outcome and generalization. Those procedures that appear to have some controlled outcome research associated with them will be discussed.

One of the most frequently discussed approaches involves the use of *parent management training* programs to modify the behavior of children having conduct problems. This approach follows from the theoretical literature on this disorder that posits that the behaviors often found in these children are developed and sustained within the family structure. Treatment, therefore, focuses on family issues, interparental conflict, child-rearing practices, family violence, child–spousal abuse, parental inconsistency, and parent psychological difficulties (see, for example, Forehand & McMahon, 1981; Kazdin, 1998; Long, Forehand, Wierson, & Morgan, 1994; Patterson, 1982; Patterson & Chamberlain, 1994; Webster-Stratton, 1993, 1994). For example, Patterson's parent training program (e.g., Patterson, 1982; Patterson & Chamberlain, 1994) involves learning: (1) how to identify and track target behaviors; (2) the use of reinforcement procedures; (3) the application of discipline practices; (4) the systematic application of monitoring and supervising of children and being sensitized regarding where the child is at when the child is/is not at home; and (5) how to problem solve situations that the parent(s) and child might find themselves in and how to negotiate with their child. The essence of this approach involves an educational/child management perspective for parents, as well as the fact that the parents are the primary target of treatment versus the child. In addition, the parent training sessions involve practice and performance feedback following the implementation of procedures in the home.

Although empirical evidence exists supporting the efficacy of parent management training procedures, certain issues arise for some parent participants (e.g., Abikoff & Klein, 1992; Kazdin, 1998; Webster-Stratton, 1993). For example, parent training programs often require that parents attend each session, be consistent in their respective applications of the management procedures, cooperate with one another in implementing the procedures, practice what they have been taught between training sessions, collect data, have frequent telephonic contact with the parent trainer(s), and read the material that has been distributed to them at the training sessions. These latter treatment conditions may not be consistent with the lifestyle and/or level of motivation of some parent participants and may contribute to resistance and even treatment drop-out. Parents therefore should be informed before treatment begins of the various demands and time commitments of this treatment procedure in order that they may make a decision regarding their participation. Child therapists should also be aware of the limited generalization of treatment effects from the home environment to other settings such as the school when parent management training is used (Webster-Stratton, 1993). If treatment gains are also expected in the school setting, for example, then additional treatment procedures need to be implemented that are specific to this other setting.

A second procedure that has ben discussed in the literature is *family therapy* (e.g., Henggeler & Borduin, 1990; Kazdin, 1998; Webster-Stratton, 1993). Although parent management training programs appear to be relatively effective in changing children's home-based conduct problems, there are some families for whom this form of treatment does not seem to work. This includes those families whose lifestyle, as described above, is not consistent with the conditions under which parent management training is conducted. It also includes families in which there is marital stress, spouse abuse, individual parent life stress, a marital partner who is not supportive of the other partner, financial difficulties, and/or psychological depression in one or both spouses (e.g., Webster-Stratton, 1993, 1994). The assumption underlying this approach is that the communication patterns and channels between family members is dysfunctional and that the family has difficulties managing stress (Dumas, 1989). The goal, therefore, is to identify various dysfunctional behaviors and alliances within the family, modify maladaptive communications, and train family members in more adaptive family functioning (e.g., Alexander & Parsons, 1982; Everett & Volgy, 1993; Henggeler & Borduin, 1990; Kazdin, 1998). Therapy often follows a family systems approach (e.g., Everett & Volgy, 1993; Henggeler & Borduin, 1990) and includes modeling and performance feedback and reinforcement on the part of both the therapist and various family members, as well as the learning of negotiation skills, more effective methods of communication, and the examination of family member's attributes and expectations regarding each other.

With regard to treatment outcome, few studies have been published that support the relative effectiveness of this procedure, although those studies that have ben performed suggest improvement in family communication patterns following treatment (e.g., Henggeler, Melton, & Smith, 1992; Kazdin, 1998; Webster-Stratton, 1993, 1994). Clearly, more research is necessary on the relative effectiveness of this procedure, but it nevertheless appears to be a viable alternative for those parents and/or families who choose not to participate in parent management training or do not improve following such training.

A third treatment approach involves *social skills training* (e.g., Gardner & Cole, 1988; Goldstein & Pentz, 1984; Goldstein, Sprafkin, Gershaw, & Klein, 1980; Kazdin,

1998; McMahon & Wells, 1989). This approach typically involves the teaching of specific social skills that are assessed as being deficient or poorly developed in the particular children being treated. Each skill is broken down into steps and then each step is taught to the child. The skills training approach uses modeling and behavior rehearsal procedures based on Bandura's social learning theory (e.g., Bandura, 1969, 1977) as well as reinforcement, performance feedback, and self-regulation methods that are consistent with Skinner's operant conditioning approach (e.g., Kanfer & Phillips, 1970; Skinner, 1938, 1953). The models that are used are often actors or cohorts of the child therapist and the child is asked to model the behavior under a variety of conditions presented by the therapist or developed by the child. Methods for enhancing transfer of training, behavior generalization, and response maintenance also are included in this treatment program to maximize the treatment gains in the child's real-life situations. Although the empirical literature suggests that social skills training is an effective method for teaching conduct disordered children prosocial behaviors, generalization of the newly learned skills to the real-life situations of these children does not appear to have been assessed on a consistent or routine basis (e.g., Gardner & Cole, 1988; Kazdin, 1991a; McMahon & Wells, 1989). This suggests that the child therapist should proceed with caution in assuming that the effects found in the treatment setting will appreciably impact the child's behavior and lifestyle in his or her everyday interactions with people.

A fourth treatment approach is *cognitive–behavioral therapy*. Since a number of studies have suggested that conduct disordered children have poor problem solving skills, this approach makes use of various self-instructional and self-regulation techniques (see, for example, Kanfer & Phillips, 1970; Kendall & Braswell, 1985; Meichenbaum, 1975; Skinner, 1953) to change the behavior of these children. Specifically, the children are taught how to generate nonaggressive alterative solutions to interpersonal or other problematic situations. This is accomplished by teaching them a step-by-step approach to analyzing the particular situation they are in and developing a response that does not involve aggression (e.g., Kazdin, Esveldt-Dawson, French, & Unis, 1987; Kendall & Braswell, 1985).

The first step involves teaching the child to recognize what is a problem and/or when he or she is in an interpersonal or other problematic situation. Next, they are taught to generate various self-instructions or self-statements that prevent them from responding immediately or impulsively with aggression. They are then taught to attend to those aspects of the problem that can lead to meaningful nonaggressive effective solutions. In this step, the children are more specifically taught to develop multiple solutions to the problem and to analyze the possible consequences of each solution. They are then encouraged to choose one solution and subsequently to evaluate how well they did with resolving the original problem (e.g., Kazdin, 1998; Lochman & Curry, 1986). Throughout this approach, the child therapist actively participates with the child in modeling the sequence of cognitive problem-solving verbal statements and self-instructions associated with finding solutions to the problematic situation. The children are also encouraged to practice the sequences in the analogue-situation, followed by gradually applying them to the real-life situations that they typically encounter. The therapist and the child also review the child's attempts at applying the problem-solving strategy, and the child receives corrective feedback, reinforcement, and encouragement from the therapist for practicing the approach.

Although outcome research on this procedure with conduct disordered children is limited, the findings are nevertheless promising. Clearly, further research is needed on this method to substantiate its effectiveness and its response maintenance and generalization effects.

In terms of other therapeutic approaches, although operant conditioning approaches have been used with success within a residential setting for conduct disordered youth, it does not appear that the gains found in the residential setting are maintained after the youth are discharged and are back in their respective community (e.g., Abikoff & Klein, 1992). Reality therapy (e.g., Wubbolding, 1993) has also been used with conduct disordered children, but research supporting its relative efficacy is lacking. Medication also has been used with this population of youth, but no drug has been found to be clearly and reliably effective in reducing the frequency, intensity, and duration of children's conduct problems (e.g., Abikoff & Klein, 1992). A few drugs, however, have been reported to be relatively effective in the reduction of aggression, namely, the neuroleptics (e.g., Pomeroy & Gadow, 1998). Inderal, lithium, and Tegretol also have "shown some early promise of efficacy" in the control of intermittent outbursts of violence (Pomeroy & Gadow, 1998).

Considerations

Since few comparison outcome studies have been published, no statement can be made about the relative effectiveness of one therapeutic procedure over the other. In addition, it should be noted that the majority of the research in this area has been conducted on preadolescent versus adolescent samples. It therefore is not clear which procedures work effectively with the adolescent population. This suggests that child therapists need to start intervention programs earlier with younger children, based on various early risk factors for the development of conduct disorder (see, for example, Short & Shapiro, 1993; Abikoff & Klein, 1992).

SUMMARY AND CONCLUSIONS

In this chapter we have presented an overview of treatment guidelines regarding the provision of psychological services to children. Clearly, much progress has been made in the past 20–25 years in identifying effective treatment procedures. What has also emerged is the fact that one particular therapeutic approach cannot be used for all childhood behavior problems under all possible conditions. Specific types of child therapy procedures are increasingly emerging as the treatment of choice for the effective treatment of particular behavior problems. This is consistent with the early adult psychotherapy research literature that suggested that treatment use or choice be determined, for example, by the client's presenting problem, family history and demographic variables, and environmental constraints on the therapist. The child therapy literature also suggests that independent of the type of therapy method chosen, the child therapist should be conducting therapy within the framework of a sound therapeutic relationship.

The literature further suggests that the child therapist needs to be sensitized to comorbidity issues, since such covariate behavior problems may interfere with the effectiveness of any planned therapy and may necessitate a change in the treatment plan for a child. One important implication of the emerging trends in practice guidelines regarding child therapy is that future child therapists will need to be trained in a variety of child therapies, not just different therapy procedures within one particular theoretical orientation. Similarly, child therapy predoctoral academic programs, predoctoral internships, and postdoctoral training programs may need to diversify in order that their respective practitioner–students are well trained for the clientele that they will be seeing in treatment.

The area of child therapy has made great progress toward the development of treatment guidelines, and we fully expect this progress to continue, especially in the area of outcome and comparison outcome research.

REFERENCES

Abikoff, H., & Klein, R. G. (1992). Attention-deficit hyperactivity and conduct disorder: Comorbidity and implications for treatment. *Journal of Consulting and Clinical Psychology, 60*, 881–892.

Alexander, J. F., & Parsons, B. V. (1982). *Functional family therapy*, Monterey, CA: Brooks/Cole.

Allen, F. H. (1942). *Psychotherapy with children*. New York: Ronald Press.

American Psychiatric Association. (APA). (1994). *Diagnostic and statistical manual of mental disorders* (4th ed.). Washington, DC: Author.

Arambula, D., DeKraai, M., & Sales, B. (1993). Law, children, and therapists. In T. R. Kratochwill & R. J. Morris (Eds.), *Handbook of psychotherapy with children and adolescents* (pp. 583–619). Boston: Allyn & Bacon.

Ayllon, T., & Michael, J. (1959). The psychiatric nurse as a behavioral engineer. *Journal of the Experimental Analysis of Behavior, 2*, 342–352.

Axline, V. (1947). *Play therapy*. Boston: Houghton Mifflin.

Azrin, N. H., & Lindsley, O. R. (1956). The reinforcement of cooperation between children. *Journal of Abnormal and Social Psychology, 52*, 100–102.

Bandura, A. (1969). *Principles of behavior modification*. New York: Holt.

Bandura, A. (1977). *Social learning theory*. Englewood Cliffs, NJ: Prentice-Hall.

Barkley, R. A. (1981). *Hyperactive children: A handbook for diagnosis and treatment*. New York: Guilford.

Barkley, R. A. (1990). *Attention-deficit hyperactivity disorder: A handbook of diagnosis and treatment*. New York: Guilford.

Beck, A. T., Rush, A. G., Shaw, B. F., & Emery, G. (1979). *Cognitive therapy of depression*. New York: Guilford.

Bergan, J. R. (1977). *Behavioral consultation*. Columbus, OH: Merrill.

Bergan, J. R., & Kratochwill, T. R. (1990). *Behavior consultation and therapy*. New York: Plenum Press.

Bernard, M. E., & Joyce, M. R. (1993). rational–emotive therapy with children and adolescents. In T. R. Kratochwill & R. J. Morris (Eds.), *Handbook of psychotherapy with children and adolescents* (pp. 221–246). Boston: Allyn & Bacon.

Bijou, S. W. (1955). A systematic approach to an experimental analysis of young children. *Child Development, 26*, 161–168.

Casey, R. J., & Berman, J. S. (1985). The outcome of psychotherapy with children. *Psychological bulletin, 98*, 388–400.

Charlop-Christy, M. H., Schreibman, L., Pierce, K., & Kurtz, P. F. (1998). In R. J. Morris & T. R. Kratochwill (Eds.), *The practice of child therapy* (3rd ed., pp. 271–302). Boston: Allyn & Bacon.

Cole, C. L., & Gardner, W. (1993). Psychotherapy with developmentally delayed children. In T. R. Kratochwill & R. J. Morris (Eds.), *Handbook of psychotherapy with children and adolescents* (pp. 426–471). Boston: Allyn & Bacon.

D'Amato, R. C., & Rothlisberg, B. A. (Eds.). (1992). *Psychological perspectives on intervention*. New York: Longman.

Dumas, J. E. (1989). Treating antisocial behavior in children: Child and family approaches. *School Psychology Review, 8*, 197–222.

DuPaul, G. L., Guevremont, D. C., & Barkley, R. A. (1991). Attention deficit hyperactivity behavior. In T. R. Kratochwill (Eds.), *The practice of child therapy* (3rd ed., pp. 115–143). Boston: Allyn & Bacon.

DuPaul, G. L., & Barkley, R. A. (1998). Attention deficit hyperactivity behavior. In R. J. Morris & T. R. Kratochwill (Eds.), *The practice of child therapy* (3rd ed., pp. 132–166). Boston: Allyn & Bacon.

Edelbrock, C., Costello, A. J., Dulcan, M. K., Kalas, R., & Conover, N. C. (1985). Age differences in the reliability of the psychiatric review of the child. *Child Development, 56*, 265–275.

Ellis, A. (1962). *Reason and emotion in psychotherapy*. New York: Stuart.

Elmslie, G. J., Kowatch, R., Costello, L., Travis, G., & Pierce, L. (1995a). *Double-blind study of fluoxetine in depressed children and adolescents*. Paper presented at the annual meeting of the American Academy of Child and Adolescent Psychiatry, New Orleans, LA.

Elmslie, G. J., Rush, H. A., Weinberg, W., Kowatch, R., Hughes, C., & Rintelmann, J. (1995b). *Efficacy of fluoxetine in depressed children and adolescents*. Paper presented at the annual meeting of the American Academy of Child and Adolescent Psychiatry, New Orleans, LA.

Evans, I. M., & Nelson, R. O. (1986). Assessment of children. In A. R. Ciminero, K. S. Calhoun, & H. E. Adams (Eds.), *Handbook of behavioral assessment* (2nd ed., pp. 601–630). New York: Wiley.

Everett, C. A., & Volgy, S. A. (1993). Treating the child in systemic family therapy. In T. R. Kratochwill & R. J. Morris (Eds.), *Handbook of psychotherapy with children and adolescents* (pp. 247–257). Boston: Allyn & Bacon.

Fauber, R. L., & Long, N. (1991). Children in context: The role of the family in child psychotherapy. *Journal of Consulting and Clinical Psychology, 59*, 830–841.

Forehand, R., & McMahon, R. J. (1981). *Helping the noncompliant child: A clinician's guide to parent training*. New York: Guilford.

Frame, C. L., & Matson, J. L. (Eds.). (1987). *Handbook of assessment in childhood psychopathology*. New York: Plenum Press.

Frame, C., Matson, J. L., Sonis, W. A., Fialkov, M. J., & Kazdin, A. E. (1980). Behavioral treatment of depression in a prepubertal child. *Journal of Behavior Therapy and Experimental Psychiatry, 3*, 329–243.

Gardner, W. I., & Cole, C. L. (1988). Conduct disorder: Psychological therapies. In J. L. Matson (Ed.), *Handbook of treatment approaches in childhood psychopathology* (pp. 163–194). New York: Plenum Press.

Gibbs, J. T., & Huang, L. N. (1989). A conceptual framework for assessing and treating minority youth. In J. T. Gibbs & L. N. Huang (Eds.), *Children of color* (pp. 1–29). San Francisco: Jossey-Bass Publishers.

Goldstein, A. P., Heller, K., & Sechrest, L. (1966). *Psychotherapy and the psychology of behavior change*. New York: Wiley.

Goldstein, A. P., & Pentz, M. A. (1984). Psychological skill training and the aggressive adolescent. *School Psychology Review, 13*, 311–323.

Goldstein, A. P., Sprafkin, R. P., Gershaw, N. J., & Klein, P. (1980). *Skillstreaming the adolescent: A structured learning approach to teaching prosocial skills*. Champaign, IL: Research Press.

Graziano, A. M. (Ed.). (1971). *Behavior therapy with children*. Chicago: Aldine-Atherton.

Henggeler, S. W., & Borduin, C. M. (1990). *Family therapy and beyond: A multisystemic approach to treating the behavior problems of children and adolescents*. Pacific Grove, CA: Brooks Cole.

Henggeler, S. W., Melton, G. B, & Smith, L. A. (1992). Family preservation using multisystemic therapy: An effective alternative to incarcerating serious juvenile offenders. *Journal of Consulting and Clinical Psychology, 60*, 953–951.

Hinshaw, S. P. (1992). Academic underachievement, attention deficits, and aggression: Comorbidity and implications for treatment. *Journal of Consulting and Clinical Psychology, 60*, 893–903.

Hightower, A. D., & Braden, J. (1991). Prevention. In T. R. Kratochwill & R. J. Morris (Eds.), *The practice of child therapy* (2nd ed., pp. 410–440). Boston: Allyn & Bacon.

Hull, C. (1943). *Principles of learning*. New York: Appleton-Century-Crofts.

Itard, J. M. C. (1962). *The wild boy of Aveyron* (*L'enfant sauvage*). (G. Humphrey & M. Humphrey, Trans.). New York: Appleton-Century-Crofts.

Jacobsen, F. M. (1988). Ethnocultural assessment. In L. Comas-Diz & E. E. Griffith (Eds.), *Clinical guidelines in cross-cultural mental health* (pp. 135–147). New York: Wiley.

Johnson, J. H., Rasbury, W. C., & Siegel, L. J. (1986). *Approaches to child treatment*. New York: Pergamon Press.

Jones, M. C. (1924). A laboratory study of fear: The case of Peter. *Journal of Genetic Psychology, 31*, 308–315.

Kanfer, F. H., & Phillips, J. S. (1970). *Learning foundations of behavior therapy*. New York: Wiley.

Kanfer, F. H., & Schefft, B. K. (1988). *The basics of therapy*. Champaign, IL: Research Press.

Kaslow, N. J., & Rehm, L. P. (1991). Childhood depression. In T. R. Kratochwill & R. J. Morris (Eds.), *The practice of child therapy* (2nd ed., pp. 43–75). Boston: Allyn & Bacon.

Kauffman, J. M. (1981). *Characteristics of children's behavior disorders*. Columbus, OH: Merrill.

Kazdin, A. E. (1989). Childhood depression. In E. J. Mash & R. A. Barkley (Eds.), *Treatment of childhood disorders* (pp. 135–166). New York: Guilford.

Kazdin, A. E. (1991a). Aggressive behavior and conduct disorder. In T. R. Kratochwill & R. J. Morris (Eds.), *The practice of child therapy* (2nd ed., pp. 174–221). Boston: Allyn & Bacon.

Kazdin, A. E. (1991b). Effectiveness of psychotherapy with children and adolescents. *Journal of Consulting and Clinical Psychology, 59,* 785–798.

Kazdin, A. E. (1993). Research issues in child psychotherapy. In T. R. Kratochwill & R. J. Morris (Eds.), *Handbook of psychotherapy with children and adolescents* (pp. 541–565). Boston: Allyn & Bacon.

Kazdin, A E. (1998). Conduct disorder. In R. J. Morris & T. R. Kratochwill (Eds.), *The practice of child therapy* (3rd ed., pp. 199–230). Boston: Allyn & Bacon.

Kazdin, A. E., Esveldt-Dawson, K., French, N. H., & Unis, A. S. (1987). Problem-solving skills training and relationship therapy in the treatment of antisocial child behaviors. *Journal of Consulting and Clinical Psychology, 55,* 76–85.

Kazdin, A. E., Siegel, T. C., & Bass, D. (1990). Drawing on clinical practice to inform research on child and adolescent psychotherapy: Survey of practitioners. *Journal of Consulting and Clinical Psychology, 21,* 189–198.

Kazdin, A. E., Siegel, T., & Bass, D. (1992). Cognitive problem-solving skills training and parent management training in the treatment of antisocial behavior in children. *Journal of Consulting and Clinical Psychology, 60,* 733–747.

Kendall, P. C. (Ed.). (1992). *Child and adolescent therapy: Cognitive–behavioral procedures.* New York: Guilford.

Kendall, P. C., & Braswell, L. (1985). *Cognitive–behavioral therapy for impulsive children.* New York: Guilford.

Kendall, P. C., & Morris, R. J. (1991). Child therapy: Issues and recommendations. *Journal of Consulting and Clinical Psychology, 59,* 777–784.

Kendall, P. C., & Sesssa, F. M. (1993). Cognitive assessment for intervention. In T. R. Kratochwill & R. J. Morris (Eds.), *Handbook of psychotherapy with children and adolescents* (pp. 58–74). Boston: Allyn & Bacon.

Kendall, P. C., Cantwell, D. A., & Kazdin, A. E. (1989). Depression in children and adolescents: Assessment issues and recommendations. *Cognitive Therapy and Research, 13,* 109–146.

Kendall, P. C., Chansky, T. E., Kane, M. T., Kim, R. S., Kortlander, E., Roman, K. R., Sesssa, F. M., & Siqueland, L. (1992). *Anxiety disorders in youth: Cognitive–behavioral interventions.* New York: Allyn & Bacon.

Kenner, L. J. (1948). *Child psychiatry.* Springfield, IL: Charles C. Thomas.

King, N. J., Hamilton, D. I., & Ollendick, T. H. (1988). *Children's phobias: A behavioral perspective.* New York: Wiley.

Kratochwill, T. R., & Morris, R. J. (Eds.). (1991). *The practice of child therapy* (2nd ed.). Boston: Allyn & Bacon.

Kratochwill, T. R., & Morris, R. J. (Eds.). (1993). *Handbook of psychotherapy with children and adolescents.* Boston: Allyn & Bacon.

Lachar, D. (1993). Symptom checklists and personality inventories. In T. R. Kratochwill & R. J. Morris (Eds.), *Handbook of psychotherapy with children and adolescents* (pp. 38–57). Boston: Allyn & Bacon.

Lochman, J. E., & Curry, J. F. (1986). Effects of social problem-solving training and self-instruction training with aggressive boys. *Journal of Clinical Psychology, 15,* 159–164.

Long, P., Forehand, R., Wierson, M., & Morgan, A. (1994). Does parent training with young noncompliant children have long-term effects? *Behaviour, Research and Therapy, 32,* 101–107.

Lopez, S., & Hernandez, P. (1986). How culture is considered in evaluations of psychopathology. *Journal of Nervous and Mental Disease, 176,* 598–606.

Lovass, O. I., & Bucher, B. D. (Eds.). (1974). *Perspectives in behavior modification with deviant children.* Englewood Cliffs, NJ: Prentice-Hall.

Marin, G. (1992). Issues in the measurement of acculturation among Hispanics. In K. F. Geisinger (Ed.), *Psychological testing of Hispanics* (pp. 235–252). Washington, DC: American Psychological Association.

Marks, I. M. (1969). *Fears and phobias.* New York: Academic Press.

Mash, E. J., & Barkley, R. A. (Eds.). (1989). *Treatment of childhood disorders.* New York: Guilford.

Matson, J. L. (Ed.). (1988). *Handbook of treatment approaches in childhood psychopathology.* New York: Plenum Press.

Matson, J. L., & Coe, D. A. (1991). Mentally retarded children. In T. R. Kratochwill & R. J. Morris (Eds.), *The practice of child therapy* (2nd ed., pp. 298–327). Boston: Allyn & Bacon.

McConaughy, S. H., & Skiba, R. J. (1993). Comorbidity of externalizing and internalizing problems. *School Psychology Review, 22,* 421–436.

McMahon, R. J., & Wells, K. C. (1989). Conduct disorders. In E. J. Mash & R. A. Barkley (Eds.), *Treatment of childhood disorders* (pp. 73–132). New York: Guilford.

McReynolds, R. A., Morris, R. J., & Kratochwill, T. R. (1989). Cognitive behavioral approaches to anxiety disorders in children. In J. Hughes (Ed.), *Handbook of cognitive behavioral approaches* (pp. 434–465). New York: Plenum Press.

Meichenbaum, D. (1975). Self-instructional methods. In F. H. Kanfer & A. P. Goldstein (Eds.), *Helping people change* (pp. 357–392). New York: Pergamon Press.

Miller, L. C., Barrett, C. L.,, & Hampe, E. (1974). Phobias in children in a prescientific era. In A. Davis (Ed.), *Child personality and psychopathology: Current topics* (pp. 89–134). New York: Wiley.

Mishra, S. P. (1980). The influence of examiner's ethnic attributes on intelligence test scores. *Psychology in the Schools, 17*, 117–122.

Morris, R. J. (1985). *Behavior modification with exceptional children: Principles and practices*. Glenview, IL: Scott, Foresman & Company.

Morris, R. J., & Collier, S. J. (1987). Assessment of attention deficit disorder and hyperactivity. In J. L. Matson & C. Frame (Eds.), *Handbook of assessment in clinical psychopathology* (pp. 271–321). New York: Plenum Press.

Morris, R. J., & Kendall, P. (1991). Clinical child psychology: Perspectives on child and adolescent therapy. *Journal of Consulting and Clinical Psychology, 59*, 763–765.

Morris, R. J., & Kratochwill, T. R. (Eds.). (1983a). *The practice of child therapy*. New York: Pergamon Press.

Morris, R. J., & Kratochwill, T. R. (1983b). *Treating children's fears and phobias. A behavioral approach*. New York: Pergamon Press.

Morris, R. J., & Kratochwill, T. R. (1998a). Fears and phobias. In R. J. Morris & T. R. Kratochwill (Eds.), *The practice of child therapy* (3rd ed., pp. 91–131). Boston: Allyn & Bacon.

Morris, R. J., & Kratochwill, T. R. (Eds.). (1998b). Historical context of child therapy. In R. J. Morris & T. R. Kratochwill (Eds.), *The practice of child therapy* (3rd ed., pp. 1–4). Boston: Allyn & Bacon.

Morris, R. J., & Kratochwill, T. R. (Eds.). (1998). *The practice of child therapy* (3rd ed.). Boston: Allyn & Bacon.

Morris, R. J., & Morris, Y. P. (1992). A behavioral approach to intervention. In R. C. D'Amato & B. A. Rothlisberg (Eds.), *Psychological perspective on intervention* (pp. 21–47). New York: Longman.

Morris, R. J., & Nicholson, J. (1993). The therapeutic relationship in child and adolescent psychotherapy: Research issues and trends. In T. R. Kratochwill & R. J. Morris (Eds.), *Handbook of psychotherapy with children and adolescents* (pp. 405–425). Boston: Allyn & Bacon.

Morris, R. J., Kratochwill, T. R., & Aldridge, K. (1988). Fears and phobias. In J. C. Witt, S. N. Elliott, & F. M. Gresham (Eds.), *Handbook of behavior therapy in education* (pp. 679–718). New York: Plenum Press.

Morse, W. C. (1993). Ecological approaches. In T. R. Kratochwill & R. J. Morris (Eds.), *Handbook of psychotherapy with children and adolescents* (pp. 320–355). Boston: Allyn & Bacon.

Mosak, H. H., & Maniacci, M. P. (1993). Adlerian child psychotherapy. In T. R. Kratochwill & R. J. Morris (Eds.), *Handbook of psychotherapy with children and adolescents* (pp. 162–184). Boston: Allyn & Bacon.

Mowrer, O. H. (1960). *Learning theory and behavior*. New York: Wiley.

Ollendick, T. H., & Cerny, J. A. (1981). *Clinical behavior therapy with children*. New York: Plenum Press.

Ollendick, T. H., King, N. J., & Yule, W. (Eds.). (1994). *International handbook of phobic and anxiety disorders*. New York: Plenum Press.

Patterson, G. R. (1982). *Coercive family process*. Eugene, OR: Casalia.

Patterson, G. R., & Chamberlain, P. (1994). A functional analysis of resistance during parent training therapy. *Clinical Psychology: Science and Practice, 1*, 53–70.

Paul, G. L. (1967). Outcome research in psychotherapy. *Journal of Consulting Psychology, 31*, 109–118.

Pavlov, I. P. (1927). *Conditioned reflexes*. (G. V. Anrep, Trans.). London: Oxford University Press.

Pomeroy, J. C., & Gadow, K. D. (1998). An overview of psychopharmacotherapy for children and adolescents. In R. J. Morris & T. R. Kratochwill (Eds.), *The practice of child therapy* (3rd ed., pp. 419–470). Boston: Allyn & Bacon.

Rehm, L. P. (1977). A self-control model of depression. *Behavior Therapy, 8*, 787–804.

Reynolds, W. M. (1990). Depression in children and adolescents: Nature, diagnosis, assessment, and treatment. *School Psychology Review, 19*, 158–173.

Rhodes, J. E., Reyes, O., & Jason, L. A. (1993). Prevention of childhood psychopathology. In T. R. Kratochwill & R. J. Morris (Eds.), *Handbook of psychotherapy with children and adolescents* (pp. 566–582). Boston: Allyn & Bacon.

Rogers, C. (1942). *Counseling and psychotherapy*. New York: Houghton Mifflin.

Short, R. J., & Shapiro, S. K. (1993). Conduct disorders: A framework for understanding and intervention in schools and communities. *School Psychology Review, 22*, 362–375.

Siegel, L. J. (1993). Psychotherapy with medically-at-risk children. In T. R. Kratochwill & R. J. Morris (Eds.), *Handbook of psychotherapy with children and adolescents* (pp. 472–501). Boston: Allyn & Bacon.

Skinner, B. F. (1938). *The behavior of organisms*. New York: Appleton-Century-Crofts.

Skinner, B. F. (1953). *Science and human behavior*. New York: Macmillan.

Sobocinski, M. R. (1990). Ethical principles in the counseling of gay and lesbian adolescents: Issues of autonomy, competence and confidentiality. *Professional Psychology: Research and Practice, 2*, 240–247.

Stark, K. D., Reynolds, W. M., & Kaslow, N. J. (1987). A comparison of the relative efficacy of self-control therapy and a behavioral problem solving therapy for depression in children. *Journal of Abnormal Child Psychology, 15*, 91–113.

Stark, K. D., Dempsey, M., & Christopher, J. (1993). Depressive disorders. In R. T. Ammerman, C. G. Last, & M. Hersen (Eds.), *Handbook of prescriptive treatments for children and adolescents* (pp. 115–143). Boston: Allyn & Bacon.

Tharp, R. G. (1991). Cultural diversity and treatment of children. *Journal of Consulting and Clinical Psychology, 59*, 799–812.

Tierney, E., Joshi, P. T., Llinas, J. F., Rosenberg, L. A., & Riddle, M. A. (1995). Sertraline for major depression in children and adolescents: Preliminary clinical experience. *Journal of Child and Adolescent Psychopharmacology, 5*, 13–27.

Vraniak, D., & Pickett, S. A. (1993). Improving interventions with American ethnic minority children: Recurrent and recalcitrant challenges. In T. R. Kratochwill & R. J. Morris (Eds.), *Handbook of psychotherapy with children and adolescents* (pp. 502–540). Boston: Allyn & Bacon.

Watson, J. B., & Raynor, R. (1920). Conditioned emotional reactions. *Journal of Experimental Psychology, 3*, 1–14.

Webster-Stratton, C. (1993). Strategies for helping early school-aged children with oppositional defiant and conduct disorders: The importance of home–school partnerships. *School Psychology Review, 22*, 437–457.

Webster-Stratton, C. (1994). Advancing videotape parent training: A comparison study. *Journal of Consulting and Clinical Psychology, 62*, 583–593.

Weiss, G., & Hechtman, L. (1993). *Hyperactive children grown up: ADHD in children, adolescents, and adults* (2nd ed.). New York: Guilford.

Weissberg, R. P., Caplan, M., & Harwood, R. L. (1991). Promoting competent young people in competence-enhancing environments: A systems-based perspective on primary prevention. *Journal of Consulting and Clinical Psychology, 59*, 830–841.

Westermeyer, J. (1987). Cultural factors in clinical assessment. *Journal of Consulting and Clinical Psychology, 55*, 471–478.

Witt, J. C., Elliott, S. N., & Gresham, F. M. (Eds.). (1988). *Handbook of behavior therapy in education*. New York: Plenum Press.

Wubbolding, R. E. (1993). Reality therapy with children. In T. R. Kratochwill & R. J. Morris (Eds.), *Handbook of psychotherapy with children and adolescents* (pp. 288–319). Boston: Allyn & Bacon.

14

Using Practice Guidelines for Quality Improvement in the Treatment of Depressive Disorders in Managed Delivery Systems

MICHAEL JOSPE

Managed care systems are increasingly shaping the ways in which behavioral and other health care services are delivered. As of this writing, about three quarters of all persons in the United States who have third-party health coverage receive treatment through some type of managed arrangement (Rosenblatt, 1997). With the growth of managed care has come a corresponding expansion in quality-related activities required (often as a result of external regulatory mandates) as a part of such arrangements. Almost a decade has passed since the first edition of the present volume was published (Stricker & Rodriguez, 1988), a time period in which the general notion of quality improvement has seen fairly widespread public acceptance and increased understanding. At the same time, the gap between quality management (QM) as a philosophy and QM as a regular practice is often quite wide. When QM programs are mandated as part of regulatory or accreditation oversight, they tend to be practiced only to the degree that service delivery organizations are required to do so.

It is not uncommon for QM programs to be based on a mistaken view that QM is defined by discrete but repetitive practices focused primarily on process- or outcome-assessment activities demonstrating compliance with mandates. In fact, QM is more correctly conceived of as a philosophical approach and organized program of ongoing activities that are essential and integral to service delivery itself. The errant view of QM may originate with the foreboding, intimidation, and resentment that many people involved in clinical service delivery feel when confronted with the reality of externally imposed, formalistic QM requirements. Such requirements may appear to have little to do with and, indeed, may be seen as antithetical to, the professional autonomy and clinical competence that practitioners seek to achieve in their day-to-day clinical work and consider the essence of their professionalism. Further, these requirements are often regarded as a hindrance to the flow of care and the ability of practitioners to make independent judgments regarding appropriate treatment for specific patients. Finally, such requirements are resented, particularly when they impose methodological or measurement-related activities intended to facilitate treat-

---

MICHAEL JOSPE • California School of Professional Psychology, Alhambra, California 91803

Handbook of Quality Management in Behavioral Health, edited by Stricker *et al.* Kluwer Academic / Plenum Publishers, New York, 2000.

ment planning and service delivery but which are regarded by practitioners as irrelevant and interfering.

WHY GUIDELINES FOR TREATING DEPRESSION ARE IMPORTANT

The following sections address simple ways in which QM principles can be integrated into the myriad clinical activities involved in the management of depression through the use of practice guidelines and the fundamental role played by such guidelines in routine service delivery in the context of a managed care program. The importance of depression guidelines is highlighted in a recent sourcebook focused on outcomes management and practice guidelines (Vibbert & Youngs, 1995). The authors state that depression

> ... appears again and again in these pages, and with good cause. Study after study shows that depression is under-recognized and under-treated, particularly by the gatekeeper [family practice or internal medicine] physicians who are now gaining so much power in managed care.... [It] is often a chronic disease.... [showing] more severe limitations of functional status than [diabetes, hypertension and chronic disease]. (p. ix)

Under this type of circumstance, particularly with regard to such a significant behavioral health disorder as depression, QM must be viewed as integral to treatment rather than as a "special" activity serving a policing function that interferes with provider autonomy. It is critical, in other words, to highlight the role of QM processes as regular, routine components of behavioral health care service delivery that improve the process of care.

Reframing QM as an organic process as integral to practice as diagnosis and treatment planning can serve to foster wider acceptance of the notions and processes of QM, feedback, and quality improvement. In fact, integration of practice guidelines can add significantly to both the cost-effectiveness and the ease of implementation of behavioral health diagnostic, treatment, and aftercare services, particularly in the context of a managed system. The aim of this chapter is to demonstrate how the strategic use of practice guidelines by behavioral health providers and care managers can help increase the likelihood that improved management of the process of care will be associated with the attainment of desired treatment outcomes.

A NEW AND BROADER DEFINITION OF PRACTICE GUIDELINES

Practice guidelines—normative statements about the process of clinical care—should, as Shueman and Troy (1994) have indicated, summarize appropriate practice. Such summaries should be based on a consideration of substantive research findings regarding intervention strategies as well as the consensus judgments of experts. Reviews of empirical research as to the efficacy of various treatments lead to evidence-based practice policies; evidence-based guidelines supplemented with quantitative estimates of the relative benefits and harms of alternative treatments lead to outcomes-based practice policies; and outcomes-based strategies that integrate data on patient preferences and attitudes lead to preference-based policies. It should be noted that this latter kind of practice policy, as yet, has found no application. Evidence- and outcomes-based policies are taken up later in the chapter.

Considerations such as these constitute only the foundation on which practice guidelines are based. An additional requirement for guidelines, necessary to make them practicable as well as salient to all concerned within the managed care context, is that they be formulated in such a way as to correspond as closely as possible to the actual process of care as manifest in both the clinical interventions of the treating practitioner and the utilization and case review activities of the specific managed care organization. This requirement allows these decision-oriented guidelines to include realistic consideration of benefit design as well as the ongoing QM needs of the managed care company.

Restricting the definition of practice guidelines to clinical interventions is too narrow a perspective for adoption in current managed care environments. The developing context means that, virtually for the first time in US history, a majority of clinical services provided by independent practitioners are being delivered in context of a system of care, however flawed. Consequently, guidelines must acknowledge and accommodate the needs of the system as well as the needs of the individual provider. This approach to guidelines leads to a new variation on Shueman and Troy's (1994) definition:

> Practice guidelines are evidence-based behavioral health service delivery policies that reflect input, process, and outcome variables which empirical evidence and expert clinical judgments indicate are significant. The guidelines are stated in ways that parallel a specific managed care organization's explicit process of care monitoring, facilitating their salience to behavioral health care professionals and, thus, their regular practical implementation in the diagnosis, treatment, and follow-up services covered by a patient's benefit plan.

Such guidelines are frequently used by providers, case management staff, and QM personnel in managed behavioral health care companies (see, for example, Kaye & Jospe, 1994, 1995; Jospe, 1997). They are written specifically to reflect not only desired clinical strategies for specific disorders but also the clinical management activities of the managed behavioral health care company. They are typically distributed to staff of these companies as well as their network providers in order to ensure that each party involved in a specific episode of care is working from a common set of principles and practices reflecting a unified approach to treatment planning and implementation.

Why Is Paralleling the Process of Care Important?

Practice guidelines should, in fact, be practiced routinely. Therefore, they should be written in a way that is useful to clinicians. Complex and highly refined practice guidelines such as the American Psychiatric Association's (1993) *Practice Guidelines for Major Depressive Disorders* are excellent examples of clinical and academic writing. So are the guidelines published by the Depression Guideline Panel (1993) of the US Department of Health and Human Services on depression in primary care. At the same time, these and many other guideline sets published to date suffer from at least four major shortcomings that make it unlikely that clinicians will be prompted to use them: they are too long; they are too complex; they do not parallel the typical flow of service delivery and care management found in clinical practice and managed behavioral health care arrangements; and they do not reflect that providers, case management staff, and quality assurance personnel require utilitarian statements that cut through the major research and clinical issues within a concise format, clearly explicating their implications for practice.

Managed care providers as well as case management staff involved in liaison, treatment review, benefit authorization, and consultation are simply too busy to read textbooklike documents and to discern how they can be applied in practice. At the same time, the continual service monitoring and collaboration between case manager and provider required with managed care arrangements cannot be effectively or efficiently implemented in the absence of clear, usable guidelines. Individuals responsible for the development and implementation of guidelines have found quite consistently that providers and case management staff in principle welcome such documents. Providers dislike guidelines that are too long and ambiguous, that complicate communications about service planning and provision by requiring reading of complex materials, or that do not acknowledge the time constraints inherent in the encounters and liaison between case managers and providers. Protracted dialogue between providers and case management staff leads to tensions and inefficiencies in the case management process.

CHARACTERISTICS OF USEFUL PRACTICE GUIDELINES

In order to maximize their usefulness to case management staff and providers alike, practice guidelines should have the following characteristics:

- They can be applied by all behavioral health care professionals, regardless of discipline.
- They are eclectic and are not written from the perspective of a single theoretical orientation.
- They are pragmatic, promoting desired actions and discouraging clinically risky or unusual practices.
- Their basis in empirical research obviates the need for individual providers and case managers to search extensively in the literature for support and guidance in their clinical actions.
- Their empirical focus is on findings relative to efficiency and cost-effectiveness in service delivery.
- They clearly convey to providers that explicit standards of care guide clinical decision making.
- They are clear and easy to use.
- Their practical utility facilitates the setting of performance standards that give case managers, providers, and others a common basis of understanding and expectations.
- They follow the specific monitoring processes of the managed care organization for which they are written.
- They allow the identification of acceptable quality.
- They encourage standardization of aspects of treatment plan formulation and implementation within the resource constraints of limited benefit plans and timelines.
- They are presented in formats (e.g., binders, software) that are immediately acceptable to providers, utilization management clinicians, and case management personnel.

- They are valued by health care professionals as assets to their day-to-day practice.
- They are aimed at improving the precision of care by eliciting a high degree of user compliance.
- They are regularly updated, increasing their usefulness to clinicians.
- They assist nonbehavioral health care providers, who frequently are also involved in care (e.g., primary care physicians), to better understand behavioral health care; they demystify issues related to collaboration and referral.

Misuse of Practice Guidelines

While practice guidelines can be useful and welcomed tools, particularly when they possess the features outlined above, they also can be misused. For example, Shueman and Troy (1994) suggest that guidelines can be mistakenly viewed as immutable, leading to implementation problems on the part of care managers (e.g., inappropriate denial of reimbursement for a technical but irrelevant deviation on a single criterion). Failure to understand either the spirit or specific focus of guidelines may also lead to problems for providers (e.g., apprehension about discussing a legitimate exception with a case manager for fear of having reimbursement denied). Clearly, rigid and inflexible use of guidelines is as problematic as failure to employ them.

Guidelines that are kept "secret" from network providers, particularly in the private sector, are worse than useless, since secrecy leads to suspicion and mistrust on the part of providers and may increase providers' sense of being "policed" by case managers. Clearly, the way to best ensure provider acceptance and use of practice guidelines is to involve those same providers in the process of guideline development, review, and revision.

Practitioners whose primary professional satisfaction comes from the "art" of care often are in particular need of support from the organizations that develop and mandate the use of guidelines. For example, it is essential for providers to receive proper training on guideline implementation to help them understand how to apply these principles in the context of their own established practice patterns (i.e., permitting providers to capitalize on the combination of "art" and "science" of care). Absent such training, providers may resent what they perceive as mandates to implement specific techniques without apparent regard for the providers' own theoretical biases, the nuances of the therapeutic relationship, and individual differences across patients. Such an attitude on the part of providers invariably leads to anger and resentment toward utilization review processes or care management staff who are responsible for evaluating compliance with guidelines.

Extending the implications of Shueman and Troy's (1994) cautions on misuse allows us to ascertain what practice guidelines are not:

- Practice guidelines are not recipes or prescriptions that dictate practice.
- They are not treatment strategies about which all providers will agree.
- They cannot, nor should they be, exhaustive treatises covering every aspect of diagnosis, treatment, and aftercare for a given condition.
- They are not rigid commands that exclude other treatment practices if those other practices can achieve similar cost-effective results.

- They are not tools for case management and quality improvement staff to police practitioner compliance.
- They are not mechanisms that inhibit or discourage clinical intuition, wise clinical practice, or the "art" of treatment.

ENHANCING QUALITY BY USING PRACTICE GUIDELINES IN TREATING DEPRESSIVE DISORDERS

Anyone attempting to ascertain current "best practices" on the diagnosis, treatment, and aftercare of depressive disorders is confronted by a host of sources—federal government guidelines, books, journal articles, workshops, pharmaceutical company publications, and continuing education courses—many of which describe conflicting theoretical and clinical approaches. The treatment of depression can be complex and difficult, and the health care organization's expectations of providers (particularly in the current practice context where the role of psychopharmacology is often debated) may be unclear. Providers may be uncertain about appropriate options in the face of the range of available treatment methodologies and the lack of clear role expectations with regard to collaborative treatment planning between medical and nonmedical providers. Early identification and treatment as well as appropriate aftercare take on increased importance with regard to this set of disorders. Misdiagnosis as well as under- or mistreatment of depressed patients may result in serious (though largely avoidable) consequences. Practice guidelines, then, assume a very powerful role because of their educational and clinical utility.

Professionals involved in the development of practice guidelines for managed care companies advocate an approach to depression guidelines that involves the whole temporal spectrum, from the initial presentation of the syndrome through the entire process of clinical care and management, and simultaneously integrates issues of quality and clinical utility. For example, Kaye and Jospe (1994) and Jospe (1997) conceptualize the flow of care, as well as the content of guidelines themselves, as follows:

1. *Access-related issues.* A sometimes complicating fact related to the treatment of behavioral health disorders is that accurate recognition of symptoms and understanding of their importance can significantly affect whether patients or those involved in their health care seek or refer for treatment and whether adequate treatment is received once help is sought. Symptomatology, therefore, is directly related to access to care. The presentation of depressive disorders can range from minor or subtle symptoms that may erroneously be assumed to be features of another condition, to serious syndromes that are both obvious in their presentation and difficult to treat if not identified and treated sufficiently early.

Variations in symptomatology among depressed patients may be more or less random or may be more systematically related to certain patient characteristics such as age. Guidelines, therefore, should specifically address systematic differences in presenting symptoms typically occurring in particular populations (for example, in the elderly) so that these symptoms will be correctly recognized as indicators of depression rather than as components of some other, perhaps medical, condition. Ethnic and cultural differences also may influence how a patient experiences and describes symptoms and, more importantly, whether and how he or she attempts to access services. Such differences in help-seeking behaviors are particularly relevant to traditionally underserved or minority populations. Their often limited financial resources may cause members of such groups to delay seeking services, and a lack of knowledge about relevant cultural factors among providers may impede their ability to accurately diagnose and appropriately treat.

An example of an access-related problem that can be obviated by proper use of guidelines is the misdiagnosis of sleep disorder in primary care. Difficulty with sleep is frequently treated in primary care by hypnotic or anxiolytic medication that can, in the presence of an actual depressive disorder, lead to an exacerbation of the problem (due to medication side effects or the failure to treat the other symptoms). The application of appropriate diagnostic guidelines can increase the probability of accurate recognition and timely intervention.

RECOMMENDATION: Practice guidelines should facilitate access to treatment by explicitly acknowledging both the factors that can interfere with recognition of the syndrome and the need to ensure referral to appropriate professionals (ideally, behavioral health specialists) for evaluation and treatment.

2. *Triage-related issues.* Given the increased risk of self-harm among people with severe depression, a critical need when dealing with patients presenting with depressive symptoms is to effectively discriminate those who require immediate, more intensive, or higher-level care. Practice guidelines, then, must focus on the assessment of established risk factors (e.g., suicidal ideation or plan; severe vegetative symptoms) and must provide protocols for making decisions regarding, for example, the need for a medication evaluation or a secure (24-hour supervised) environment and the need to involve a physician in the disposition when a patient has attempted suicide by an overdose of medication. Conversely, the existence of guidelines can help ensure that a patient who does not need immediate or higher-level care is offered access to appropriate, "routine" care, thereby preventing the use of unnecessarily costly resources.

RECOMMENDATION: Practice guidelines for depressive disorders should include information that facilitates appropriate triage decisions, regardless of the level and intensity of care required for the particular patient.

3. *Referral issues.* Appropriate treatment of depressive disorders may involve the integration of multiple treatment modalities and multiple providers. For example, certain features of depressive disorders frequently present as features of other psychological or physical disorders, and vice versa. Psychotic features in the presentation of some depressions also may be mistaken for features of other diagnoses (including organic conditions), and the diagnostic picture can be clarified significantly by practice guidelines.

For depressed patients with a coexisting medical problem (particularly the elderly), coordination of care with a specialist physician is essential. For others, a psychologist or social worker who is providing psychotherapy may need to decide if and when to refer for a medication evaluation and subsequently how to coordinate his or her services with those of the medical professional. The challenges of professional collaboration and coordination of care under such circumstances historically have tested service delivery in the private sector. That is, practitioners have not been particularly eager to refer their patients to other behavioral health professionals or to coordinate care with other professionals, either behavioral health or medical. A critical role, then, of practice policies is to address referral issues such as when to refer a patient for medication evaluation, when to involve a physician, and how to ensure coordination of care.

RECOMMENDATION: Practice guidelines should advocate restricting the referral of patients to those providers who have the competence and qualifications to treat the disorders in cost-effective ways. These guidelines should also indicate when collaborative care with other providers is critical, especially when considering pharmacotherapy and the treatment of depression in patients with medical conditions.*

4. *Assessment-related issues.* Because of the potential challenges in the differential diagnosis of depression, depressed patients should be referred to behavioral health professionals who have the skills and knowledge to address the spectrum of assessment-related issues particular to depression (see footnote). These include knowledge of culture- (when relevant) and age-related aspects of presentation; ability to discriminate between symptoms reflecting medical conditions and symptoms of depression; and knowledge of organically based neurological or general systemic conditions that directly or indirectly affect or mimic the symptoms of depression. In addition, providers should be sensitive to the need to assess the family's role in the problem of the identified patient, particularly when a family member denies the severity of the patient's condition or when family dynamics may be an exacerbating factor. Providers also must be able to discern stages of depressive disorders, particularly in cases where previous treatment has not been effective. Finally, practitioners doing assessments must be sensitive to issues related to the need for timely referrals for psychological testing, for medication evaluation with a psychiatrist, and for other medical consultation when symptoms may have a medical etiology.

RECOMMENDATION: Practice guidelines related to the treatment of depressive disorders should explicitly address the assessment issues involved, particularly in cases presenting complex assessment and differential diagnostic challenges.

5. *Diagnostic issues.* Providers commonly avoid using the *Diagnostic and Statistical Manual of Mental Disorders*, 4th edition (DSM-IV) (American Psychiatric Association, 1994) or other diagnostic systems, and may lack the knowledge or experience necessary to make valid diagnoses. Guidelines therefore can serve a particularly important function in facilitating communication between providers and the case management organization. They serve to focus the provider and the case manager on the most critical aspects of the clinical situation and highlight areas most likely to lead to diagnostic confusion. They can guide providers in the gathering of critical information from patients, family members, and medical providers. Finally, they can help ensure that all the potentially relevant diagnostic indicators have been considered and, as a consequence, assist the clinician in avoiding the more common diagnostic errors.

RECOMMENDATION: Practice guidelines for depression must include diagnostic justification criteria.

6. *Treatment issues: diagnosis specific.* Depressive disorders continue to be a focus of disputes about the relative efficacy of psychotherapeutic and pharmacological approaches, alone and in combination (Jarrett, 1995; also see Fava & Rosenbaum,

*In the case of severe depression there is compelling evidence that the early involvement of a behavioral health specialist is associated with improved outcome.

1995). Guidelines can promote an objective, empirically based determination of a patient's need relative to this question and avoid the traditional disagreements between provider and case manager that tend to be based on theoretical or discipline-specific biases. Guidelines should specify the treatments of choice and their role vis-à-vis individualized treatment plan development. They should also address the broad psychosocial issues that require consideration when formulating a comprehensive treatment plan, especially when incorporating the services of other health care practitioners in a collaborative way. The context in which symptoms occur and environmental and situational factors that need to be considered in the treatment plan can also be addressed in the guidelines.

While indications for the prescription of as well as contraindications for the use of medications are essential components of guidelines, they should also address other medication-related issues. Examples include the length of time typically required for patient response (a factor frequently related to patient noncompliance and treatment failure) and for continuation of maintenance medication. Treatment of the complex issues inherent in professional collaboration around the joint clinical management of depressed patients by providers (commonly, the physician–nonphysician dyad) is a central task of guidelines designed to advance the precision of intervention with such targets.

Since patient compliance is a critical variable affecting the treatment of depression, efficacious guidelines address issues of patient education as well as education of family members or carers and nonpsychiatric medical practitioners involved in the treatment of the patient. Guidelines need not prescribe specific educational interventions or foci. Rather, these should be determined by the provider, perhaps with case manager assistance.

7. *Treatment issues: generic.* Almost all managed care companies provide network practitioners with generic guidelines for the development and modification of treatment plans—initial, concurrent, discharge and follow-up. Issues typically addressed by guidelines at these four treatment stages include:

Initial treatment plan review: A range of critical issues need to be addressed early in treatment to help ensure that the provider makes effective use of the available benefit resources from the outset. These include:

- Thoroughness of the assessment (inclusion of all issues that can reasonably be known at a particular point in treatment).
- Extent to which diagnostic criteria for the specific depressive condition have been met.
- Evidence for medical necessity at prescribed level and intensity.
- Consideration of risk factors.
- Extent to which the treatment plan is feasible given the parameters of the benefit plan.

Concurrent review: One of the most important issues that guidelines can address is the provision of decision parameters addressing ways in which patient improvement will be assessed. Managed behavioral health care organizations vary in their requirements for this feature, but at all costs guidelines should emphasize how critical it is to avoid judging progress merely on the basis of statements such as "I feel better and less depressed," rather than assessing targeted changes on a mix of objective indicators. Specific issues addressed by concurrent review guidelines include:

- Evaluation of progress relative to indicators established at the beginning of treatment.
- Evaluation of patient compliance.
- Plans for discharge or referral to lower level of care.

The major risk areas at the point of concurrent review are undertreatment, particularly when depressed patients taking medication begin experiencing symptom relief; the increased risk of self-harm when patients who were previously emotionally and behaviorally disabled regain a sense of competence and direction; and, finally, the risk of noncompliance because of medication side effects and unrealistic expectations about both the efficacy and course of psychopharmacological treatments.

Discharge management and monitoring: Efficacious guidelines invariably address strategies to ensure maintenance of progress made in the active phase of treatment. Critical issues to be adduced at discharge include dealing with future stresses, the importance of medication compliance, and procedures for accessing care in the future.

RECOMMENDATION: Practice guidelines for treatment of depressive disorders should contain information concerning criteria supporting the development of individualized treatment plans (including the role of pharmacotherapy), collaborative care with other health care providers, establishing and monitoring realistic treatment goals, performing concurrent reviews that accurately identify hindrances to treatment, and ensuring high-quality discharge and follow-up care.

CONCLUSION

Practice guidelines will be of little consequence if providers are not trained in their rationale, their structure and format, and how they will be applied by the managed care organization. The same injunction applies to case managers: giving case managers guidelines to be used as tools but not training them in their rationale and use almost guarantees either resistance to using them or, more likely, misuse. Well-constructed practice guidelines, if accepted by both providers and managed care staff, can ultimately help to define a common base for collaboration in the interest of the patient. Failure to attend to the critical issues of implementation, however, increases the probability that these documents will be no more than a cause for disagreement and contention between the two parties.

The treatment of depressive disorders is an area of behavioral health care rife with risk, lack of knowledge on the part of providers, and significant inter- and intraprofessional disagreement about appropriate treatment. It is also an area, however, in which relatively recent empirical research has much to say about the contingencies associated with patient improvement. Consequently, the potential for empirically informed practice guidelines to advance the precision of depression management across the disciplinary spectrum is significant. The challenge for both providers and managed care organizations is to put aside the traditional conflicts and adopt a more collaborative approach to treatment planning and development based on these guidelines.

REFERENCES

American Psychiatric Association. (1993). *Practice guidelines for major depressive disorders*. Washington, DC: Author.

American Psychiatric Association. (1994). *Diagnostic and statistical manual of mental disorders* (4th ed.). Washington, DC: Author.

Depression Guideline Panel. (1993). *Depression in primary care: Vol. 1. Detection and diagnosis. Clinical practice guideline, Number 5* (AHCPR Publication No. 93-0550). Rockville, MD: US Department of Health and Human Services, Public Health Service, Agency for Health Care Policy and Research.

Fava, M., & Rosenbaum, J. F. (1995). Pharmacotherapy and somatic therapies. In E. E. Beckham & W. R. Leber (Eds.), *Handbook of depression* (2nd ed., pp. 280–301). New York: Guilford.

Jarrett, R. B. (1995). Comparing and combining short-term psychotherapy and pharmacotherapy for depression. In E. E. Beckham & W. R. Leber (Eds.), *Handbook of depression* (2nd ed., pp. 435–464). New York: Guilford.

Jospe, M. (1997). Practice guidelines for depressive disorders. In M. Jospe, *Plan 21 provider/case manager treatment reference guide*. Houston: Plan 21 Behavioral Health.

Kaye, D., & Jospe, M. (1994). *CMG clinical management guidelines*. Owings Mills, MD: CMG Health.

Kaye, D., & Jospe, M. (1995). Depressive disorders. In S. Vibbert & M. T. Youngs (Eds.), *The 1996 behavioral outcomes and guidelines sourcebook* (pp. E20–E54). New York: Faulkner & Gray.

Rosenblatt, R. (1997). Cost of health care for state's big firms falls 2.5% in 1996. *Los Angeles Times*, January 21, 1997.

Shueman, S. A., & Troy, W. G. (1994). The use of practice guidelines in managed behavioral health programs. In S. A. Shueman, W. G. Troy, & S. L. Mayhugh (Eds.), *Managed behavioral health care: An industry perspective* (pp. 149–164). Springfield, IL: Thomas.

Stricker, G., & Rodriguez, A. R. (Eds.). (1988). *Handbook of quality assurance in mental health*. New York: Plenum Press.

Vibbert, S., & Youngs, M.T. (1995). Introduction. In S. Vibbert & M. T. Youngs, (Eds.), *The 1996 behavioral outcomes and guidelines sourcebook* (pp. ix–x). New York: Faulkner & Gray.

IV

FOR THE GOOD OF THE PUBLIC

Regulating Bodies and Their Roles

15

Governmental Initiatives in the Area of Quality Assurance

Patrick H. DeLeon, Nancy K. Gilmore-Lee, Stephen A. Ragusea, and Paul A. Eckert

In addressing and conceptualizing the issue of quality assurance from a public policy frame of reference, it is important to appreciate the fundamentally different roles that the government (federal and state) can appropriately play in ensuring the delivery of *quality* health care. Few would disagree that both the federal government and the various state entities have a clear and distinct responsibility for ensuring that their direct beneficiaries receive necessary and appropriate health care. And many, but admittedly not all, of our colleagues also appreciate that the government does possess the authority, if it decides to utilize it, to explore (i.e., support) demonstration projects to ensure that within the health care system at large (including the private sector) services being provided within its geographic jurisdiction are of the highest quality possible.

At its conceptually cleanest extreme, since its creation in 1906 [PL 59-384], the federal Food and Drug Administration (FDA) has sought to ensure that drugs and later medical devices are safe and effective. At the state level, licensing boards seek to ensure that practitioners and facilities meet certain minimum educational and experiential standards and function competently. Nevertheless, as one reflects upon governmental efforts in this area over the past two decades, there clearly are signs of considerable policy ambivalence. Should health care practitioners be held to objective guidelines (i.e., standards), or should practitioners instead be "urged" to conform to subjective peer determinations of appropriateness? Should the government attempt to "mandate" clinician expectations and behaviors, or should individual patients be held "accountable" (after being provided with relevant information) for determining quality? Admittedly, many legislative and administrative steps have been taken; however, often in seemingly contradictory directions. Throughout, however, a fundamentally

The views expressed are those of the authors and do not represent the position of the US Government.

PATRICK H. DeLEON • American Psychological Association, Washington, DC 20002-4242. NANCY K. GILMORE-LEE • Office of Senator Inouye, Washington, DC 20510. STEPHEN A. RAGUSEA • Child, Adult, and Family Psychological Center, State College, Pennsylvania 16801. PAUL A. ECKERT • Office of Senator Breaux, Washington, DC 20510.

Handbook of Quality Management in Behavioral Health, edited by Stricker *et al.* Kluwer Academic / Plenum Publishers, New York, 2000.

educational (rather than prescriptive) approach seems to have prevailed in policy deliberations (DeLeon, Willens, Clinton, & VandenBos, 1988).

THE DEMONSTRATION APPROACH

Historically, the federal government and numerous private foundations have been quite active over the years in sponsoring demonstration projects focusing on ensuring that health services that are provided in this country are fundamentally safe and most recently cost-effective. Interestingly, with some notable exceptions, the various states have generally not been particularly active in this area. Perhaps this lack of state activity is due to the importance of having sufficient numbers of experiences from which to draw reasonable policy conclusions (i.e., access to patient "incidents"). In our judgment, however, this demonstrated hesitancy at the local level is more likely a direct result of the considerable political turmoil that often results whenever "scope of practice" findings are addressed.

An Example of a State Demonstration Initiative

An example of a state health professions demonstration initiative with far-reaching implications for quality mental health care was the effort by the California Office of Statewide Health Planning and Development in the late 1970s, to explore the efficacy of having various nonphysicians make medication determinations (State of California, 1982). Since this was a state-sponsored demonstration project, pursuant to a specific legislative directive, the usual limitations on scope of practice activities under already-enacted licensing acts were not applicable. The project covered 10–13 geographic sites. Eventually, over 1,000,000 patients were seen by the nonphysician prescribers, over a 3-year period of time. The principal teaching methods used were lectures and seminars, which varied from 16 hours to 95 hours in length. As an aside, only 56% of the participating trainees possessed baccalaureate or higher academic degrees. Patients and the supervising physicians and pharmacists expressed considerable satisfaction. Most importantly, no adverse clinical consequences were reported. The recommended modifications for expansion of the relevant state practice acts were ultimately not implemented by the California legislature. However, nearly two decades later, the successful findings do represent a significant building block in professional psychology's efforts to obtain prescription privileges (DeLeon & Wiggins, 1996). The State of California had clearly demonstrated that nonphysician providers could be readily trained to safely and competently prescribe, thus, providing "real-life" data directly contradictory to the alleged "public health hazard" arguments that medicine always seems to raise whenever nonphysicians attempt to expand their clinical responsibilities (DeLeon, Sammons, & Fox, in press).

FUNDAMENTAL DEFINITIONAL DIFFERENCES

Over the years, our collective observation has been that most health care practitioners (including professional psychologists) come from the frame of reference that once they have obtained licensure from their state professional licensing board, that individual practitioner judgments should be given considerable weight, except in the most aggrieved situations. From a health policy frame of reference, licensing boards are established to protect the public by ensuring that at least minimum standards are met. From the practitioner's frame of reference, however, these boards typically ensure sufficient standards. No one, and particularly not our colleagues, appreciates being "second guessed" by one's peers. The emotions that one quickly encounters in even attempting to establish consensus surrounding what might serve as fundamental parameters for systematic discussion are extraordinary (DeLeon, VandenBos, & Cummings, 1983). And for mental health practitioners in particular, the historical importance of ensuring absolute patient confidentiality further compounds the underlying complexity. Conceptually, it is very difficult, if not impossible, to assess the quality or appropriateness of care being provided without access to a significant number of comparative records. The essence of determining and ensuring "quality care" is accountability, disclosure, and ready access to accurate and comparable data.

Without question, "quality" is a multidimensional concept. Although experts in the field may often seem to agree on its components, they often disagree strongly on the significance of each of the proposed elements. The Institute of Medicine (IOM), a major health policy "think tank" for the Administration and Congress, has defined "quality" as: "... the degree to which health services for individuals and populations increase the likelihood of desired health outcomes and are consistent with current professional knowledge" (Lohr, 1990, p. 128). This definition would specifically exclude financial constraints as an entity of quality.

The IOM definition is considered by many to be inadequate precisely because it apparently fails to recognize the impact of resource constraints on quality. Some argue that putting a price on quality care, particularly for a significant other or family member with a life-threatening diagnosis, is analogous to putting a price on the quality of their loved one's life.

Many arguments also ensue among health policy experts on exactly how to measure quality, what data are appropriate for use in measuring quality, the impact of financial arrangements on quality of care, and even how quality should be defined (Chassin, 1997; Darby, 1998).

While few would disagree that the health care delivered in this country is of "high quality," variations in the meaning of quality exist as do significant variations in what is actually being provided. And, with the many issues surrounding quality care delivery in managed care organizations recently surfacing within the popular and professional media, this has become a major political issue for the Clinton Administration. Further, as political rhetoric has escalated, it has become increasingly difficult for political and health policy experts to determine whether the public's alleged anxiety over the quality of health care provided by managed care will ultimately translate into action-oriented policy agendas designed to improve quality, or will the process instead degenerate into highly partisan debates between elected officials, competing health care professions, and those who provide care versus those who ultimately "pay the bill" for services rendered.

POLICY DEBATES SURROUNDING MANAGED CARE

In many ways, managed care's emerging dominance in the health care industry has changed the organization, financing, and the actual delivery of health care (Copeland, 1998; Wilensky, 1997). Today, nearly 164 million Americans (approximately 57%

of the US population) obtain their health coverage through some form of managed care. The year 1996 represented the first time in our nation's history that enrollment in health maintenance organizations (HMOs) exceeded that in indemnity plans. And, according to the congressionally established Prospective Payment Assessment Commission (PPAC), even indemnity insurers have now adopted some managed care techniques such as precertification of hospital admissions (PPAC, 1997).

In the mid-1990s, increasing numbers of health consumers and providers began voicing concerns about plans that restricted access to specialty providers, emergency room care, clinical trials, and the ability to dispute denials of claims or services (i.e., calling for a "Patients' Bill of Rights"). Consumers and their providers complained about the alleged "gag rules" and network participation rules that potentially undermine the integrity of the traditional provider–patient relationship. Basic to these concerns is the perception that economic factors are steadily taking precedence over clinical factors in determining what care is actually to be provided; that is, that insurance company personnel were making "medical decisions" (Cantor, 1998).

As a direct response to these reactions and concerns, state legislators began proposing and enacting numerous bills that attempt to offer reasonable protections for managed care plan consumers and that theoretically increase the overall quality of care being provided. These measures are commonly referred to as "anti-managed care legislation" by the managed care industry, because they place constraints on or ban certain activities used by the plans to reduce costs. It has been estimated that during the 1997–1998 legislative session, approximately 1000 broadly defined anti-managed care bills were introduced at the state level. In 1997 alone, 18 states enacted comprehensive patient protection acts, with an additional six states doing so the following year. Several states have taken the approach of forming health data commissions that collect and report outcome data on managed care plans, including measures of performance, quality, and cost. These have been enacted in Pennsylvania, Minnesota, and Maryland. Public health agencies in Missouri have collaborated with managed care plans, providers, and purchasers to develop the Missouri Health Indicator Set for assessing quality. Their data are being collected from births, deaths, hospital discharges, and tumor registries. The primary drawback to these state efforts is the general lack of consistency of effort between states in developing one agreed upon set of standards for quality assurance; that is, to what extent can these findings be accurately generalized.

In his January 1998, State of the Union Address, President Clinton, as he has done each year, demonstrated his continuing personal commitment to the importance of all Americans having ready access to high-quality health care:

> We have to make it possible for all hard-working families to meet their most important responsibilities. Two years ago, we helped guarantee that Americans can keep their health insurance when they changed jobs. Last year, we extended health care to up to 5 million children. This year, I challenge Congress to take the next historic steps. A hundred and sixty million of our fellow citizens are in managed care plans. These plans save money, and they can improve care. But medical decisions ought to be made by medical doctors, not insurance company accountants. I urge this Congress to reach across the aisle and write into a law a consumer bill of rights that says this: You have the right to know all your medical options, not just the cheapest. You have the right to choose the doctor you want for the care you need.... You have the right to keep your medical records confidential. (Clinton, 1998, p. A24).

The underlying policy foundation for the President's recommendation was developed by his 34-member Advisory Commission on Consumer Protection and Quality in the Health Care Industry, which was co-chaired by Secretaries Herman (Department of Labor) and Shalala (Department of Health and Human Services). Beverly Malone, President of the American Nurses Association (ANA) and a member of American Psychological Association (APA), served as one of the Commissioners. The Commission's report proposed eight areas of consumer "rights and responsibilities" (Advisory Commission, 1997):

1. *Information disclosure*. Consumers have the right to receive accurate, easily understood information and assistance in making informed health care decisions about their health plans, professionals, and facilities.
2. *Choice of providers and plans*. Consumers have the right to a choice of health care providers sufficient to ensure access to appropriate high-quality health care.
3. *Access to emergency services*. Consumers have the right to access emergency health care services when and where needed. Health plans should provide payment when a consumer presents to an emergency department with acute symptoms of sufficient severity—such that a prudent layperson could reasonably expect the absence of medical attention to result in serious jeopardy, serious impairment to bodily functions, or serious dysfunction of any bodily organ or part.
4. *Participation in treatment decisions*. Consumers have the right and responsibility to fully participate in all decisions related to their health care. Consumers who are unable to fully participate in treatment decisions have the right to be represented by parents, guardians, family members, or other conservators.
5. *Respect and nondiscrimination*. Consumers have the right to considerate, respectful care from all members of the health care system at all times and under all circumstances. An environment of mutual respect is essential to maintain a quality health care system. Consumers must not be discriminated against in the delivery of health care services consistent with the benefits covered in their policy or as required by law based on race, ethnicity, national origin, religion, sex, age, mental or physical disability, sexual orientation, genetic information, or source of payment. Consumers who are eligible for coverage under the terms and conditions of a health plan or program or as required by law must not be discriminated against in marketing and enrollment practices based on race, ethnicity, national origin, religion, sex, age, mental or physical disability, sexual orientation, genetic information, or source of payment.
6. *Confidentiality of health information*. Consumers have the right to communicate with health care providers in confidence and to have the confidentiality of their individually identifiable health care information protected. Consumers also have the right to review and copy their own medical records and request amendments to their records.
7. *Complaints and appeals*. All consumers have the right to a fair and efficient process for resolving differences with their health plans, health care providers, and the institutions that serve them, including a rigorous system of internal review and an independent system of external review.
8. *Consumer responsibilities*. A health care system that protects consumers' rights should expect and encourage consumers to assume reasonable responsibilities. Greater individual involvement by consumers in their care in-

creases the likelihood of achieving the best outcomes and helps support a quality improvement, cost-conscious environment.

The Commission consciously sought to chart a course for the continued enhancement of health systems that would serve to protect consumers and ensure quality. The bulk of their recommendations are expected to be in place within three years with three major goals: (1) To strengthen consumer confidence by assuring the health care system is fair and responsive to consumers' needs, to provide consumers with credible and effective mechanisms to address their concerns, and to encourage consumers to take an active role in improving and assuring their health; (2) to reaffirm the importance of a strong relationship between patients and their health care professionals; and (3) to reaffirm the critical role consumers play in safeguarding their own health by establishing the rights and responsibilities for all participants in improving health status.

The guiding principles for the Administration's Consumer Bill of Rights and responsibilities include: (1) All consumers are created equal; (2) quality comes first; (3) preserve what works; and (4) costs matter. The Commission took the far-reaching policy position that the American people should have access to health care that is of high quality, evidence-based, safe, free of errors, and available to all Americans regardless of ability to pay. Progress over time will require changes that must be made prudently, realistically, and with due regard to the needs of all stakeholders in the system. The Consumer Bill of Rights and responsibilities specifies improvements that are potentially achievable now and over the next several years. It acquires even more meaning in the context of a broader overarching commitment to ensure that full access to high-quality health care will eventually be available to all Americans.

During the closing weeks of the 105th Congress (1997–1998), there was a flurry of legislative activity surrounding the possible enactment of a Patients' Bill of Rights. The Patient Access to Responsible Care Act of 1997 (PARCA), introduced by Senator D'Amato (S. 644) and Representative Norwood (H.R. 1415), became the major legislative focus for what quickly turned into a highly partisan debate. This legislation has been a very high priority for APA's legislative and state grassroots efforts.

Just prior to the August 1998 recess, the House of Representatives narrowly passed the Republican leadership bill by a vote of 216 to 210. The House Minority Leader proclaimed: "This is bill with rhetoric, but not a remedy." The Administration stated: "It covers too few people, it provides too few patient protections and it contains unnecessary and irrelevant provisions that undermine the chances for a bipartisan agreement...." (Health, 1998, p. 2007). In contrast to the Republican proposal, the Democratic legislation would allow individuals to sue their health plans under state law for personal injury or wrongful death; ensure that patients have continuity of care if their employers change health plans or their doctors leave their plan; and insure greater access to necessary specialist care. The initial Republican leadership proposal would have also expanded the availability of medical saving accounts (MSAs), a particularly partisan issue. Conceptually, throughout this debate the key to ensuring quality centered around the notion of timely access and the informed judgment of individual patients and clinicians, not around reviewing objective data.

Not surprisingly, the underlying policy question for the Administration, the Congress, and the nation continues to be: How exactly is this laudable goal to be accomplished? And, given the extent to which it is the strongly held view of some credible health policy experts that it is really the various health care professions that are instigating and continuing the policy debate rather than consumers, to what extent is the current debate surrounding managed care really about quality or perhaps instead about professional autonomy and economic stability (DeLeon, Bulatao, & VandenBos, 1994)?

THE AGENCY FOR HEALTH CARE POLICY AND RESEARCH

The Agency for Health Care Policy and research (AHCPR) was established by the Congress as a provision of the Omnibus Budget Reconciliation Act of 1989 on a truly bipartisan basis. The IOM subsequently estimated that AHCPR saves Medicare at least $200 million annually. However, during its deliberations on the concurrent budget resolution (which proposed that the federal budget be balanced by the year 2002), the US Senate specifically recommended that the agency's budget be reduced by 75% (Gaus & DeLeon, 1995).

AHCPR's fiscal year 1999 budget justification requested approximately $171.4 million, and noted that the underlying mission of AHCPR is to:

> ... generate and disseminate information that improves the delivery of health care. This mission is unique. AHCPR's research goals are to determine what works best in clinical practice; improve the cost-effective use of health care resources; help consumers make more informed choices; and measure and improve the quality of care. These goals were developed to explicitly address the major changes affecting health care and the role of government (US Department of Health and Human Services, 1998, p. 27).

Institutionally, AHCPR has been acutely aware of the rapid changes that are evolving in our nation's health care system, how these are dramatically altering the services available to both publicly and privately insured patients, and the extent to which the Congress, practitioners, public health experts, and the public at large have strongly held views:

> ... [M]anaged care is restructuring delivery to rely more heavily on primary care services and providers with largely unknown impact on cost and quality. The increasing complexity of the choices facing patients, physicians, health plans, and purchasers has resulted in an explosion in the need for the knowledge, measures, and tools of health service research. Patients, providers, purchasers and plans that make decisions about health care services in an increasingly market-sensitive health care system require information about their options to improve health outcomes and effectiveness. In addition to informing decision makers about the effectiveness, outcomes, and quality of clinical services, health services research also informs decision makers about the impact of changes in the organization and financing of health care. This is particularly relevant today, when competition is altering the nature and content of primary care services. Thus the science base developed by AHCPR serves as the key navigational tool for decisions at each of these levels of decision making about health care. (US Department of Health and Human Services, 1998, p. 27)

The Administration's vision for AHCPR includes: (1) improving clinical practice—clinicians, patients, and health care institutions need information about what works, for whom, when, and at what cost; (2) improving health care systems—medical practices, hospitals and other institutions, health networks, and plans need information to improve the health care system's capacity to deliver quality care; (3) tracking the nation's progress—policymakers need more information to monitor and evaluate the impact of system changes on access, cost, and use of health care; and (4) improving activities that support all areas of research including dissemination, cost-effectiveness analysis, priority populations including minority and ethnic groups, women, children, and the elderly, and health services research training.

In 1997, AHCPR launched a new initiative to actively promote evidence-based practice in everyday care, through the establishment of 12 "evidence-based" practice centers. These centers are expected to develop evidence reports and technology assessments on clinical topics that are common, expensive, and/or are significant for the Medicare and Medicaid populations, for which the federal government has considerable direct clinical responsibility. It is the Administration's vision that this particular programmatic vehicle would allow AHCPR to become a "science partner" with both private and public organizations in their efforts to improve the quality, effectiveness, and appropriateness of clinical care by facilitating the translation of evidence-based research findings into clinical practice.

The agency expects that this approach will provide the potential users of this research (i.e., private and public entities) with the foundation necessary for developing and implementing their own practice guidelines, performance measures, review criteria, and other clinical quality improvement tools. Further, the findings from these evidence-based practice centers should provide health plans and payers with information they will find necessary to make informed decisions about coverage policies for new and changing medical devices and procedures. Professional associations, such as the APA, are viewed as definite potential users of these evidence reports and technology assessments.

AHCPR also has announced that nominations for topics for the evidence-based practice centers would be solicited routinely through public notices in the *Federal Register* on an ongoing basis. Professional associations, health plans, providers, and others that nominate topics are expected to serve as active partners with the centers, providing technical expertise and serving as peer reviewers of the final product. Those serving as partners are then expected to assist in translating the findings from the reports and assessments into practice guidelines or other implementation tools in order to effectively improve quality of care within their respective organizations. Of direct relevance to professional psychology, included in the initial topics selected for the 12 centers were: depression treatment with new drugs, pharmacotherapy for alcohol dependence, rehabilitation of persons with traumatic brain injury, and treatment of attention deficit-hyperactivity disorder. The agency has further indicated that it expected to support future evidence focuses on the broad topic areas of child and adolescent health, mental health and substance abuse, rehabilitation, and preventive care. How relevant and timely for professional psychology is this approach? We would note that in the summer of 1998, the APA Practice Directorate placed upon their website the APA Guidelines for Child Custody Evaluations in Divorce Proceedings, the APA Guidelines for Psychological Evaluations in Child Protection Matters, and the APA Guidelines for the Evaluation of Dementia and Age-Related Cognitive Decline.

Another Example of a Timely State Initiative

The Pennsylvania Psychological Association's Practice–Research Network

History teaches us that some professions have not survived the test of time as well as the profession of psychology. One example of a failed discipline is the antique "science" of phrenology, the study of skull protuberances. Phrenology posited that skull characteristics reveal a person's character and mental capacity. Only 200 years ago there were departments of phrenology at some of the world's major universities. However, practitioners of phrenology extended their practice too far beyond the available scientific data, which resulted in phrenologists developing a well-justified reputation as charlatans. Their profession eventually withered and all the departments of phrenology vanished from the universities. Who knows, perhaps if phrenologists had based their work on research, they would have developed neuropsychology 100 years before psychologists did! But they did not, and phrenology was eliminated as a science and as a profession; thus, proving that natural selection works in various venues. Professional psychology must be careful not to repeat the phrenologists' errors. Psychology must continually renew its foundation in quality scientific research.

With financial support from APA's Committee for the Advancement of Professional Practice (CAPP) and the Pennsylvania State University, in 1995, the Pennsylvania Psychological Association established a unique network of practitioners and researchers at the state level who were interested in the application of outcome and other clinical research. The Practice–Research Network is led by an executive committee, chaired by coauthor Stephen Ragusea. Other members of the executive committee include Thomas Borkovec and Ruben Echemendia. The network grew out of a desire to strengthen the ties between psychology's practice and research communities.

The Pennsylvania Psychological Association is committed to developing a way to reunite psychology's practice and research communities, which have been drifting apart for decades. It is critically important that all of professional psychology support the underlying concept that science and practice must advance hand in hand for either to survive into the 21st century. Psychology's research heritage has provided the scientific foundation that allowed psychology to leap ahead of psychiatry over the past 50 years, and all of psychology must continue to nurture the dynamic interaction between practice and research, in order for the field to thrive as a viable science and profession.

In addition, third-party payers and consumers today are vitally interested in demonstrations of the effectiveness of the psychological services they pay for. Furthermore, individual practitioners are interested in demonstrating and quantifying the effectiveness of their work, as well as utilizing feedback from outcome studies to improve the quality of their future efforts. Finally, every psychologist should be interested in furthering the science and profession of psychology to the benefit of all of society. The Pennsylvania Psychological Association's Practice–Research Network is now linking practitioners with researchers in a mutual enterprise, to share expertise and resources. Immediate goals are to collect basic outcome data from practitioners, allow the development of more specialized research projects involving both practitioners and researchers, and to focus on research questions of direct relevance to clinical practice.

At present, an adult battery has been developed, under the direction of Ruben Echemendia, that utilizes several new and established clinical instruments including sections of Ken Howard's COMPASS Battery. This 30-minute battery is administered to therapy patients after the first, seventh, and termination sessions. It is again administered 6 months after termination. Independent assessments of each patient are conducted on a parallel basis by the clinician. Feedback is provided to clinicians following each evaluation. In order to minimize cost and clinician time commitments, the entire project is self-contained and distributed through the mail. A child and adolescent battery that uses Tom Achenbach and Craig Edelbrock's Youth Self-Report and Child behavior Checklist is also in current use.

Any Pennsylvania psychologist can participate in the Practice–Research Network after signing an agreement to accept the basic ground rules established for the project. These rules include guidelines for ethical collection and utilization of the data. All Practice–Research Network projects must be reviewed by the Pennsylvania State University's human subjects' committee and the Practice–Research Network's own ethics committee, which is chaired by Thomas Borkovec. All data are coded so that only the individual clinician can identify his or her own patients. All outcome measures are analyzed through the research center at Pennsylvania State University and the data are only to be published or shared as aggregate data from the entire group or subgroup of providers, thus ensuring individual patient confidentiality. Turnaround time between receiving patient assessments from a clinician and the mailing of a scored report back to the clinician (including COMPASS scoring) averages 14 days.

Individual data will only be shared with the treating psychologist. The aggregate data will be distributed to all participating clinicians, as well as through normal publication channels. The data are being analyzed from a number of different perspectives, including the analysis of such variables as length of treatment, psychologist's level of training, amount of insurance copayment, theoretical orientation, patient health issues, medication utilization, and so forth.

Data collection began in 1996. By September 1997, 151 clinicians agreed to participate and recruitment continues. Seventy-one clinicians have submitted the required letter of agreement and therapist demographic information in preparation for their active participation. Of these 71, 60 clinicians enrolled 101 patients in the project with completed pretherapy measures. Patient gender is 61% women, 14% are ethnic minority, and 78% have been diagnosed with mood or anxiety disorders. Seventy-seven percent of the psychologists have doctoral degrees, 45% are women, and 88% work in individual or group practice. The therapists typically see 21.9 patients per week and average 16.3 years of clinical experience. Forty patients thus far have completed posttherapy assessment.

The preliminary data suggest that psychologists working in private practice offices are producing substantial therapeutic change on standardized test instruments and that these measured changes are consistent with the psychologist's subjective rating of their patient's progress. These data are important because they represent the ultimate in realistic setting measures of therapeutic effectiveness. While most clinical research is of questionable generalizability, this type of research represents the true test of psychology's effectiveness in the real world and complements traditional, well-controlled laboratory studies (Seligman & Levant, 1998).

In addition to this pilot study (now 2 years into data collection), which serves to establish an infrastructure for future research, other projects are envisioned by the Pennsylvania Psychological Association to assess a wide range of interest areas. These projects may include child custody evaluation, geropsychology, school psychology, prison psychology, and so on. However, the project will always remain focused on the primary goals of developing clinically useful knowledge while encouraging the interaction of researchers and practicing clinicians.

The existence and success of the Pennsylvania Practice–Research Network is important for several reasons. First, it provides a channel for unification of the practice and research communities in the birth of a newly defined scientist–practitioners model. Second, the Practice–Research Network will begin to generate uniquely practical research results from entirely naturalistic settings. Third, the basic model can be replicated anywhere (and by any discipline) in response to a wide variety of critical clinical questions. Imagine the potential inherent in the data that can come from 100 practicing psychologists, with 500 patients from across Pennsylvania. Now, imagine the data that can grow from an additional 1000 psychologists from throughout North America, with 5000 of their patients. Psychology has over 80,000 licensed practitioners. Imagine a series of such practice–research networks, over a decade of practice. Allow the imagination to consider the potential for the rebirth of professional psychology.

We would suggest, however, that for the Pennsylvania Psychological Association's vision to ultimately come to fruition, one absolutely critical step is for organized psychology (i.e., the APA) to become more active participants in shaping the Agency for Health Care Policy and research's priorities and programmatic agenda. It has been our observation that throughout the federal government's quality efforts to date, mental health care and particularly psychological care, is at best, an afterthought. At the public policy level, very rarely is psychology's potential contribution to our nation's health care system seriously appreciated. Psychology should be a leading voice in this arena. Such active public policy involvement is, in fact, a societal responsibility for every one of the "learned professions" (DeLeon, 1988; Lorion, Iscoe, DeLeon, & VandenBos, 1996).

Historical Perspective

In many ways, the need for this particular agency grew out of Congressional hearings on the variations in medical practice that existed in the mid-1980s. The US Senate Appropriations Committee, for example, held a special hearing in November 1984, at which time Charles Kiesler, former Executive Officer of the American Psychological Association, participated. Witnesses testified that their research into geographic patterns of health care delivery revealed extensive variation in the use of hospital services from one community to another. For many medical or surgical conditions, the variations suggested opportunities to considerably reduce expenditures under Medicare and Medicaid, without reducing the clinical benefits. For other conditions, the variations suggested a very real, if not critical, need to evaluate the outcomes of different approaches to treatments. The need to systematically balance and evaluate cost concerns and clinical concerns was evident, as well as the underlying notion that more services did not necessarily mean better clinical outcomes.

Reflecting several of the critical themes that have constantly reoccurred over the past decades during national policy debates surrounding the importance of ensuring quality care, the American Medical Association testified:

> The AMA applauds the work of Dr. Wennberg, and we recognize three significant strengths to the activity he is encouraging: The dependence on local and regional initiatives; the use and reliance on peer influence among physicians to bring about changes; and the primary focus on quality of care. The American Medical Association recognizes that variations in practice patterns constitute a challenge that needs to be addressed aggressively.... The AMA is also undertaking efforts to eliminate inappropriate variations in medical practice. We have under-

> way several projects aimed at providing practicing physicians with information to aid them in making appropriate patient care decisions. In the area of medical education, the provision of appropriate high-quality care in a cost-effective way is facilitated by physicians educated and sensitized to cost considerations. (Davis, 1984, p. 136)

At approximately the same time, professional psychology was also institutionally struggling with the very same clinical policy issues in the form of developing proposed clinical standards (i.e., guidelines) for the delivery of quality mental health care under the Department of Defense CHAMPUS program (Willens & DeLeon, 1982). In this situation, the federal government had contracted with several national professional mental health associations, including the APA, to develop objective peer review processes for their practitioners, with the hope of eventually developing national criteria that might be utilized through the health care system. Considerable organizational time and energy was exerted. In the end, however, the increasingly vocal concerns of association practitioners led to the diminishing participation of the various national organizations. Restated from a different perspective: Everyone agrees that only high-quality health care should be provided. However, practitioners of all disciplines have considerable concern about how this laudable goal might be accomplished and what if any role their professional association should play.

At the US Senate Appropriations Committee hearings, Charles Kiesler testified directly to some of the difficulties one must expect by relaying exclusively on clinician judgments, as demonstrated within the mental health arena.

> Many people believe, and this includes the general public and mental health professionals, that mental hospitalization is the most effective treatment for the people who utilize the service. That is, the few people we are hospitalizing are correctly placed, because no alternative exists to treat them more effectively. The data seem clear on this last issue: Traditional inpatient care for mental disorders is neither the most effective nor the most cost-effective method of treatment.... In every study, differences favored the alternative care rather than mental hospitalization, in terms of psychiatric symptomatology, ratings by family, probability of being able to locate or maintain a job, subsequent hospitalization, and the like. In every case where there has been systematic calculation, the alternative care was less expensive.... Our national policy of increasing mental hospitalization flies in the face of available scientific evidence (Kiesler, 1984, pp. 141–142)

Further, we would note that the Department of Defense Fort Bragg Child and Adolescent Mental Health Demonstration Program, after a multiyear expenditure of $80 million and extensive evaluation, strongly suggests similar conclusions: that is, that within the mental health arena, more care does not necessarily result in better clinical outcomes, notwithstanding practitioner expectations (DeLeon & Williams, 1997).

LEGISLATIVE RESPONSE

During the closing months of the 105th Congress (1997–1998), the Chairman of the Senate Labor and Human Resources Subcommittee on Public Health and Safety, which has jurisdiction over AHCPR, introduced legislation to refocus the agency and to rename this element of the Department of Health and Human Services as the Agency for Health Care Quality (AHQ). The chairman and the only physician serving in the US Senate stressed that the AHQ would be built on the platform of the current AHCPR but would be refocused on quality in order to become the central figure in the federal government's efforts to improve the overall quality of health care. He made clear that the role of the AHQ would *not* be to mandate national standards of clinical practice. Rather, his proposed legislation was based on the premise that definitions and measures of quality are an evolving science, a science critically important to making educated and appropriate choices in a rapidly changing and dynamic health care system. The promotion and support of health services research would lead to greater determination, which would ensure that prudent decisions could be made by families, patients, employers, and practitioners.

The chairman's introductory remarks on the floor of the US Senate at the time of the introduction of his bill (S. 2208) provide a sense of the intensity of the ongoing debate within the health care arena about how to accomplish the underlying policy objectives:

> ... All Americans want better health care and the federal government must respond by offering helpful information on quality, channeling scientific evidence to clinicians, and investing in research on improving health services.... Health care quality is a matter of personal preference—it means different things to different people. We all remember when health care quality became a political showdown, the low back pain guidelines backfired because they were viewed as an attempt to mandate "cook book" medicine, and the Agency for Health Care Policy and Research had a near death experience.
>
> Over the past three years, since I first came to the United States Senate, I have looked very closely at this agency. The Subcommittee on Public Health and Safety, which I chair, has held three hearings to invite public input on this agency. As a result, this legislation responds to many of the past criticisms of the agency. This legislation will take AHCPR—under a new name—to new heights and will establish it as the center of health care quality research for the country.
>
> The new Agency for Health Care Quality will:
>
> 1. Promote quality by sharing information. While proven medical advances are made daily, patients are waiting too long to benefit from these discoveries. We must get the science to the people by better sharing of information and more effective dissemination. In addition, the Agency will develop evidence-rating systems to help people in judging the quality of science.
>
> 2. Build public–private partnerships to advance and share true quality measurers. Quality means different things to different people. In collaboration with the private sector, the Agency shall conduct research that can figure out what quality really means to patients and to clinicians, how to measure quality, and what actions can improve the outcome of health care.
>
> 3. Report annually on the state of quality, and cost, of the nation's health care. Americans want to know if they receive good quality health care. But compared to what? Statistically accurate, sample-based national surveys will efficiently provide reliable and affordable data—without excessive, overly intrusive, and potentially destructive mandatory reporting requirements.
>
> 4. Aggressively support improved information systems for health quality. Currently, quality measurement too often requires manual chart reviews for such simple data as frequency of procedures, infection rates, or other complications. Improved computer systems will advance quality scoring and facilitate quality-based decision-making in patient treatment.
>
> 5. Support primary care research and address issues of access in underserved areas. While most policy discussions this year are targeting managed-care, quality improvement is just as important to the sole practitioner. The Agency's authority is expanded to support health care improvement in all types of office practice—not just managed care. The agency shall specifically address quality in rural and other underserved areas by advancing telemedicine services which share clinical expertise with more patients.
>
> 6. Facilitate innovation in patient care with streamlined evaluation and assessment of new technologies. Patients should benefit from proven breakthrough technologies sooner, while inefficient methods should be phased out faster. Today, manufacturers and distributors of new technologies face major hurdles in trying to secure coverage. The Medicare technology committee has ben particularly criticized for its process. Criteria are unclear, delays are long,

> and decisions are unpredictable. The Agency will be accessible to both private and public entities for technology assessments and will share information on assessment methodologies.
>
> 7. Coordinate quality improvement efforts of the government. Most of the many federal health care programs today support some kind of health services research and conduct various quality improvement projects. The Agency shall coordinate these many initiatives to avoid disjointed, uncoordinated, or duplicative efforts.
>
> In summary, we need to practice, not just publish, better patient care. We all want to see better quality. Real improvement can come from progress in health sciences, from promoting innovation in patient care, and from better practical application of new scientific advances. The Agency for Health Care Quality will focus on overall improvement in health care and enable us to judge the quality of care we receive. Americans want better health care and the federal government shall respond by offering helpful information on quality, channeling scientific evidence to clinicians, and investing in research on improving health services. Mr. President, the "Health Care Quality Enhancement Act of 1998" will reduce the gap between what we know and what we do in health care. The refocused Agency for Health Care Quality is the right step forward and I urge my colleagues to support this legislation to improve health care for all Americans. (Frist, 1998, p. S.6888–S.6889)

MENTAL HEALTH PARITY

As professional psychology has become a more active participant within our nation's overall health care delivery system, rather than relying on its traditional narrower focus as exclusively being a mental health specialty, it has become increasingly evident to the profession that ensuring access to quality mental health care must become an integral component of society's fundamental definition of "quality care" (DeLeon et al., 1996; DeLeon & VandenBos, 1983). That is, regardless of the nature of the physical symptom that initially brings an individual into the health care system, without ready access to psychological care, the care that is ultimately provided may very well not be of the quality desired.

One of managed care's principal tools for cost reduction has been the limitation of access to mental health services, when compared to physical health services. This has been of particular concern to professional psychology because it reveals an undervaluing of mental health care. During the 104th Congress (1995–1996), a major new federal policy initiative was put in place to address this problem (Sleek, 1996). The Mental Health Parity Act, signed into law in September 1996 [PL 104–204], removed inequitable annual and lifetime limits on mental health coverage. This act was actually a somewhat truncated version of the Domenici–Wellstone amendment, which passed the US Senate in April of that year but was unresolved in House–Senate conference negotiations.

Since September 1996, efforts have continued at the federal level to implement more comprehensive parity. "Full" parity would mean that coverage of mental health services (including substance abuse) could not be more limited than coverage for physical health services. Coverage would include both inpatient days and outpatient visits, both copayments and deductibles (out-of-pocket costs), and both annual and lifetime benefits. Insurance plans could still use preadmission screening and restrict coverage to medically necessary services. Specific benefits would not be mandated. The parity requirement would include both group and individual health coverage offered under self-insured Employee Retirement Income Security Act (ERISA) plans, HMOs, and traditional insurance plans.

A number of compelling clinical and public policy arguments have been advanced by professional psychology and the other mental health disciplines in favor of comprehensive parity (Eckert, 1994);

- Parity improves the quality of patient care (APA, 1996b). The efficacy of treatment for mental illness is well established. Parity encourages treatment based on medical necessity and appropriateness, rather than on adherence to arbitrary limits in insurance benefits. Inefficiencies in service delivery that are driven by benefit design, such as overutilization of hospital care, will be eliminated.
- Parity maintains control of both public and private sector medical costs. Parity will lower the overall national cost for mental health care by $5.5 billion (7.6% of mental health care costs and 0.5% of total health care costs), according to Coopers and Lybrand (Bachman, 1996). This reduction will result from allowing more people to be treated in the private sector rather than the less cost-effective public sector. Increased private sector care will result in only a very small increase in private sector insurance premiums (no more than 3.2%, as estimated by Coopers and Lybrand). Business lobby claims of much larger increases (8% to 11%) are based on studies making questionable assumptions (Watson Wyatt Worldwide, etc.), such as exaggeration of increases in consumer demand for mental health services (EBRI, 1997). In fact, an improved benefit structure might eliminate the need for premium increases altogether. For example, Milliman and Robertson estimated that use of a $50 deductible on all health care would eliminate the small premium increase that parity might otherwise cause (15 cents per covered person per day) (Melek & Pyenson, 1996). According to the Bazelon Center for Mental Health Law, the private sector cost-effectiveness of parity is already evident at the state level (Judge David L. Bazelon Center for Mental Health Law, 1996). Minnesota and Maryland, where existing parity laws are quite similar to the proposed federal parity law, have not experienced any major increases in private health care expenses. In some cases, costs have actually decreased.

  Parity preserves the availability of health insurance. Countering claims that parity might deprive many employees of health benefits, the Congressional Budget Office (CBO, 1996) concluded that mental health parity might actually have no effect at all on access to health insurance. Even if increased costs did lead to reduction in availability of insurance, the CBO estimated that this would affect less than one half of 1% of the insured workforce (400,000 employees, as well as an equal number of their dependents). This analysis helped discredit a business-sponsored study that predicted an effect of more than twice that size (Price Waterhouse, 1996).
- Parity saves private sector medical dollars by improving benefits management and access to care (APA, 1996a,c). Primary care patients with diagnosable mental disorders consistently average twice as many visits to their primary care physicians as those without a mental disorder. Consequently, improved access to mental health care can decrease inappropriate use of physical medicine services, thereby reducing overall medical care expense. Major corporations such as BellSouth, Digital, and First Chicago have removed limits on mental health benefits and lowered costs through reasonable

and responsible benefits management. Similarly, Aetna found that overall medical costs dropped by up to 33% per insured person over a 3-year period, when mental health treatment was made available.

- Parity increases business cost-effectiveness by improving productivity, reducing absenteeism, and decreasing disability. The Mental Health Liaison Group observed in 1996 that mental disorders cost over $130 billion a year in lost productivity, absenteeism, disability, and early death (Mental Health Liaison Group, 1996). For depression alone, the MIT Sloan School of Management estimated in 1993 that the business cost was $22 billion. The Washington Business Group on Health (WBGH), representing many of the nation's largest corporations, acknowledged that mental health care can yield major cost savings, given that over 80% of depression cases can be rapidly and effectively treated (England, 1997). WBGH reported growing corporate recognition of evidence that mental health treatment saves money by alleviating a wide variety of employee performance problems.
- Parity standardizes insurance policy at the federal level. Decades of uncertainty and neglect have created considerable inconsistency in mental health insurance coverage. Federal standards are needed because the free market has failed to provide a "level playing field" among all types of health insurers. Some employers cannot get adequate mental health coverage in the market, and state legislation is insufficient because of the exemption of ERISA plans (which insure up to 60% of all employees in many states). A "level playing field" protects responsible insurers and employers from attracting poor risks, increasing their costs, and being placed at a competitive disadvantage. In short, supporters of full mental health parity have convincingly argued that it would have a number of very positive effects, including closing current gaps in the national health care system, improving workforce productivity, and removing insurance barriers to cost-effective care.

Unfortunately, efforts to implement parity are currently stalled at the federal level, due in part to the ever overcrowded congressional agenda and more importantly, we suspect, to a reluctance on the part of many legislators to implement an expanded parity statute before learning the results of the more limited legislation already enacted. At the state level, however, efforts are proceeding actively across the nation. Supporters of comprehensive parity believe that, through a combination of state and federal efforts, the battle for appropriate access to mental health services will eventually be won.

THE FEDERAL GOVERNMENT AS A PROVIDER OF CARE

THE DEPARTMENT OF VETERANS AFFAIRS

The Department of Veterans Affairs (VA) has long been the single largest employer and trainer of professional psychologists. The VA's primary mission is:

> ... to serve America's veterans and their families as their principal advocate in ensuring that they receive the care, support, and recognition they have earned in service to the Nation. The VA's operating units include the Veterans Health Administration, Veterans Benefits Administration, National Cemetery System, and staff offices. The Veterans Health Administration

> develops, maintains, and operates a national health care delivery system for eligible veterans; carries out a program of education and training of health care personnel; carries out a program of medical research and development; and furnishes health services to members of the Armed Forces during periods of war or national emergency. A system of 172 medical centers, 673 outpatient clinics, 134 nursing homes, and 40 domiciliaries is maintained to meet the VA's medical mission. (US Congress, Senate Committee of Veterans' Affairs, 1997, p. 6)

For fiscal year 1999, the Administration recommended $17.027 billion for the VA health account.

As is the case for the rest of the nation, the VA's health care system is evolving in a dramatic and unprecedented fashion. It is the largest fully integrated health care system in the world because of the multitude of missions, which include providing medical care to veterans with service-connected disability, continuing health professional education and training, conducting research that directly benefits veterans, and providing contingency support to the Department of Defense and the US Public Health Service during times of disaster or national emergency.

In its efforts to ensure the highest possible quality of care, the VA health care system has initiated several reengineering efforts over the past 3 years, with the goal of improving the consistency and predictability of the quality of care provided by systematically comparing its clinical efforts with verifiable national standards. For example, the VA Preventative and Chronic Disease Index, a tool developed based on the Health Plan Employment Data and Information Set (HEDIS), an instrument used in the private sector (minus the pediatrics and obstetrical care indices), consists of nine quality outcome indicators that measure how well VA follows national prevention and early detection recommendations for diseases having significant social impact, such as cancer, smoking, and alcohol abuse. By specifically making an institutional effort to comply with these recommendations, the VA reports obtaining almost a doubling of success in fiscal year 1997, from a low of 34% to almost 68%. The agency reports that on average, the VA health systems exceed the private sector on all comparable indicators, ranging from 5% to 69% better on individual quality indicators. The VA also has exceeded the US Public Health Service *Healthy People 2000* goals for five indicators: immunizations for pneumonia and influenza and cancer screening for colorectal, breast, and cervical cancer (US Department of Health and Human Services, 1991).

The chronic disease care index (CDC index), the primary quality care measuring mechanism within the VA system, consists of 14 quality indicators measuring how well the VA is following national guidelines for such high-volume diagnoses as ischemic heart disease and diabetes. Percentages reflect the number of patients who actually received a required medical intervention. The CDC index in aggregate rose 73% in fiscal year 1997. Again, the data indicate that the VA consistently outperforms the private sector, with ranges from 21% to 124% better compliance on individual quality indicators. Examples of VA versus private sector performance include the rate of aspirin therapy for patients with documented heart disease (92% versus 76%), and the percentage of diabetics whose blood glucose levels are monitored annually by a blood test (85% versus 38%).

As part of the VA's health reengineering efforts, officials also have systematically tracked the 1-year survival rates for high-volume medical conditions that affect the most vulnerable veteran subpopulations. Survival rates for several of these important conditions (i.e., congestive heart failure, chronic obstructive pulmonary disease, pneumonia, and chronic renal failure) have increased by 4 to 9% over 1992 baseline data. Other clinical conditions of direct relevance to professional psychology, such as major depressive disorder, bipolar disorder, and schizophrenia survival rates, have remained stable at 98% to 99%. The VA clinical programs, an initiative established in 1997 by the VA health system, attempts to formally recognize "the best practices" in American health care, as demonstrated by clinical outcomes, processes, resource utilization, and service satisfaction. As of October 1997, 36 such clinical programs across the nation have been formally designated as programs of excellence. From a public policy frame of reference, what one observes within the VA is a systematic effort at the highest administrative level to hold health care providers to observable and objective standards of care (Valentine, 1998).

And yet, a special staff report developed by the minority staff of the US Senate Committee on Veterans Affairs in its oversight role found that:

> Staff has found that many of VA's quality management programs had potential, but were terminated rather than being modified to overcome any noted deficiencies. Staff has also found that many programs currently in operation have not been adequately monitored, do not gather data systematically in an integrated and coordinated manner, and do not effectively track and trend the information gathered. This results in data which has little or no applicability to repairing system faults. Other programs are not all universally implemented, are not adequately monitored at the headquarters' level, or are too new to have demonstrated substantial, documented benefits.... Staff found that VA has had numerous opportunities to improve its management of quality, but has squandered many good ideas in this field. VA headquarters does not require that its hospitals and clinics use uniform methods for collecting data. This severely limits the ability of one facility to compare itself to another or to an outside benchmark. If data are not uniformly collected, it is impossible to raw definitive conclusions and give guidance for the improvement of patient care that is based on documented evidence. Other programs and activities were discontinued, leaving gaps which were never closed.... Throughout the organization and within its various programs, VA has not sufficiently emphasized quality concerns. Examples of this exist in VA's organizational structure, which places the office responsible for quality management three bureaucratic levels down from the Under Secretary for Health and the lack of emphasis on quality management issues in VA's research program and strategic plan.... (US Congress, Senate Committee on Veterans' Affairs, 1997, p. iii–v)

The staff recommendations include: (1) the VA should establish an advisory board to direct the development of an integrated and coordinated quality management program; (2) the VA's quality management program should be the direct responsibility of, and should report directly to, the Undersecretary for Health; and (3) the VA should increase education and training in quality management practices and activities. In conclusion,

> Staff wishes to emphasize that VA has many good programs, and many dedicated personnel. What is needed is strong, central leadership, and the commitment from VA headquarters to develop a national system devoted to managing quality of care issues, with the resources and organizational prominence needed to carry out this important mission. (US Congress, Senate Committee on Veterans' Affairs, 1997)

The January 13, 1998 response to the staff report by the VA Undersecretary for Health noted, in part:

> I think it is important to also acknowledge that no one has yet established the definitive approach to quality management in health care or the best method of deploying quality improvement through large health care systems. As a member of the Institute of Medicine's (IOM) National Roundtable for Health Care Quality, I certainly have been impressed by the

> knowledge gaps in this regard, as well as the variance in opinion about the preferred strategies to achieve the best outcomes. In this vein, I recognize that similarly intended people can have differing views on the best tactics to achieve a shared goal. Some of the comments in the staff report appear to reflect these types of differences. Notwithstanding this, when we reviewed the staff report we were struck by the conspicuous absence of any mention of the notable improvement in VA quality of care that has been achieved in the past two years.... In closing, let me again emphasize that I believe we are both very committed to improving the quality of VA health care and that we welcome your review and criticism of our efforts. Through such dynamic tension I believe VA will build on its already notable success and provide critical experiential information for other health care systems as they increasingly become subject to the same type of expectations and scrutiny that exist for VA ... (Kizer, 1998

Medicare and Medicaid

Historically, the federal government's quality assurance efforts have primarily centered on Medicare, with the states assuming the primary responsibility for Medicaid. As the APA Practice Directorate matured, significant efforts were soon made to have psychology included as an autonomous profession under Medicare, given the extent to which it became evident that Medicare's rules and regulations dramatically affected all aspects of health care, including the private sector (DeLeon & VandenBos, 1980; Uyeda, DeLeon, Perloff, & Kraut, 1986). Accordingly, in developing materials for this chapter, we were genuinely surprised to realize the extent to which during the recent past there has been very little congressional or administrative focus on Medicare's quality assurance efforts.

The Medicare Utilization and Quality Control Peer Review Organization program was established by Congress in 1982, building upon the former Professional Standards Review Organizations (PSROs) (US Congress, House Committee on Ways and Means, 1998). The new Peer Review Organizations (PROs) were charged with reviewing services furnished to Medicare beneficiaries to ensure that they met professionally recognized standards of care, were "medically necessary," and were delivered in the most appropriate setting. In many ways, this latter charge reflects the beginning of today's maturing interest by Congress to ensure the provision of cost-effective care. Most PRO review is focused on inpatient hospital care; however, there is limited review of ambulatory surgery, postacute care, and services received from Medicare HMOs; again, a recent evolution.

Presently there are 53 PRO areas, incorporating the 50 states and territories. Organizations eligible to become PROs include physician-sponsored and physician access organizations and in limited circumstances, Medicare fiscal intermediaries. Those selected receive contracts through a competitive proposal process. As of October 1996, each of the PROs were operating under their fifth round of contracts.

Each PRO has a medical director and staff of nurse and other technical reviewers. The PRO's board of directors is physician dominated; however, by statute each must possess a consumer representative. Since the board is usually consulted before a case is referred to the department's inspector general for possible sanction, the board tends to play a major role in the PRO review process. Only physician advisors can make initial determinations about services furnished or proposed by another physician.

PROs conduct both utilization (usually retrospectively) and quality review. If the PRO determines that the case was of poor quality, steps must be taken to correct the problem. Specific sanctions are required if "grossly substandard" care was provided or if there is found to be a pattern of substandard care by the practitioner. Although authority exists for the PRO to deny payments for substandard quality care, this provision of the law has never been used. Under the department's newest review strategy, the Health Care Quality Improvement Initiative, PROs are required to use explicit, nationally uniform criteria to examine patterns of care and outcomes using detailed clinical information on providers and patients. Instead of focusing on unusual deficiencies in care, the PROs were instructed to focus on persistent differences between actual indications of care and outcomes from those patterns of care and outcomes considered achievable. The current emphasis is on continuous quality improvement, with each PRO being required to conduct 4 to 18 quality improvement projects each year, depending on the size of their beneficiary populations. The various states are required to ensure similar "appropriateness and quality" review for Medicaid beneficiaries.

The Balanced Budget Act of 1997 (PL 105-33) stressed that states entering into Medicaid contracts with managed care entities would be required to establish a quality assurance program, consistent with departmental standards. Further, state quality assurance programs are required to include standards for access to care, examination of aspects related to the improvement of quality of care, and procedures for monitoring and evaluating quality of care. The statute directed the secretary to:

> in consultation with States, managed care organizations, the National Academy of State Health Policy, representatives of beneficiaries with special health care needs, experts in specialized health care, and others, [to] conduct a study concerning safeguards (if any) that may be needed to ensure that the health care needs of individuals with special health care needs and chronic conditions who are enrolled in Medicaid managed care organizations are adequately met. (PL 105-33, Section 4705(c)(2))

We would reiterate: Medicare (and Medicaid) has traditionally represented the federal government's primary quality assurance effort, and yet, surprisingly, there has been very little recent public attention paid to this aspect of the program. At the public policy level, cost concerns seem to have taken precedence over access and quality of care concerns.

THE FUTURE—TELEHEALTH

In our judgment, the most exciting development occurring today within health care is the exponential growth in the computer (and related technological) arena and its increasing direct applicability to health care. Telehealth (i.e., telemedicine), computerized patient records, and related technological advances are rapidly reshaping our expectations for (and ability to ensure) quality health care. Computer technology, including interactive patient records that can constantly respond to modifications in laboratory results or patient input via modems, can drastically alter how care is provided. With readily accessible data and instant virtual consultation ability, the importance of standardized reporting becomes critical (DeLeon, Sammons, Frank, & VandenBos, in press b).

The General Accounting Office (GAO) has identified nine federal departments and independent agencies that have invested at least $646 million in telehealth projects from fiscal year 1994 to 1996, with the Department of Defense providing over one third of the funding. In 1994, the Congress established the ad hoc Steering

Committee on Telehealth and Health Care Informatics. By the end of the first session of the 105th Congress (1997), impressive reports had already been issued by the Institute of Medicine, the former Office of Technology Assessment, the General Accounting Office, and the US Department of Commerce. The federal government had established a Federal Interagency Joint Working Group on Telemedicine, which among other responsibilities has been tasked with establishing a worldwide web-accessible inventory of federally sponsored telemedicine projects. The Balanced Budget Act of 1997 (PL 105-33) directed that Medicare reimburse for professional consultations under Part B, no later than January 1, 1999. By the end of 1997, 15 states had decided to offer some telemedicine coverage under their Medicaid programs and the states of California and Louisiana had enacted legislation mandating coverage for telehealth consultation services under private insurance plans.

The Commerce Department report expressly addressed the potential applicability of telehealth for mental health services:

> Unlike some specialties such as cardiology, mental health telemedicine applications do not require a high degree of image specificity, thus the technology can be simpler and costs can be lower. Moreover, initial evidence indicates that telemedicine works well for group therapy as well as individual consults. (US Department of Commerce, 1997, p. 19).

Some of the major policy issues being addressed include confidentiality of patient records, insurance reimbursement, interstate licensure decisions, malpractice liability, and the potential for "cookbook medicine" or requiring predetermined algorithms of care. Many of these policy issues eventually will be decided at the state level, both in the legislature and by administrative agencies.

To again focus on the federal government's role as a provider of health care and thereby to give another perspective of the extent to which telehealth has already matured: In 1996, the health officials of the Department of Defense testified before the Senate Appropriations Committee. The witnesses described their considerable enthusiasm for the clinical and teaching potential inherent in the technology revolution. Medical digital technology, telemedicine, advanced computer-based medical expert systems, and information management—for combat as well as for day-to-day business and clinical practice—were explicitly addressed. Allowing attending providers on board ships to transmit real-time ultrasound videos and full color images back to specialists at major treatment facilities hundreds of miles away was clearly doable. By 1998, the Navy Surgeon General reported that on board ship telehealth mental health consultations were standard operating procedure and that he was able to reduce MEDEVACS by 28%, 40% of which are traditionally mental health related.

CLOSING REFLECTIONS

The issue of ensuring high-quality health care is extraordinarily important for all Americans. Very few practitioners or health policy experts would disagree. And yet, over the years there has been considerable policy disagreement as to how to accomplish this laudatory goal and equally importantly how to fundamentally define "quality care." A review of the government's efforts in this arena indicates considerable policy ambivalence.

The key to ensuring high-quality health care is ready access to objective measures of what clinical services are being provided, under what conditions, and a systematic evaluation of how particular clinical protocols compare with treatment being rendered for similar cases elsewhere. Yet, for anyone other than the patient's own practitioner to possess this information definitely would seem to violate practitioner–patient confidentiality, which is particularly critical in mental health. Further, as the behavioral sciences have matured, there has been growing consensus that their input should be reflected in the underlying definition of quality. Similar inclusive attitudes also have been evolving regarding more broadly defined quality of life indicators.

At the same time, it also has become quite evident that any proposed modification in the traditional hierarchial status quo is very unsettling. Practitioners appear to be particularly concerned that their individual clinical judgments might be "second guessed" and that various third-party payment mechanisms (such as Medicare or CHAMPUS) might become conditioned upon their following national standards or guidelines (i.e., requiring cookbook medicine). Nevertheless, recent exponential advances within the computer and related technological fields (including interactive computerized records and telehealth) are rapidly moving the health professions toward accountability and verifiability.

Since President Clinton was elected to office, there has been unprecedented political activity surrounding the issues of increased access and most recently increased consumer accountability. The impact of managed care and other cost-containment efforts without question have revolutionized the delivery of health services. In its role as a direct provider of health care, the federal government has been exploring various approaches to ensuring quality care, and also, how these might eventually become applicable to the private sector. For the 105th Congress, quality care seems to mean patient choice, not objective measures of clinical services.

It is clear that at this point in our nation's history there is not genuine consensus about the ultimate goal, let alone how to achieve it. There does seem to be the general recognition that change is coming, and further, that an educational (rather than prescriptive) approach by government and those who ultimately pay the bill for health services has the greatest likelihood of ensuring a positive maturation.

REFERENCES

Advisory Commission on Consumer Protection and Quality in the Health Care Industry. (1997, November). *Consumer bill of rights and responsibilities: Report to the President of the United States*. Washington, DC: Author.

American Psychological Association (APA). (1996a). *Case studies illustrate cost savings resulting from appropriate mental health intervention* (Issue Brief). Washington, DC: Author.

American Psychological Association (APA). (1996b). *Mental health benefit is cost-effective* (Issue Brief). Washington, DC: Author.

American Psychological Association (APA). (1996c). *The costs of failing to provide appropriate mental health care* (Issue Brief). Washington, DC: Author.

Bachman, R. E. (1996, April). *An actuarial analysis of the Domenici–Wellstone amendment to S. 1028 "health insurance reform act" to provide parity for mental health benefits under group and individual insurance plans*. Washington, DC: Coopers & Lybrand.

Cantor, D. W. (1998). News from Washington, DC—Achieving a mental health bill of rights. *Professional Psychology: Research and Practice, 29*(4), 315–316.

Chassin, M. R. (1997, May/June). Assessing strategies for quality improvement. *Health Affairs, 16*, 151–161.

Clinton, W. J. (1998, January 28). The State of the Union. *The Washington Post*, p. A24.

Congressional Budget Office (CBO). (1996, May 13). *CBO's estimates of the impact on employers of the mental health parity amendment in HR 3103*. Washington, DC: US Government Printing Office.

Copeland, C. (1998, April). *Issues of quality and consumer rights in the health care market* (Issue Brief No. 196). Washington, DC: Employee Benefit Research Institute.

Darby, M. (1998, February). *Health care quality: From data to accountability.* (Background paper). National Health Policy Forum: The George Washington University.

Davis, J. E. (1984, November). Testimony before the US Senate Appropriations Committee. *Variations in medical practice* (S. Hrg. #98-1239), 124–138.

DeLeon, P. H. (1988). Public policy and public service: Our professional duty. *American Psychologist, 43,* 309–315.

DeLeon, P. H., & VandenBos, G. R. (1980). Psychotherapy reimbursement in federal programs: Political factors. In G. R. VandenBos (Ed.), *Psychotherapy: Practice, research, policy* (pp. 247–285). Beverly Hills, CA: Sage.

DeLeon, P. H., & VandenBos, G. R. (1983). The new federal health care frontiers—Cost containment and "wellness." *Psychotherapy in Private Practice, 1*(2), 17–32.

DeLeon, P. H., & Wiggins, J. G. (1996). Prescription privileges for psychologists. *American Psychologist, 51*(3), 225–229.

DeLeon, P. H., & Williams, J. G. (1997). Evaluation research and public policy formation: Are psychologists collectively willing to accept unpopular findings? *American Psychologist, 52*(5), 551–552.

DeLeon, P. H., VandenBos, G. R., & Cummings, N. A. (1983). Psychotherapy—Is it safe, effective, and appropriate? The beginning of an evolutionary dialogue. *American Psychologist, 38,* 907–911.

DeLeon, P. H., Willens, J. G., Clinton, J. J., & VandenBos, G. R. (1988). The role of the federal government in peer review. In G. Stricker & A. R. Rodriguez (Eds.), *Handbook of quality assurance in mental health* (pp. 285–309). New York: Plenum Press.

DeLeon, P. H., Bulatao, E. Q., & VandenBos, G. R. (1994). Federal government initiatives in managed mental health. In S. A. Shueman, S. L. Mayhugh, & B. S. Gould (Eds.), *Managed behavioral health care: An industry perspective* (pp. 97–112). Springfield, IL: Charles C. Thomas.

DeLeon, P. H., Howell, W. C., Newman, R. S., Brown, A. B., Keita, G. P., & Sexton, J. L. (1996). Expanding roles in the twenty-first century. In R. J. Resnick & R. H. Rozensky (Eds.), *Health psychology through the life span: Practice and research opportunities* (pp. 427–453). Washington, DC: American Psychological Association.

DeLeon, P. H., Sammons, M. T., & Fox, R. E. (in press a). Prescription privileges. In A. E. Kazdin (Ed.), *Encyclopedia of psychology.* Washington, DC: American Psychological Association.

DeLeon, P. H., Sammons, M. T., Frank, R. G., & VandenBos, G. R. (in press b). Changing health care environment in the United States—Steadily evolving into the 21st century. In A. N. Wiens (Ed.), *Professional issues (Vol. 8): Comprehensive clinical psychology.* New York: Elsevier Science.

Eckert, P. A. (1994). Cost control through quality improvement: The new challenge for psychology. *Professional Psychology: Research and Practice, 25*(1), 3–8.

Employee Benefit Research Institute (EBRI). (1997, February). *Issues in mental health care benefits: The costs of mental health parity* (Issue Brief No. 182). Washington, DC: Author.

England, M. J. (1997, January). The mental health parity act: Lifting benefit plan limits. *HIU Magazine.*

Frist, W. H. (1998, June 23). Introduction of S. 2208, the healthcare quality enhancement act of 1998. *Congressional Record, 144*(3), S.6888–S.6889. Washington, DC: U.S. Senate.

Gaus, C. R., & DeLeon, P. H. (1995). News from Washington, DC—Thinking beyond the limitations of mental health care. *Professional Psychology: Research and Practice, 26*(4), 339–340.

Health: GOP's managed care bill rushes through House. (1998, July 25). *Weekly Report,* p. 2007. Washington, DC: 1998 Congressional Quarterly.

Judge David L. Bazelon Center for Mental Health Law. (1996, May). *Paying for parity: A review of costs in two states with health insurance laws mandating equal coverage of mental health care.* Washington, DC: Author.

Kiesler, C. A. (1984, November). Testimony before the US Senate Appropriations Committee. *Variations in medical practice* (S. Hrg. #98-1239), 138–164. Washington, DC: US Government Printing Office.

Kizer, K. W. (1998, January 13). Letter response to John D. Rockefeller IV, ranking minority member, Committee on Veterans' Affairs, United States Senate, unpublished correspondence.

Lohr, K. N. (Ed.). (1990). *Medicare: A strategy for quality assurance, Vol. II.* Institute of Medicine. Washington, DC: National Academy Press.

Lorion, R. P., Iscoe, I., DeLeon, P. H., & VandenBos, G. R. (Eds.). (1996). *Psychology and public policy: Balancing public service and professional need.* Washington, DC: American Psychological Association.

Melek, S. P., & Pyenson, B. (1996, April 12). *Premium rate estimates for a mental illness parity provision to S. 1028: "The health insurance reform act of 1995."* Milliman & Robertson.

Mental Health Liaison Group. (1996). *equal treatment of mental health services in health plans: Facts about the*

Domenici–Wellstone amendment to Senate bill S. 1028. (Issue Brief). Washington, DC: American Psychological Association.

Price Waterhouse, LLP. Health Policy Economics Group. (1996, May 31). *Analysis of the mental health parity provisions in S. 1028.* Washington, DC: Author.

Prospective Payment Assessment Commission (PPAC). (1997, June). *Medicare and the American health care system. Report to Congress.* Washington, DC: US Government Printing Office.

Seligman, M. E. P., & Levant, R. F. (1998). News from Washington, DC–Managed care policies rely on inadequate science. *Professional Psychology: Research and Practice, 29*(3), 211–212.

Sleek, S. (1996, December). Psychology continues call for equity. *APA Monitor, 27*(12), 28, 30.

State of California, Office of Statewide Health Planning and Development, Division of Health Professions Development. (1982, November). *Prescribing and dispensing pilot projects* (Final report to the legislature and to the healing arts licensing boards). Sacramento, CA: Author.

US Congress. House Committee on Ways and Means. (1998). *1998 green book: Background material and data on programs within the jurisdiction of the Committee on Ways and Means* (WMCP 105-7). Washington, DC: US Government Printing Office.

US Congress. Senate. Committee on Veterans' Affairs. (1997, December 19). *Staff report on quality management in the veterans health administration department of veterans affairs: Prepared by the minority staff of the Committee on Veterans' Affairs.* Washington, DC: US Senate.

US Department of Commerce. (1997, January). *Telemedicine report to Congress.* (#1997-418-626/42023). Washington, DC: Government Printing Office.

US Department of Health and Human Services (HHS). (1991). *Healthy people 2000: National health promotion and disease prevention objectives.* (DHHS Pub. No. (PHS) 91-50212(3)). Washington, DC: US Government Printing Office.

US Department of Health and Human Services (HHS). (1998). *Fiscal year 1999 justification of estimates for Appropriations Committees: Agency for health care policy and research.* Washington, DC: US Government Printing Office.

US Department of Veterans Affairs and Housing and Urban Development, and Independent Agencies appropriations bill, 1999. (S. Rpt. #105-216). Washington, DC: US Senate.

Uyeda, M. K., DeLeon, P. H., Perloff, R., & Kraut, A. G. (1986). Financing mental health services: A comparison of two federal programs. *American Behavioral Scientist, 30,* 90–110.

Valentine, N. M. (1998). Quality measures essential to the transformation of the veterans health administration: Implications for nurses as co-creators of change. *Nursing Administration Quarterly, 22*(4), 76–87.

Wilensky, G. R. (1997, May/June). Perspective—Promoting quality: A public policy view. *Health Affairs, 16,* 77–81.

Willens, J. G., & DeLeon, P. H. (1982). Political aspects of peer review. *Professional Psychology, 13,* 23–26.

16

The Role of External Entities in the Quality Management Process

The National Committee for Quality Assurance

MAUREEN MANGOTICH

> Notions about accountability are more than descriptions of the current system; they are also normative guides to determine the institutional structures for health care organizations and the type of health care delivery system we should have. Emanuel and Emanuel (1996, p. 229)

During the 1980s, the first managed behavioral health care organizations emerged as a mechanism for providing cost predictability and cost stabilization for purchasers of mental health and chemical dependency services. Today, more than 120 million Americans receive mental health services through more than 300 managed behavioral health care organizations (MBHOs). Thus far, these organizations have focused primarily on serving the commercial market, but there is increasing momentum for public purchasers to move beneficiaries into managed care systems. At least 17 states have received waivers from the Health Care Financing Administration for Medicaid managed care that includes mental health and chemical dependency services.

Accountability has become the dominant theme in managed health care in the 1990s. Consumers and purchasers are now demanding formal documentation of the quality and value of health services purchased. Much of the recent ad hoc legislation relating to managed care, such as mandated maternity length of stays, represents attempts (whether meritorious or not) to better define the accountability of managed care systems. Managed care quality initiatives such as performance report cards and formal accreditation programs have developed significantly over the last several years as a response to the market need for ways of promoting functional accountability.

Emanuel and Emanuel (1996) describe three sectoral models of accountability in health care: professional, economic, and political. The professional model of accountability treats health care as a service rather than a commodity, with a primary focus on accountability in professional competence and ethical conduct. The economic model of accountability is commodity-based, with individual patients viewed as consumers

The views expressed in this article are solely those of the author, and do not represent the opinions of Pfizer or Pfizer Health Solutions.

MAUREEN MANGOTICH • Pfizer Health Solutions, Santa Monica, California 90404.

Handbook of Quality Management in Behavioral Health, edited by Stricker *et al.* Kluwer Academic / Plenum Publishers, New York, 2000.

or customers, and clinicians, facilities, and managed care organizations (MCOs) as suppliers of goods and services who compete for market share. Under this model there is a role for regulators to ensure fair and efficient operation of the market and to supply information about price and quality to guide consumer decision making. The political model of accountability views stakeholders as "citizen members" of a community who appoint or elect representatives to operate the health care system and represent their interests. Mechanisms for achieving patient well-being are defined in the context of the overall needs of the community. Managed care systems must make decisions about allocation of resources, which necessarily involve moral decisions about relative needs.

Emmanuel and Emanuel (1996)suggest that an optimal accountability system would incorporate aspects of all three models: the professional model to guide provider–patient interactions, the economic model for MCOs and integrated delivery systems, and the political model for relations between MCOs and purchasers.

Accreditation (usually voluntary) has long been used as a mechanism for adjudging the "quality" of educational institutions, health care service facilities, and professional education and training programs across the health care disciplines. It is, nonetheless, a rather blunt instrument for the designation of quality in the public interest. Health care accreditation bodies such as the National Committee for Quality Assurance (NCQA) and the Joint Commission for Accreditation of Healthcare Organizations (JCAHO) function as "appointees" of purchasers to evaluate the quality of managed care delivery systems on behalf of service users.

The National Committee for Quality Assurance (NCQA) is a private, not-for-profit organization that focuses on the assessment of general medical health maintenance organizations (HMO)—referred to by NCQA as managed care organizations, or MCOs—certain provider organizations, and specialty managed behavioral health organizations (MBHO). Since 1991, about half of the nation's 550 HMOs have participated in NCQA accreditation reviews. Accreditation of the other two categories of organizations was initiated in 1997. The following section provides a general outline of the essentials of the process used by NCQA for managed behavioral health care organizations seeking accreditation (NCQA, 1997).

DEVELOPMENT OF ACCREDITATION STANDARDS FOR BEHAVIORAL HEALTH ORGANIZATIONS

In developing new accreditation programs, NCQA solicits input from purchasers, providers, and consumers (typically in the form of representative consumer organizations) who will be affected by the program. In 1995, NCQA convened a 22-member Behavioral Health Task Force, with representatives from employers, unions, public purchasers, consumers, managed care organizations, managed behavioral health care organizations, and mental health and substance abuse experts. This work group used the 1995 Standards for MCO Accreditation (NCQA, 1995) as the starting point for development of MBHO standards.

NCQA released the draft standards for public comment in April 1996. The task force used these public comments and results from pilot testing of the draft standards in two MBHOs and one MCO during the second half of 1996, to further develop these draft standards. Examples of modifications include the addition of standards to assess cultural competence, requirements for inclusion of input from the MBHO's members, clarification of standards for access, and delineation of an MBHO's accountability for collaboration and coordination with providers of medical services.

NCQA Accreditation Categories and Standards

The first standards for MBHO accreditation (NCQA, 1997) were released in February of 1997 and represent an ambitious set of operational objectives for quality improvement in managed behavioral health care as established by a consensus of stakeholders. There are approximately 50 standards for behavioral health quality organized within seven categories (see Table 1). The accessibility category of standards, which is unique to the MBHO program, was added to address the triage and assessment functions that are so integral to the provision of behavioral health services within managed systems.

Managed behavioral health organizations must meet NCQA-specified eligibility criteria in order to apply for a behavioral health care review (see Table 2). For now, MCOs that manage their own behavioral healthcare programs will continue to be reviewed using NCQA standards for MCO accreditation, but have the option of also seeking MBHO accreditation for their behavioral programs. NCQA has proposed that by the year 2000, all managed behavioral health programs, whether operating as independent organizations or as part of a larger MCO, will be assessed using the MBHO standards.

Survey Process and Procedures

Organizations wishing to be accredited by NCQA must complete an application and pay a $7500 application fee. After the application is processed and a survey (site visit) date is set, NCQA estimates the actual survey fees based on the size, complexity, and structure of the organization. A fact-finding survey team composed of at least one physician reviewer and one administrative surveyor with experience in quality management spends between 2 and 4 days on site to review the organization's quality systems and assess the level of compliance with NCQA standards. Surveyors review

Table 1. Categories of NCQA Standards for MBHO Accreditation

Quality management and improvement: Ensure establishment and monitoring of structures, processes, and outcomes of care
Accessibility, availability, referral, and triage: Ensure accessibility and availability of behavioral health services and network adequacy
Utilization management: Support appropriate procedures for obtaining authorization for behavioral health standards
Credentialing and recredentialing: Ensure that all licensed behavioral health practitioners have appropriate training and experience
Member rights and responsibilities: Promote open communication with members
Preventive behavioral health standards: Ensure prevention and early detection of behavioral health problems
Clinical evaluation and treatment records: Ensure providers maintain current, comprehensive, and organized treatment records

TABLE 2. Eligibility Requirements for MBHO Accreditation by NCQA

The MBHO:
- Has been in operation for at least 18 months
- Provides defined benefit package that includes child and adolescent mental health services, adult mental health services, substance abuse and chemical dependency services, and preventive behavioral health standards
- Provides inpatient, residential, partial hospitalization, and outpatient services
- Maintains organized quality management process

written documentation and records provided by the organization, interview staff and network practitioners, and audit a random sample of treatment records.

Following the site visit, the survey team prepares a detailed written report outlining findings; this report is reviewed by executive-level NCQA staff for clarity and consistency. The organization may be contacted at this point to provide additional documentation in support of on-site team findings or to clarify outstanding issues. The organization then receives a copy of the draft report detailing findings and recommendations, and may submit comments regarding factual errors or omissions. These comments are in turn considered by NCQA and incorporated into the report as appropriate. The Review Oversight Committee (ROC) reviews the preliminary report and associated documentation, considers the recommendations of the survey team, and either renders one of five possible accreditation decisions or defers a decision pending additional fact finding (see Table 3). Reconsideration procedures have been established to resolve disagreements between the organization and NCQA about accreditation decisions.

When it is deemed that a sufficient number of MBHOs have undergone accreditation reviews, NCQA will make the review results available to the public in the form of an Accreditation Status Report (sample in Appendix 1) which can be viewed at the NCQA website or ordered through the committee's publications department. Organi-

TABLE 3. NCQA Accreditation Decisions

Finding	Decision	Duration
Full accreditation	Full/substantial compliance	3 years
Accreditation with recommendations	Full/substantial compliance One or more issues warranting action Remediable within 90 days	3 years
One-year accreditation	Significant compliance Further action needed Remediable within one year	15 months
Provisional accreditation	Partial compliance No risk to patient care	15 months
Denial of accreditation status	Minimal compliance *or* Potentially significant risk to patient care	1 year
Deferral of accreditation status	Additional information needed *or* Issues of concern to NCQA	60 days maximum

zations that have never been surveyed or accredited by NCQA may elect initially to submit to a practice accreditation review (PAR) before applying for a full survey. On the basis of the PAR, NCQA prepares a detailed report describing performance against the standards, areas of strength, and opportunities for improvement. No accreditation decision is made on the basis of the PAR. Rather, it is used by the MBHO as a guide to system improvement in preparation for the actual site visit.

NCQA: AN ASPIRATIONAL FORCE FOR BEHAVIORAL HEALTH

The 1997 MBHO standards for accreditation define characteristics of an optimal managed behavioral health care system. The system of accreditation is thus aspirational. Some of the goals set for MBHOs represent significant departures from current operations of most if not all of these organizations, and will only be met incrementally over time. NCQA has established tiered performance levels for 1997 in the three areas judged most likely to require significant development on the part of MBHOs: coordination of behavioral health with medical care; implementation of population-based, quality improvement systems; and implementation of preventive behavioral health programs.

Coordination of Care

NCQA aims to strengthen coordination of behavioral and medical care in two ways. The committee requires evidence that care is coordinated among providers across medical and mental health delivery systems and that the behavioral and medical systems share data on quality initiatives and performance measurement. Communication is a two-way process and MBHOs cannot necessarily control the flow of information from MCOs to them. The 1997 standards, therefore, require only that the MBHO have mechanisms in place to support effective interorganizational communication.

Quality Improvement

Improvement in population-based service planning is heavily emphasized in NCQA standards, since managed care systems are increasingly associated with defined populations. MBHOs, however, may be required only to have the capacity to identify only those members who have actually used services. NCQA has identified four population groups that are meaningful to MBHOs. Level 1 includes all members using or having used behavioral health services. Level 2 includes level 1 members together with members receiving behavioral health care services from primary care physicians. Level 3 includes level 2 as well as members requiring behavioral health care who are not already receiving it. Level 4 represents all members who could potentially seek services (the entire covered population). For 1997, however, the MBHO is held accountable only for level I members, with the expectation that over time, as communication and coordination between mental health and medical care systems improve, MBHOs and MCOs will jointly share accountability for the behavioral health of the entire covered population

Preventive Health

In keeping with NCQA's emphasis on prevention in its MCO accreditation standards, there is an entire section devoted to preventive behavioral health standards for MBHO accreditation. Preventive activities can be primary (to prevent a condition), secondary (to minimize morbidity from a known condition), or tertiary (to manage manifestations of an existing condition). Predictably, NCQA standards require that the organization formally assess the needs of its covered population as an initial step in planning prevention programs. For 1997, only the needs of level 1 members will be assessed.

CATEGORIES FOR NCQA ACCREDITATION

As noted above, the NCQA standards are organized into seven discrete but somewhat overlapping categories. These functional categories subsume virtually all areas deemed to have a direct impact on a member's access to appropriate care and services.

Quality Improvement

The organization must have a clearly defined quality improvement (QI) program with active oversight by its governing body, dedicated staff and resources sufficient to meet the program's short- and long-range quality goals, and involvement of practitioners and members in activities aimed at improvement of clinical care and service. Program scope and content should be comprehensive, reflecting the organization's delivery system and population demographics, and should address clinical and service quality, practitioner and provider relations, and member services.

The organization also must assess and evaluate at least three clinical issues relevant to its membership, using appropriate methods for data collection and analysis. Actions must be taken to improve quality, with an assessment of the effectiveness of the interventions through systematic follow-up. If any quality activities are delegated,* the organization must oversee the performance of the entity to which the delegated responsibility is given.

Contracts with providers must include provisions requiring the providers to cooperate with QI activities, comply with quality standards, and allow access to member records in accordance with state and federal confidentiality laws. To ensure member satisfaction, the organization must have systematic procedures for identifying and addressing sources of dissatisfaction with the full range of operations, including access, providers, utilization management procedures, quality of care, quality of member services, claims payment procedures, and benefits provided under their health plan.

*Delegations is a formal process wherein the MBHO requires an entity with which it contracts to take responsibility for some aspects of service delivery or monitoring normally assumed by the MBHO itself. For example, the MBHO might have an arrangement under which a behavioral health practice group is responsible for specific aspects of quality or utilization monitoring. Alternately, the group practice may be required to formally credential its own providers. Delegation may occur under any of the seven standard categories.

The NCQA also requires the particular MBHO to conduct a member satisfaction survey and to evaluate, at least annually, member complaints, appeals, and requests to change practitioners. Providers and members must be notified of the results of surveys and activities to improve satisfaction. To promote best practices, the organization must adopt, distribute, and periodically update evidence-based clinical practice guidelines. It must also measure adherence to at least two guidelines on an annual basis. In order to achieve full accreditation, the organization must demonstrate at least three meaningful improvements in clinical care or service.

Accessibility, Availability, Referral, and Triage

To ensure that members have prompt access to behavioral health services and information about those services and the service system, NCQA has defined accessibility standards for behavioral health care services, including routine services as well as services of a more urgent nature and member (i.e., customer) services. The organization must undertake to measure its performance against the standards, take actions to improve when necessary, and notify providers and members of the results. Availability is the extent to which the organization has an appropriate provider network (with consideration given to professional discipline, specialty, number, cultural diversity, and geographic distribution of practitioners) to meet the needs of its membership. The organization must establish standards to ensure availability, measure performance against the standards, and initiate actions for improvement when necessary. Referral and triage functions must be appropriately implemented, monitored, and professionally managed using evidence-based protocols and the appropriate level of staff for decision making.

Utilization Management

The goal of the utilization management (UM) program is to effectively manage the allocation of available resources to ensure that necessary and appropriate care and services are delivered. NCQA requires a written UM program description with mechanisms for decision making that are explicitly defined and consistently applied, standards for timeliness of review, and written descriptions of information to be collected to support UM decisions. Licensed behavioral health practitioners must assess the clinical information used to support UM decisions. Practitioners and members are required to be given written notification of denials that include the reason for the denial and the process for appealing the decision. There must be a process in place to evaluate new technologies and new applications of existing technologies for inclusion in the benefit package. The organization must survey members and practitioners at least every 2 years about their level of satisfaction with the UM program and procedures and effectively address sources of dissatisfaction.

Credentialing and Recredentialing

Because members receiving services through an MBHO are generally required to use network or contracted practitioners, these organizations have the responsibility periodically to verify education, training, and clinical qualifications and assess practitioner performance using explicit criteria and a systematic process for credentials review. NCQA requires "primary source"* verification of professional license; hospital privileges, Drug Enforcement Agency (DEA) certificate, education, and training; board certification (if applicable); work history, sanctions or limitations placed on license' malpractice insurance coverage' and malpractice claims history (through a query to the National Practitioner Data Bank). Practitioners sign a statement describing any physical or mental impairments that interfere with their ability to perform essential job functions; in addition, they must attest to lack of present illegal drug use and describe any current or prior loss of license, hospital privileges, sanctions, or disciplinary actions.

The MBHO is required to conduct an initial site visit to any new provider's office and conduct a review of his or her medical record-keeping practices prior to accepting the provider onto the network. At least every 2 years, practitioners are recredentialed. Data reviewed during the recredentialing process relate to provider-specific member complaints, identified quality issues, UM performance, and results of satisfaction surveys, site visits, and medical record reviews. The organization must maintain policies and procedures for altering the conditions of a practitioner's participation (e.g., placing limitations on the types of patients the provider may treat) based on issues of quality of clinical care and service and for reporting on identified quality issues as required by state and local authorities. When practice limitations are imposed on a provider or when the organization terminates the practitioner from the network because of quality of care concerns, the practitioner must be offered an opportunity to appeal the decision. Facility credentialing must occur prior to contracting and at least every 3 years using defined standards for participation.

Member Rights and Responsibilities

When an organization clearly communicates its expectations of the rights and responsibilities of members, these members are better equipped to use the service system effectively. NCQA requires that organizations define member rights and responsibilities in writing and distribute the policy to members, participating behavioral health providers, and primary care physicians.

The handling of member complaints and grievances is generally regulated by state and federal agencies. NCQA looks for evidence of a structured process for registering and responding to complaints and appeals that includes standards for timeliness, investigation of the substance of the issue, and written notification to the member of the outcome as well as procedures for appealing the decision. Written materials describing benefits and charges (copayments, deductibles, noncovered services), procedures for accessing services, and instructions on initiating complaints are to be provided to all members. These materials must be member tested for readability and comprehension. For example, a typical requirement is that member materials be written such that they can be understood by someone with an eighth grade reading level.

*Primary source verifications is the practice of directly consulting the appropriate regulatory, educational, or other agency or organization to verify a professional's credentials, for example, contacting a state licensing board to verify that a professional holds a current, active license to practice, or a university to verify that a professional actually earned the degree that he or she claims to possess.

Preventive Health

NCQA expects organizations to distribute information about preventive behavioral health programs at least annually and to identify and engage in outreach to members who may be at risk for behavioral health problems. The organization should annually monitor and evaluate at least two age-appropriate preventive behavioral health screening and educational interventions based on an assessment of the needs of its covered population. Examples of types of preventive behavioral health interventions include identification of learning and behavioral problems in preschoolers, adolescent eating disorders, early onset serious mental illness (schizophrenia), adult mood disorders, and organic brain syndromes in the elderly, as well as parent training or domestic violence programs made available to the community.

Treatment Records

Treatment records communicating patients' clinical history, health status, treatment plans for current and future clinical care, and plans for coordination of care are essential tools for the delivery of coordinated and high-quality behavioral services. Organizations are required to establish standards for treatment records, to review records for conformity with the standards, and to institute corrective actions when standards are not met. The record content should reflect adherence to national standards of practice and clinically appropriate patient management protocols. Organizations should have in place policies for ensuring patient confidentiality that are consistent with applicable state and federal regulations.

FUTURE DIRECTIONS FOR BEHAVIORAL HEALTH ACCREDITATION

With the establishment of its new managed behavioral health accreditation program, NCQA has defined a comprehensive quality agenda for managed behavioral health systems in the 21St century. It will take a number of years for MBHOs to meet these ambitious standards. Essential ingredients for implementing effective quality improvement systems are committed trained staff, accessible clinical information systems, and valid, reliable standardized performance measures.

It is interesting to note that in the fee-for-service system that (with the exception of Kaiser and several other group or staff model HMOs) dominated health care until the 1980s, there were virtually no applicable quality standards outside of institutions, such as hospitals, and certain organized care settings, such as community mental health centers. In these settings JCAHO (in those earlier days named the Joint Commission for Accreditation of Hospitals, or JCAH) and the Commission on Accreditation of Rehabilitation Facilities (CARF) were the dominant standard setters. It is only with the advent of managed health care that the administrative and management structures exist outside of facilities and organized care settings to allow implementation of organized programs for improving quality. During the entire period of its ascendency, the fee-for-service "system" supported no such programs.

Few people within the health services industry would argue the desirability of developing the types of accountability and quality improvement systems called for by NCQA. At the same time, an open question regarding these standards is whether the significant costs associated with their implementation will prove to be justified in terms of the benefit accruing to patient care and health outcomes. Development and maintenance of the structures and processes mandated by the NCQA behavioral health standards constitute sometimes significant departures from the way these companies have traditionally done business and, more importantly, require a significant commitment in the form of financial resources. For example, for a large MBHO, credentialing a provider network according to the standards of NCQA is a multimillion dollar activity. At the same time, the credentialing process for an individual practitioner, program, or facility is independently repeated by every MBHO with which that provider contracts. Further, a single written communication to all subscribers of a medium-sized MBHO (e.g., information on a preventive health topic) would cost several hundred thousand dollars. Such expenses will surely add to the costs of health care premiums paid by employers and other purchasers of care. Most certainly, then, the cost-benefit issues will need to be addressed in the years to come as MHBOs gain experience with the standards and as the true costs of compliance become known.

Conclusion

A set of general characteristics or trends can be discerned in the current and emerging context of behavioral health service system accreditation. These are identified below and offered as rudimentary signposts along a road with many forks in rough terrain. While the particular mission, mechanisms, and standards associated with behavioral health systems accreditation by the NCQA by no means account for all the variance within the field, it is reasonable to draw from these some general inferences.

1. *Accountability to multiple stakeholders.* This emerges as a central normative tenet driving the accreditation of behavioral health service delivery systems. Payers and purchasers as well as the population at large now join the consumer as entities to which accountability is owed and directed.

2. *Manifest accountability "rules" in behavioral health.* This is novel in the extreme and currently more the exception than the rule. Nonetheless, the long-touted aphorism—competition on the basis of quality as well as cost—has begun to find operational forms. This same development will increasingly be the death knell of the independent and small group practice in the behavioral professions. It is only functionally integrated systems that possess the infrastructure and other means to meet the criteria for effective quality management. Accreditation entities now recognize this.

3. *Accountability pressures, including accreditation, will drive the integration of behavioral and general health services.* Before the end of this century the NCQA will require medical HMOs offering behavioral health services to meet the MBHO as well as the MCO (general medical) standards. The increasing use of population-based services planning will also fortify this trend.

4. *Improved communication between purchasers and MBHOs.* Purchasers and payers will not long be able to play both ends against the middle. That is, they will not be able to claim that they are the protectors of consumers while continuing to exercise their purchasing power in the cause of cost-containment in a buyer's market. Pur-

chasers must be led to understand that effective quality management does not come cheap and that what truly matters is cost-effective care rather than care that is cost-contained. Accreditation, albeit in indirect ways, supports the development of effective and enduring quality management systems.

5. *The face of accountability will change.* As noted earlier in this chapter, accreditation is a very blunt instrument indeed in the service of quality improvement. It does possess, however, a "sentinel" effect. That is, it keeps the players on notice that there is an (more or less vigilant) external watchdog. Again, the traditional voluntary nature of accreditation becomes increasingly meaningless in operational terms if such status is inextricably linked with the capacity of an MCO or MBHO to become or remain a player in the competitive marketplace.

6. *The power and efficacy of external regulation as a quality improvement tool is on the wane.* This seems paradoxical in light of the prevailing increase in regulatory pressures on managed care and particularly on HMOs. Yet this upsurge of ad hoc initiatives is largely the consequence of stakeholders' confusion about their role in an industry whose rapid and essentially chaotic growth is beyond their control. While entities such as NCQA may be an effective political stimulus for the development of quality management programs, enduring quality improvement will only be the result of forces and a commitment internal to the service delivery system.

APPENDIX

Below is a sample of an Accreditation Summary Report (ASR). This report is the vehicle through which NCQA makes public how a health plan performed on its accreditation survey. The report is posted on the NCQA website. (http://www.ncqa.org/)

Providence Health Plan - Oregon

PORTLAND, OREGON

June 12, 1998 - June 12, 2001

NCQA Standards cover the following areas: | *The plan achieved the following scores:**

In **Quality Management and Improvement,** NCQA evaluates:
- how effectively the plan works to continuously improve the quality of care and service
- how the plan makes sure that members have access to the care they need
- the improvements in quality the plan can show

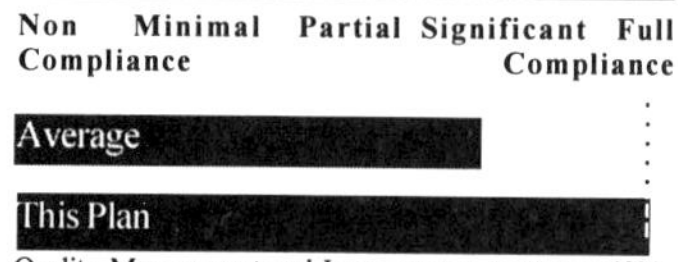

Quality Management and Improvement counts as 40% of the overall accreditation decision.

In **Members' Rights and Responsibilities,** NCQA evaluates:
- how clearly the plan informs members about how to get care and use services
- how well the plan responds to members' complaints and concerns
- what actions the plan takes to measure and improve members' satisfaction

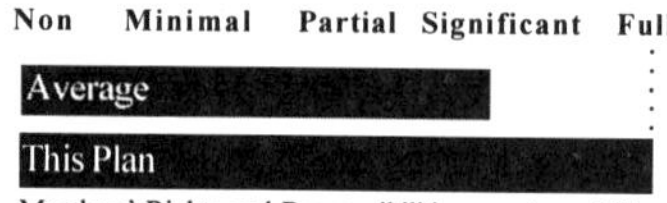

Members' Rights and Responsibilities counts as 10% of the overall accreditation decision.

In **Physician Qualifications and Evaluation** for physicians in the network, NCQA evaluates:
- how fully the plan investigates each physician's qualifications and practice history, before letting the physician into the network
- how the plan assesses physicians in its network on an ongoing basis

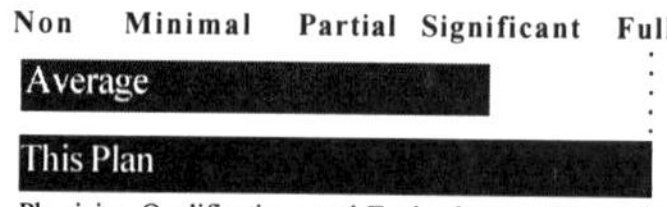

Physician Qualifications and Evaluation counts as 20% of the overall accreditation decision.

In **Preventive Health Services,** NCQA evaluates:
- how well the plan promotes health and encourages members to use preventive services such as immunizations and mammograms
- how well the plan can show that members receive preventive services

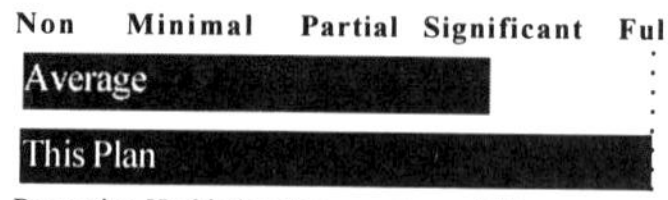

Preventive Health Services counts as 15% of the overall accreditation decision.

In **Utilization Management** (making decisions about approving services), NCQA evaluates:
- how fair, consistent, and prompt the plan is in making decisions
- how the plan ensures that the approval process does not cause unnecessary problems for members or providers

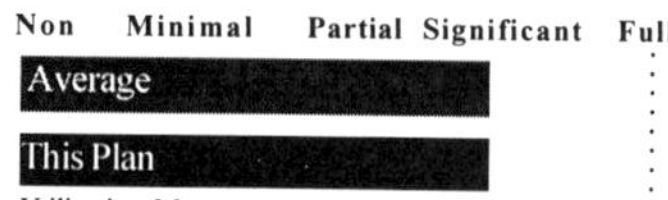

Utilization Management counts as 10% of the overall accreditation decision.

In **Medical Records** for physicians in the plan's network NCQA evaluates a number of factors such as:
- the standards that the plan sets for medical records and medical care
- how complete the medical records are
- how well the records show coordination between primary

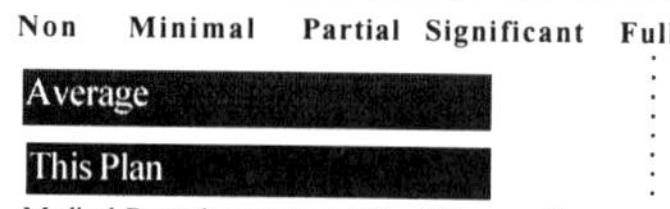

Medical Records counts as 5% of the overall accreditation decision.

*LEGEND

Average bar shows the level of performance against each category of NCQA Standards achieved by all plans evaluated to date against the same Standards.

This Plan bar shows the level of performance against each category of NCQA Standards that this plan achieved.

The levels are:

Full compliance:	met all of the requirements	*Minimal compliance:*	met few of the requirements
Significant compliance:	met most of the requirements	*Noncompliance:*	met none or almost none of the requirements
Partial compliance:	met about half of the requirements		

For more information about NCQA or its work, please call 202/955-5697, or to order additional reports 202/955-3510.

NCQA ID Number: JUL1598-OR00802; PMDS-10029R284

REFERENCES

Emanuel, E. J., & Emanuel L. L. (1996). What is accountability in health care? *Annals of Internal Medicine, 124,* 229–239.

National Committee for Quality Assurance (NCQA). (1997). *1995 surveyor guidelines for the accreditation of managed care organizations.* Washington, DC: Author.

National Committee for Quality Assurance (NCQA). (1997). *1995 surveyor guidelines for the accreditation of managed behavioral healthcare organizations.* Washington, DC: Author.

17

Licensing and Credentialing as Quality Management Tools in Behavioral Health Care

JUDY E. HALL

Professional licensing in health services has very little to do with the assurance of quality. While people assume it does, or wish it did, knowing that a provider is licensed assures us only that the state has determined him or her to possess a minimum level of competence. Minimum competence is typically defined as the provider having completed a defined sequence of education, training, and experience followed by successful performance on an independent examination of knowledge and skills.

EVOLUTION OF STANDARDS OVER TIME

Notwithstanding the definition of licensing as a minimum standard, over time there is a tendency in professional regulation to raise eligibility standards. In effect, by closing off a grandparent or waiver period, the minimum standard for eligibility to practice is raised. Then, as a profession matures, mechanisms develop in nongovernmental sectors that are often adopted as standards by states, for example, accreditation of medical residency programs. The newer standard them becomes the minimum accepted for admission to the licensing process. It is this gradual accretion process that many point to when attributing improvement in quality to the licensing process.

Credentialing organizations rely on licensing authorities to determine that a professional practitioner has met the foundation requirements for entry-level, generic practice. (In this chapter the professionals discussed include physicians, psychologists, social workers, and nurses.) The license, then, is often a prerequisite for acquisition of voluntary credentials whose standards are national and may be at a higher level than those required for state licensing*. Therefore, the goal of licensure—to serve the public need—is furthered by credentialing organizations' assessment of specialized education and training and specialty competence. At the same time, these voluntary certification bodies are dependent on licensing for certain state-level protec-

*In some of the newer, emerging professions, such as marriage and family therapy, the voluntary credential substitutes for a license in those jurisdictions without statutory recognition of those practitioners.

JUDY E. HALL • National Register of Health Service Providers in Psychology, Washington, DC 20005.

Handbook of Quality Management in Behavioral Health, edited by Stricker *et al.* Kluwer Academic / Plenum Publishers, New York, 2000.

tions such as the investigation of complaints of professional misconduct. While licensure is distinctly a state responsibility, certification involves national standards. It is from this perspective that this chapter is written: Neither licensing nor certification alone is sufficient as a mechanism to protect the public and ensure minimum competence; both are needed.

LICENSURE

Licensing laws are proposed by the professions that they are intended to regulate. Once in statute, these laws are protected by those same professionals and act as powerful tools contributing to the continuing growth of these professions. The primary purpose of such laws, however, is not to ensure growth of a profession, but rather to protect the public from unqualified, unscrupulous, unethical, or incompetent practitioners. The underlying assumption is that the public is incapable of determining who is qualified to practice. Therefore, legal jurisdictions provide mechanisms, typically licensing (protection of the practice) but occasionally certification (protection of the title) or registration (designation of individuals eligible to use the title), through which the evaluation of behavior and performance is conducted by the state on behalf of the consumer or user. The practitioner who meets the standard is given the imprimatur of the state and is authorized to practice, theoretically for a lifetime or until the license is revoked or surrendered.*

State licensing boards are concerned not only about the entrance to professional practice but also about the licensees' continuing adherence to ethical, professional, and legal standards related to the practice of the profession. Therefore, the state assumes the responsibility for monitoring the practice of that professional through various means and providing the consumer an avenue that may be used to complain about a professional considered to have deviated from appropriate conduct or legal standards. The regulatory process presents significant challenges to a consumer wishing to pursue a complaint against a licensed practitioner. Perhaps the most frustrating of these challenges from the consumer's perspective is the amount of time required for the process to be completed. As a consequence, many consumers are hesitant to pursue the regulatory remedy.

INPUTS TO LICENSING—PRE AND POST

Historically, more attention has been directed at evaluating education through the application of accreditation standards and licensing examinations than on assessing the benefits of training and continuing education or relating input criteria to outcome variables. What exactly are the inputs to behavioral health care regulation? The inputs that help determine initial eligibility for licensure include: (1) professional education; (2) on-the-job experience that is documented or supervised, or an organized program of training such as an internship or residency; (3) examination procedures, assembled or unassembled; and (4) high moral character or judged fitness to practice. The inputs used to determine continuing eligibility to maintain a license

*In this chapter, the term *license* is used to refer to any type of regulation of a profession by a state, provincial, or territorial government.

include: (1) continuing education or other means of competency assurance; (2) a process of relicensure or reexamination; and (3) evidence of adherence to professional rules of conduct or disciplinary actions (Hall, 1988, 1993). While each variable may itself contribute to service quality, several of them also provide potentially useful outcome measures. For example, the effectiveness of knowledge or skill acquisition in an educational or training program can be ascertained partly by the performance of its graduates on the licensing examination.

In recent years, the focus of regulation has shifted to what happens after a license is obtained. This takes the form of monitoring to ensure safe and effective practice. Disciplinary activity is an important measure and deserves particular attention here.

DISCIPLINARY PROCESS AND STRUCTURE

In the past 15 years, increasing public scrutiny of professional conduct and behavior has forced state and federal legislators to place more emphasis on disciplinary activity. Finding the "bad docs" is the tag line for several mechanisms established in the 1980s: (1) disciplinary databases maintained by the respective professions; (2) inclusion of laypersons or consumers on professional licensing boards; (3) the National Practitioner Data Bank (NPDB); and, more recently, (4) the Health Insurance Portability and Accountability Act of 1996 (HIPAA).

Cumulative compilations of disciplinary actions against individual practitioners are found in the disciplinary databases maintained by the organization representing each profession's state licensing boards. These include the Federation of State Medical Boards of the United States (FSMB), the National Council of State Boards of Nursing (NCSBN), the American Association of State Social Work Boards (AASSWB), and the Association of State and Provincial Psychology Boards (ASPPB). These databases, maintained either in hard copy or electronic format, are operated primarily for the benefit of the state boards themselves. They also may be made available, however, to relevant credentialing organizations.

Private credentialing organizations are not required to take disciplinary actions against their own listees, but many do. Some go further and publish their actions. The National Register of Health Service Providers in Psychology, for example, reports the delisting of registrants to (1) state or provincial boards where the individual is licensed, (2) the American Psychological Association (APA) or state association of which the person is a member, and (3) the American Board of Professional Psychology (ABPP) if the person is credentialed by that body. In addition, a summary of each action is published in the quarterly newsletter, *Register Report*, or the yearly *Register*. Efforts such as these by public and private credentialing bodies can assist the public in identifying errant practitioners and in preventing those same practitioners from acquiring additional credentials in new states or from other credentialing bodies without review of prior disciplinary actions.

During the 1980s, mandating public (consumer) representation on state licensing boards was promoted as a mechanism for addressing a perceived "conspiracy of silence," in which professionals were seen as reluctant to criticize their colleagues. It was assumed that consumer representatives would challenge the professionals by questioning the bases of their decisions. During the past decade and a half, adjudication of licensing complaints has also improved, that is, regulatory board members began to be trained in the administrative legal process and were provided legal assistance and counsel. The result of these efforts has been more effective detection and enforcement and increased awareness on the part of the public of their right to appropriate health service provision. As a result of the growing sophistication of the public and the better funded and developed structure for competency assurance, the number of health care providers disciplined has continually increased. Despite this, however, from the public's perspective, the low absolute number of professionals who are disciplined suggests that licensing boards are not fulfilling their obligation to protect the public.

Typically, consumers seek specific information about the health care professional from whom they seek such information. Increasing use of the Freedom of Information Act (FOI), for example, has made specific information on disciplinary actions of state regulatory bodies more available to the public. Further, the advent of internet home pages operated by governmental licensing authorities (see, for example, New York State's Home Page at <http://www.nysed.gov>) has made information on disciplinary activity much more easily and readily available.

OTHER SOURCES OF DISCIPLINARY ACTION

The National Practitioner Data Bank (NPDB), authorized by the Health Care Quality Improvement Act of 1986 and implemented in September 1, 1990, maintains records of both disciplinary actions taken against health care practitioners and malpractice payments made on their behalf. The data bank contained more than 120,000 disciplinary actions and malpractice payments involving more than 86,000 practitioners as of December 31, 1995. Almost 82% of these reports relate to malpractice payments. Of the individual practitioners reported to the databank, 75.2% were physicians and 15.5% were dentists. All other types of practitioners made up 9.3% of the listings (NPDB, 1995).

The NPDB reports are available electronically for $4.00 per query to hospitals, health maintenance organizations (HMOs) state licensing boards, professional societies engaged in professional peer review, and other quality assurance and credentialing authorities. Hospitals are required to query the NPDB for information on all new applicants for staff privileges, for new staff appointments, and once every 2 years for their entire staff as part of the recredentialing process. Failure to query the NPDB at those times subjects the hospital to potential loss of legal immunity for peer review functions as well as potential liability if a practitioner whose record was not checked is found guilty of malpractice or incompetence. In the near future, an NPDB record on a practitioner will also indicate whether that professional is listed on the Medicare and Medicaid sanctions list.

The NPDB has not been popular with professional associations who particularly object to its inclusion of malpractice actions in perpetuity. The Federation of State Medical Boards, for example, takes the position that malpractice claims are not

> accurate measures of a physician's competence or violation of the law. The reasons are twofold: (1) anyone can file a malpractice suit without showing evidence of damage, and (2) often malpractice insurance carriers decide to settle out of court rather than incur the expense of a court appearance. Many times the physician's guilt, innocence, or preference is not a factor in this decision (Federation of State Medical Boards of the United States, 1997).

There are ways of protecting practitioners who are guilty of malpractice from being reported to the NPDB. Organized care systems, in particular, may engage in such practices. For example, a "corporate shield" may be used in a settlement wherein the hospital rather than the staff practitioner is named as the defendant. A hospital may also choose to suspend a practitioner's privileges for less than 30 days, and thereby avoid the necessity to report the action to the NPDB.

When the new Health Insurance Portability and Accountability Act of 1996 (HIPAA) is implemented, there will be a new all-payer Fraud and Abuse Control Program established to identify, investigate, and prosecute those who commit fraud against the nation's health care delivery system. HIPAA regulations were to have been issued in July of 1997. The program covers both public and private health plans. It also mandates a broader group of organizations, including state licensure boards, to report on all health care providers and includes the establishment of a national database (the Adverse Action Data Bank) to record final adverse actions against health care providers and supply reports on them in response to a proper queries. This database is intended to complement rather than duplicate the NPDB. Although its purpose is primarily to combat fraud and abuse in the Medicare and Medicaid programs, it will be open to queries by private third-party payers.

CRITICISMS OF THE LICENSING PROCESS

As the public has become more sophisticated about issues related to health practitioner competence, licensing has come under increasing scrutiny and criticism. As early as 1977, a proposal was made for the creation of a National Commission on Health Certifying Agencies, a private organization promoted by the federal government for the purpose of setting national standards for the credentialing of health professionals. Most recently, the Pew Health Professions Commission (1995) released a report containing proposals for licensing reform. Stimulated by changes in health services organization and financing, the commission proposed policy considerations for the 21st century, stating that "the regulatory system.... [has] an equivocal relationship to quality."

While criticisms of the licensing process may be quite compelling, it is critical to note that the primary purpose of licensing is not to ensure quality. Rather, as stated earlier, it is to protect the public by ensuring that professionals licensed to practice possess a minimum level of competence.

CREDENTIALING ORGANIZATIONS

Strategic alliances between credentialing* organizations and licensing boards would seem to offer significant potential for raising the level of quality in health services. Although licensing is a state function and independent of any private entity (except in rare circumstances where licensing functions have been privatized), private credentialing builds on and complements licensing. By recognizing and capitalizing

*Instead of the more generic term *certification*, which can apply to a governmental or private association process, the term *credentialing* is used to describe the efforts of voluntary organizations that award practitioners a credential.

on this complementary relationship, opportunities are created for both protecting the public and improving the overall quality of services provided by health service professionals.

For each of the major licensed professions in behavioral health care—medicine (psychiatry and addiction medicine), psychology, social work (clinical social work), and nursing (psychiatric nursing)–multiple national credentialing bodies exist. Not all of these organizations, however, restrict their credential to professionals holding a license. Clearly, those that do not cannot be seen as contributing to protection of the public.

Credentialing bodies do not directly regulate professional practice. If a credentialed professional fails to adhere to a particular credentialing organization's ethical or practice standards or mandated reporting requirements, loss of the voluntary credential is virtually the only consequence. Such a loss does not affect the professional's right to practice. Although state licensing boards are free to review actions taken by credentialing organizations, they rarely do.

Some credentialing organizations have multiple pathways to qualify for a credential and accept any individual who meets the standards of any single pathway. For example, the American Board of Quality Assurance and the National Registry of Group Psychotherapists encourage applications from physicians, psychologists, social workers, and nurses. Other organizations, such as the National Board of Certified Counselors, offer certification in specialty areas to a range of licensed professionals. These multidisciplinary organizations are clearly more difficult to assess vis-à-vis their contributions to quality because of the variation in education, training, experience, and license deemed as acceptable from candidates.

In a recent review of credentialing organizations that accept psychologists as listees, 42 such organizations were identified (Hall & Sales, 1997). Many of them, however, either did not require a license as a prerequisite for the awarding of the credential or did not monitor whether the license is maintained while the credential is active. Those credentials for which professional licensure is not required for eligibility are sometimes referred to as "vanity" credentials, and as such are not seen as being positively associated with service quality. Gaining consensus on what is or is not a vanity credential is not always easy, however, even among professionals. It is no surprise, therefore, that consumers are often unable to ascertain the extent to which a credential is associated with higher quality services or even with a legal right to practice. That is, a naïve consumer may make the mistaken assumption that a credential, even one that would be recognized by a professional as "vanity," gives its holder a legal right to practice his or her trade. Such ignorance on the part of consumers makes it easier for unlicensed professionals to practice illegally.

Credentialing organizations that require listees to possess a license to practice and annually verify the existence of an active, unrestricted license contribute to the protection of the public. If such organizations have access to the disciplinary databases maintained by the associations of state boards, they can more effectively identify errant providers and assist regulatory agencies in enforcing professional disciplinary actions.

QUALITY ASSURANCE IN CREDENTIALING

From the consumer's perspective, the more consistency and uniformity that exists within a profession in the definition and application of standards for credentialing, the easier it is to understand and have faith in the process. Since 1934, the American Board of Medical Specialties (ABMS) and the American Medical Association Council on Medical Education (AMA/CME) have reviewed and approved specialty boards in medicine in an attempt to ensure quality control of the credentialing process. Certification by one of these 24 approved specialty boards is rapidly becoming the standard for the practice of medicine. In contrast to the low numbers of certificate holders in other health service professions, approximately 80% of licensed physicians (518,705 of approximately 650,000) hold ABMS certificates. The existence of the ABMS, however, has not prevented approximately 125 other certification bodies from being organized. A member of the public can determine whether a physician credentialing board is "approved" by ABMS by accessing the Internet website for that organization at <http://www.abms.org>.

In nursing, the emergence of recognized specialty boards is more recent. Although the American Nurses Association (ANA) established the ANA Certification Program in 1973, it was not until 1989 that the ANA Commission on Organizational Assessment and Renewal voted to establish the American Nurses Credential Center (ANCC) as a separately incorporated entity (American Nurses Credentialing Center, 1997). The standards for certification were established by the ANA Congress for Nursing Practice. The functions of the ANCC are carried out through ten separate certification boards.

Social work and psychology lag behind medicine and nursing with regard to developing an integrated, interorganizational system of credentialing licensed practitioners. Three credentials are offered by the National Association of Social Workers (NASW), the main professional membership body for social workers. Only one of these, the Diplomate in Clinical Social Work (DCSW), requires that the candidate possess a license to practice. This credential is reported to be held by approximately 22,000 licensed practitioners. A competing credential, the Board Certified Diplomate (BCD), is awarded by an independent credentialing organization, the American Board of Examiners in Clinical Social Work (ABECSW). This latter credential is possessed by approximately 15,000 social workers. Since NSAW membership is approximately 150,000, it is clear that, relative to medicine, the penetration of credentialing of licensed practitioners within the social work profession is quite low.

The first independent credentialing organization for psychologists, the American Board of Professional Psychology (ABPP), was established in 1947. Building on its own work as well as the work of two APA work groups, the Subcommittee on Specialization (SOS) (Sales et al., 1984) and the Task Force on Specialty Criteria, ABPP assumed the responsibility for recognizing emerging specialty areas in psychology by applying the SOS identification criteria to specialty credentialing boards. As of this writing, approximately 3200 diplomas have been awarded by 12 specialty examining boards in psychology.

In 1995, APA created a Commission for the Recognition of Specialties and Proficiencies in Professional Psychology to determine which additional areas of practice warrant recognition by the association as specialties or proficiencies (American Psychological Association, 1995). These identification criteria do not require the prior existence of a credentialing organization to examine the candidates. To date, one new area of practice, clinical neuropsychology, has received specialty recognition. This specialty was already recognized by ABPP, however.

A different approach to credentialing is offered by the National Register of Health Service Providers in Psychology. This independent national organization identifies licensed psychologists who are qualified on the basis of education and experience to provide health services to the public (Council for the National Register of Health Service Providers in Psychology, 1996). The psychologists credentialed as health care providers represent many different specialties. Perhaps because the register criteria are not restricted to a particular specialty, it has become the most successful credentialing organization in psychology.

The National Register and ABPP, both of which are independent of the APA, are the two major credentialing organizations in psychology. The former is the larger in terms of professional membership but the latter is older. The APBB Board of Trustees recently decided that doctoral psychologists listed in the *National Register* meet the common eligibility requirements for recognition as a specialist by ABPP (American Board of Professional Psychology, 1997). This establishes a complementary relationship within the profession between the two largest credentialing organizations.

Recommendations have been made for establishment of a cross-professional organization dedicated to quality control of credentialing activities. One such entity exists. This organization, the National Commission for Certifying Agencies (1996) argues that its standards for accreditation are "nationally recognized principles utilized by a variety of certification organizations for certification programs in diverse professions and occupations" (p. 1). Although this entity has accredited 34 organizations, none of the 34 is related to social work, psychology, or medicine. Two certification boards within nursing are accredited by this commission, but neither is ANCC sanctioned.

MEASURE OF QUALITY

In theory, voluntary organizations, through their ability to impose standards over and above those required by licensing boards, have the potential to contribute to the quality of services. Is a higher standard in education or training, however, correlated to higher service quality? In 1983, Carroll and Gaston studied measures of "quality" used by three professions, law, pharmacy, and optometry, to determine whether such a correlation exists. For lawyers, the authors used peer ratings, malpractice insurance rates, and disciplinary actions as measures of quality. They found that for each measure greater quality control (higher levels of education and training) was associated with a higher average quality for the licensed practitioners. Similar measures were used and similar outcomes observed for pharmacy and optometry: that is, there was a direct association between standards and service quality as it was defined for the study. The authors concluded that higher licensing standards yielded "an enhanced quality of a practitioner" (Carroll & Gaston, 1983, p. 141).

VIABILITY OF CREDENTIALING ORGANIZATIONS

If the results of Carroll and Gaston (1983) can be generalized to all professions, it would follow that, to help ensure a higher level of service quality, credentialing agencies should set eligibility standards over and above those required for state licensing. This does not always happen, however. One reason for this is that private credentialing organizations are financially dependent on the application and renewal fees of their listees. If they set their standards too high, they receive fewer applicants and fewer fees. If, on the other hand, standards are set too low, the credibility of the credentialing organization is undermined. Further, if credentialing standards are no higher than those required for licensing, few benefits would seem to accrue to listees. In today's competitive health care market place, practitioners are more likely to seek credentials that are likely to result in increased third-party reimbursement.

Typically, credentialing organizations are not profitable, and if a credentialing organization operates independently of the principal membership organization for the profession (e.g., in the case of psychology this would be the American Psychological Association), it may be unable to survive financially. At the same time, a legal affiliation between a professional membership organization and a credentialing entity brings to the former organization potential liability for the acts of the latter.

If a credentialing organization is financially viable and independent of the membership organization, it is better able to insulate itself from the political forces that inevitably affect governmental regulation and membership associations whose decisions are driven by a voting constituency. To the degree that the decision-making process of a credentialing organization is free from political pressures, its effectiveness and credibility are increased. To the degree that this is not true, the capacity of the credentialing organization to contribute to protection of the public or quality improvement is vitiated.

REGULATION OF MEDICAL PROFESSIONALS

Each of the behavioral health professions and their associated credentialing organizations and licensing authorities endorse a range of activities intended to improve the quality of services provided by their members. These activities, which are particularly well developed in medicine, underscore the value of interrelationships between licensing and credentialing.

Psychiatry and Addiction Medicine

The American Board of Psychiatry and Neurology (ABPN), the ABMS entity that credentials psychiatrists, defines those criteria over and above a medical license that are required for a physician to define him- or herself as a psychiatrist. Qualifications include completion of an internship and a 4-year organized psychiatric residency program. To be credentialed by ABPN, a physician also must pass an examination. While ABPN is rapidly becoming the minimum standard for a physician to hold him- or herself out as a psychiatrist, no law or regulation prohibits a physician who has not passed the ABPN exam from doing so.

In 1988, there were 29,531 (ABPN or self-designated) psychiatrists in the United States, while in 1995, the number had grown to 33,486 (Peterson,et al., 1996). Some of these physicians who specialize in the treatment of addictions seek a secondary credential in addiction medicine. This credential is awarded by the American Society of Addiction Medicine (ASAM), an organization not currently approved by ABMS. More than 3000 physicians currently possess the ASAM credential.

General Medicine

Postgraduate professional experience is a universal requirement for a state license to practice medicine. States vary in this requirement from one (n = 41 states) to three (n = 3 states) years (Federation of State Medical Boards of the United States, 1995). Many states also require applicants to answer questions that are presumed to reflect their fitness to practice. Such questions include history of psychiatric treatment and drug or alcohol abuse.

Two examinations are currently used by medical licensure boards. The first of these is the recently introduced United States Medical Licensing Examination (USMLE), a three-step exam taken during medical education and training. Steps I and II of this exam are also taken by international medical graduates as part of the certification by the Educational Commission for Foreign Medical Graduates (ECFMG), which allows them to seek residency training in the United States.

The second examination used by medical licensure boards is the new Special Purpose Examination (SPEX). The SPEX may be used by states to reexamine a physician who is applying for endorsement/reciprocity several years after initial examination or when the physician is seeking reinstatement or reactivation of his or her license following a period of professional inactivity. Although not required for all endorsement candidates at this time, SPEX is required in 12 jurisdictions for physicians applying for a second license 10 years or more after being originally examined for licensure. In an additional 28 jurisdictions the examination may be used at the discretion of the state board (Federation of State Medical Boards of the United States, 1995).

As an examination used to determine continuing competence of health services professionals, the SPEX is unique. It is too soon to determine whether the SPEX will serve as an effective measure for ensuring continuing competence. Currently, a majority of jurisdictions require evidence of continuing education for this purpose, in spite of the lack of evidence that the quality of services improved by such experiences.*

Medical disciplinary activity has increased steadily in the last decade, with the number of actions from 1991 to 1996 now available on the Federation of State Medical Boards of the United States home page (<http://www.fsmb.org>). The FSMB data bank currently contains 70,000 actions on 25,000 physicians out of an estimated 650,000 physicians nationwide. This database does not allow public access, however. For a member of the public to obtain specific information about actions against an individual physician, he or she would need to either request it directly from a state licensing board, invoking the Freedom of Information Act, or access the information through a medical board's Internet home page. For example, the home page of the Association of State Medical Board Executive Directors has this type of information for five state medical boards (<http://www.aimdocfinder>).

REGULATION OF PSYCHIATRIC AND MENTAL HEALTH NURSING

Certification for nurses specializing in mental health is conducted by the ANA's American Nurses Credentialing Center (ANCC). Beginning in 1998, a nurse wishing

*A study of the impact of continuing education (CE) on public accountancy by the New York State Licensing Board for Certified Public Accountants revealed that knowledge proficiency increased with participation in CE, higher levels of participation produced higher levels of knowledge, and concentrated study in a specific area was a more powerful predictor of increased knowledge than general study in a wider area. However, the relationship between CE and professional behaviors was not studied (see Hall, 1993).

to gain a credential for the general practice of psychiatric nursing must possess a baccalaureate or higher degree (American Nurses Credentialing Center, 1997). To be eligible for an advanced practice credential (APN), a candidate must possess a master's degree in psychiatric nursing.

All states except Illinois have regulations applying specifically to advanced practice nurses, 33 regulate clinical nurse specialists in psychiatric/mental health nursing, and 23 states regulate nurse practitioners in the area of psychiatric/mental health nursing. Twenty-eight states accept the certification as clinical nurse specialist (without regard for specific specialty area) as a qualification for advanced practice, while 37 states accept the nurse practitioner national credential (also without regard for specialty area) for advanced practice (National Council of State Boards of Nursing, 1996).

The right to prescribe medications is automatically granted to certified nurse specialists in 11 states and to nurse practitioners in 24 states (American Nurses Credentialing Center, 1997). These privileges may be collaborative (requiring medical supervision) or substitutive (not requiring supervision of a physician), although the latter is less prevalent.

According to the ANA home page, there are approximately 2.2 million registered in the United States. As of April 1997, 19,001 nurses were credentialed in psychiatric and mental health nursing, 6,453 held a credential as a clinical specialist in adult psychiatric and mental health nursing, and 822 were credentialed in child and adolescent mental health nursing.

The National Council of State Boards of Nursing (NCSBN) disciplinary data bank was established in 1981, but it was not until June 1996 that all state boards reported their disciplinary actions to NCSBN. Currently, approximately 40,000 actions, a high percentage of which are disciplinary actions related to chemical dependency,* are registered with the NCSBN. These records, however, are currently not publicly available, even to nursing credentialing organizations.

REGULATION OF PSYCHOLOGY

The standard for the independent practice as a psychologist is the doctoral degree and 2 years experience, including 1 year in an internship or organization training program (for those providing direct services) and 1 year of supervised postdoctoral experience. All states except Vermont and West Virginia hold to the doctoral standard for independent practice, but approximately 30 states allow masters-level practice under supervision of a doctoral-level psychologist. Several Canadian provinces (Alberta, Newfoundland, Quebec) also license masters-level professionals for independent practice.

The two major credentialing organizations in psychology (the National Register and ABPP) require the doctorate. At the same time, the APA itself supports a proficiency certificate program in alcohol and substance abuse treatment that accepts masters-level applicants, and the Canadian Register of Health Service Providers in Psychology currently accepts registered psychologists at the masters level. This will

*Thirty-two states have implemented formal nondisciplinary diversion programs for nurses abusing alcohol or drugs (National Council of State Boards of Nursing, 1996). It is expected that disciplinary actions related to substance abuse will decrease with the advent of such programs.

continue, however, only until the expiration of a waiver period in the year 2000 (Canadian Register of Health Service Providers in Psychology, 1997).

Of the 70,000 licensed psychologists in 1995 (Peterson et al., 1996), it is estimated that approximately 50,000 possess the doctoral degree. Of these, approximately 37,500 may be involved in the direct provision of clinical services, and therefore would be eligible for listing in the National Register or ABPP. The numbers of psychologists who are credentialed by these organizations are 16,000 and 3,200, respectively.

The largest credentialing organization in psychology (the National Register) is not technically a specialty certification organization. Rather, this organization determines whether a licensed psychologist satisfies national criteria related to education (an acceptable doctoral degree in psychology) and experience (provision of services in an organized health services setting). There is no parallel organization in any other health services profession. With a majority of psychology graduates being educated with a specialty emphasis in their doctoral program (clinical, counseling, school, clinical neuropsychology, etc.), an apt description of the registrant is that he or she has been educated as a specialist but has been trained as a health service provider (G. Hurley, personal communication, June 2, 1997).

In 1980, the National Register developed internship criteria for internal use in selecting candidates for credentialing. These criteria, identified as "Guidelines for Defining an Internship or Organized Health Service Training Program," were subsequently adopted as standard criteria for internships in professional psychology by the APA and the Association of Postdoctoral Internship Centers (APIC). Because internships are intended to provide a breadth of training, they are not labeled as or considered to be a specialty in, for example, clinical or counseling.

Both the National Register and ABPP facilitate movement of psychologists between states. ABPP is currently used by 34 state boards as a means of facilitating endorsement for licensure. Further, since both organizations receive quarterly disciplinary database reports from ASPPB, they are able to assist states in monitoring actions taken against psychologists who may move from one state to another.

REGULATION IN SOCIAL WORK

It is estimated that there are 190,000 clinical social workers in the United States, an estimate that comes from doubling the number of clinical social workers who are members of NASW (Peterson et al., 1996). Licensure is available for social workers in all states except Michigan where a registration process still exists. Although there is variation across states, licensure is available at four levels: bachelors degree, masters degree in social work (MSW), MSW with 2 years postmasters experience, and MSW with 2 years postmasters direct clinical social work experience. Because of the multiple levels of licensure in some states, the American Association of State Social Work Boards (AASSWB) offers four examinations that assess the basic, intermediate, clinical, and advanced levels.

AASSWB established a disciplinary database, the disciplinary action reporting system, in the early 1990s. As of June 1997 this database had recorded 631 actions on 504 social workers (C. Getty, personal communication, June 9, 1997). Although information is provided only to member state boards every other month, "an annual subscription contract will soon be available to related social work organizations, third party payors of social work services, and other interested entities" (AASSWB, June 1997). Continuing education is required for renewal of the license to practice in approximately 34 states.

After licensure, a masters-level social worker may pursue multiple credentials, only two of which require a license to practice as a prerequisite. Three are available through NASW and one through the American Board of Examiners in Clinical Social Work (ABECSW). The oldest certification is that granted by the Academy of Certified Social Workers (ACSW). It was initiated in 1962 by NASW; it applies to individuals practicing in any area of social work and has the largest number of credentialed professionals (approximately 55,000). A license to practice is not required for the ACSW.

After obtaining the ACSW a social worker may apply for the qualified clinical social worker (QCSW) credential, which also does not require a license to practice. The highest credential offered by NASW is the diplomate in clinical social work (DCSW). This credential requires the candidate to hold "the highest level of social work license or certification available in their state." The NASW *Register of Clinical Social Workers* lists individuals with QCSW and DCSW credentials. Although there are reportedly 22,000 NASW diplomates, the June 1997 edition of the register contains approximately 10,000 professionals (either QCSW or DCSW) who have complied with the renewal requirements (A. Ricks, personal communication, June 1997).

The American Board of Examiners in Clinical Social Work (1997) offers the other credential available to social workers (the BCD). This organization was incorporated in 1987 based on an agreement between NASW and the National Registry of Health Care Providers in Clinical Social Work (initiated in the 1980s and modeled after the National Register of Health Service Providers in Psychology) to cease issuing separate credentials. When the time lines on that agreement expired, however, NASW reinstituted its own diplomate (February 1992), which put it into direct competition with the ABECSW.

Differences exist between the two systems of awarding a diplomate in clinical social work. They include both eligibility criteria (e.g., an examination was introduced only recently for the DCSW but eliminated for the BCD) and criteria for maintaining the advanced credentials (e.g., hours of clinical practice, continuing education). On-line access to the names, addresses, and practice characteristics of those possessing a BCD soon will be available through ABECSW's home page at <http://www.abescw.org>. While competition is generally considered healthy, the competing diplomate credentials in social work may confuse both the public and new graduates in social work. Further, since AASSWB does not release the disciplinary information to credentialing organizations, its capacity to promote quality is compromised.

RESTRICTING PRACTICE TO A SPECIALTY

Most licensure is generic. This is based on the assumption that a broad foundation is necessary to practice any profession. Most credentialing organizations are more restrictive, being concerned either with a particular specialty area or health services provision. For specialists in medicine, nursing, and psychology, credentialing may be used to support the regulatory process by substituting for certain licensure requirements. Examples in which specialty certification may substitute for some element in licensure are listed below (Hall & Ames, 1991, p. 2):

- When a licensed professional is required by statute to have taken the licensure examination within 10 years of application for licensure (but has not done so), specialty certification may be accepted by the licensing board as a substitute for the exam. For example, state medical boards accept specialty certification or recertification in 11 jurisdictions.
- When a license is or can be specialized, as opposed to generic, jurisdictions may accept the specialized examination in place of the generic examination administered by the licensing board.
- When the licensure examination includes an oral component, the specialty examination may be substituted for this component.
- When the specialty area is used to limit the scope of practice, the specialty examination may be accepted.
- When the right to advertise is tied to the definition and title of a specialty, the specialty designation may be accepted.
- When a question of negligence arises in professional disciplinary or malpractice hearings, the specialty may be used to define the standard used in assessing negligence.
- The definition of the specialty may be used to define specifically delineated privileges at a hospital or other facility.

CONCLUSION

If state and federal agencies, in collaboration with relevant professional associations, were to adopt uniform standards for professional practice and specialty, implementing them consistently and sharing information on professional disciplinary actions, all stakeholders would benefit. The consumer of services could with more confidence select a service provider who is appropriate to his or her needs, who possesses the competencies necessary to be an effective helper and who has not been guilty of malpractice or professional incompetence. For the professional practitioner, national standards would translate into greater mobility across states and a reduction in costs associated with maintaining a variety of credentials. For third-party payers, identifying appropriate service providers would be simplified and the costs of credentialing would be reduced. For the various regulatory bodies, enforcement of regulations and disciplinary actions would be greatly simplified and probably more effective.

Even if cooperation of the scope described above does not occur, consumers as well as the professions themselves could still benefit from more limited collaboration. For example, professions might establish interorganizational bodies to establish standards for credentialing, much as has been done in medicine. While the existence of such entities cannot prevent the emergence of nondesignated credentialing organizations, it can still provide purchasers with a benchmark for such organizations.

Nursing has consolidated many but not all of its credentialing bodies into a certification center, permitting some measure of oversight and quality control. While not as well organized in this regard, psychology established a psychology executive roundtable for the purpose of facilitating communication among the national organizations engaged in credentialing-related activities. Following this, other vehicles for interorganizational cooperation have emerged (Drum & Hall, 1993). It would seem, however, that social work has made only limited progress in consolidating or achieving a significant level of cooperation from its two primary credentialing bodies.

Even if credentialing organizations across the behavioral health disciplines continue independently to pursue their own initiatives, they should seek to inform one another of the potential impact of any significant change in the same way that licensing boards hold public hearings and seek consumer input on proposed regulatory changes. While this has not been accepted practice for voluntary credentialing organizations, it would seem an appropriate responsibility for entities such as ABMS, ABPP, or ANCC.

Interdisciplinary collaborative efforts have the potential to improve the licensing and credentialing processes for all professions. For example, an innovative quality management mechanism such as the SPEX in medicine might be equally well applied in other practice areas. It could be used both to periodically assess the competence of licensed professionals and to facilitate professional mobility across states. In addition, substituting specialty certification for some aspect of licensing would advance much needed simplification in the licensing process for many professionals.

Clearly, a balance must occur between a profession's pursuit of what it considers to be its own interests and the needs of the health care system as a whole. Elsewhere in health care, consolidation has become the rule; it is difficult to believe that the same development is not inevitable in the areas of licensing and credentialing (indeed, the indicators of such change are already apparent). At the same time, however, in view of the complexity of the context in which professional associations and credentialing organizations operate, consolidation and uniformity may not be deemed desirable options. Organizations that have invested many years and significant resources in systems to recognize and credential specialties will be reluctant to abandon these efforts and the prestige and control that accompany them. Further, if professionals believe it will translate to marketplace advantage for them, they will continue to seek new credentials, whether or not these credentials are valid reflections of special competence. Barring some unforeseen external event (such as a cataclysmic kind of regulatory intervention), enduring changes that show promise of advancing quality in behavioral health will, as with all things, likely proceed slowly.

REFERENCES

American Board of Examiners in Clinical Social Work. (1997). *ABECSW home page*. [On-line] Available: http://www.abecsw.org

American Board of Medical Specialties. (1997). *ABMS home page*. [On-line]. Available: http://www.abms.org

American Board of Professional Psychology. (1997, May). *Board of trustees minutes*. (Available from ABPP, 514 E. Capitol Ave., Jefferson City, MO 65101.)

American Nursing Association. (1997). *ANA home page*. [On-line]. Available: http://www.ana.org

American Nurses Credentialing Center. (1997). *Advanced practice certification catalog*. Washington, DC:Author.

American Psychological Association. (1995, February). *Council of representatives minutes*. (Available from APA, 750 E. First Street, NE, Washington, DC 20002.)

Association of State Medical Board Executive Directors. (1997). *Home page.* [On-line]. Available: http://www.aimdocfinder

Canadian Register of Health Service Providers in Psychology. (1997). *Canadian register of health service providers in psychology.* Ottawa, ON: Author.

Carroll, S. L., & Gaston, R. J. (1983). Occupational licensing and the quality of service: An overview. *Law and Human Behavior, 7,* 139–146.

Council for the National Register of Health Services Providers in Psychology. (1996). *National register of health service providers in psychology.* (rev. ed.). Washington, DC: Author.

Drum, D. J., & Hall, J. E. (1983). Psychology's self regulation and the setting of professional standards. *Applied and Preventive Psychology, 2,* 151–161.

Federation of State Medical Boards of the United States. (1995). *The exchange: Section 1, USMLE and M.D. Licensing requirements.* Euless, TX: Author.

Federation of State Medical Boards of the United States. (1997). *FSMB home page* [On-line]. Available http://www.fsmb.org

Hall, J. E. (1988). The role of the state. In G. Stricker & A. Rodriguez (Eds.) *Handbook of quality assurance in mental health* (pp. 331–362). New York: Plenum Press.

Hall, J. E. (1993). The role of the state in ensuring quality in health care service delivery and its linkage with the private and public sectors. In P. Wohlford, H. F. Myers, & J. E. Callan (Eds.), *Serving the seriously mentally ill: Public-academic linkages in services, research, and training* (pp. 195–205). Washington, DC: American Psychological Association.

Hall, J. E., & Ames E. (1991, February). The impact of specialty certification on professional licensing efforts. Presented at a meeting of the Federation of Associations of Regulatory Boards, Albuquerque, NM.

Hall, J. E., & Sales, B. D. (1997). Credentialing organizations that recognize psychologists. In B. D. Sales & J. E. Hall (Eds.), *Specialty recognition in psychology.* Manuscript in preparation.

Health Care Quality Improvement Act of 1986, Title IV of P.L. 99-660. (42 U.S.C. 11101 et. seq.).

Health Insurance Portability and Accountability Act of 1996, P.L. 104-191, Title XI. (41 U.S.C. 1301 et. seq.), §221.

National Association of Social Workers. (1997). *NASW home page.* [On-line]. Available: http: //www.nasw.org

National Commission for Certifying Agencies (1996, December 5). *NCCA accredited certification organizations.* (Available from NCCA, 1200 19th Street, NW, Ste. 300, Washington, DC 20036.)

National Council of State Boards of Nursing (1996). *Profiles of member boards.* Chicago, IL: Author.

National Practitioner Data Bank (1995). *annual report.* (Available from U.S. Department of Health and Human Services, Health Resources and Services Administration, Bureau of Health Professions, Dividion of Quality Assurance, 5600 Fishers Lane, Suite 8-A-55, Rockville, MD 20857).

New York State Education Department. (1997). *NYSED home page.* [On-line]. Available: http://www.nysed.gov

Peterson, B. D., West, J., Pincus, H. A., Kohout, J., Pion, G. M., Wicherski, M. M., Vandivort-Waren, R., Palmiter, M., Merwin, E. I., Fox, J. C., Clawson, T. W., Rhodes, K. K., Stockton, R., Ambrose, J. P., Blankertz, L., Dwyer, K. P., Stanhope, V., Fleischer, M. S., Goldsmith, H. F., Witkin, M. J., Atay, J. E., & Manderscheid, R. W. (1996). An update on human resources in mental health. In R. W. Manderscheid & M. A. Sonnenshein (Eds.), *Mental health, United States, 1996* (pp. 168–190). (DHHS Pub. No. (SMA) 96-3098). Washington, DC: Center for Mental Health Services.

Pew Health Professions Commission. (1995). *Reforming health care workforce regulation: Policy considerations for the 21st century.* (Available from UCSF Center for the Health Professions, 1388 Sutter Street, STE 805, San Francisco, CA 94109.)

Sales, B. D., Bricklin, P., & Hall, J. E. (1984, November). *Specialization in psychology: Principles.* (Available from American Psychological Association, Board of Professional Affairs, 750 First Street, NE, Washington, DC 20002-4242.)

18

Legal and Quality of Care Issues for Providers in Managed Behavioral Health Care Arrangements

SHIRLEY ANN HIGUCHI, J.D. AND CHERIE JONES, J.D.

OVERVIEW

Over the last two decades, Americans have witnessed a dramatic increase in enrollment in privately insured managed care plans. For example, in 1970, there were 33 health maintenance organizations (HMOs) covering 3 million persons, whereas by 1980, there were 236 HMOs serving 9.1 million persons (DeLeon, VandenBos, & Bulatao, 1991). Between 1980 and 1992, the number of privately insured managed care enrollees grew to more than 90 million (Rosenbaum, Serrano, Wehr, & Spernak, 1995). In the mid-to-late 1980s, many HMOs began contracting with specialized companies to provide managed behavioral health care services, and by 1994, 106.6 million were enrolled in over 300 plans that offered some type of program for managed behavioral health care* (Iglehart, 1996). Including Medicare, this 106.6 million represents 48.7% of the insured population (Sipkoff, 1995).

As a result of the expansion of managed care arrangements for mental health coverage, providers are increasingly dealing with legal and business issues unknown to them 20 years ago. Most providers have had some contact with the primary managed care arrangements, which are described in the following section. These arrangements include the HMO, the preferred provider organizations (PPO), utilization review (UR) programs, and employee assistance programs (EAP).

Although each type of arrangement has its own benefits and limitations, providers must be cognizant of legal issues that may arise in any managed care situation and that ultimately may have an impact on the quality of care that they can deliver.

*These mental health management firms such as HAI, Merit Behavioral Care, Value Behavioral Health, and Green Spring Health Services, typically enter into "carve-out" arrangements, either directly with self-insured employers or as subcontractors to HMOs or other insurers. Under such arrangements, the mental health management firm assumes financial and/or administrative responsibility for the mental health services required by persons covered by a particular benefit plan.

SHIRLEY ANN HIGUCHI, J.D. AND CHERIE JONES, J.D. • American Psychological Association, Washington, DC 20002-4242.

Handbook of Quality Management in Behavioral Health, edited by Stricker *et al.* Kluwer Academic / Plenum Publishers, New York, 2000.

The issues include problematic clauses in managed care contracts, potential for conflicts of interest, limitations on treatment, confidentiality concerns, and issues relating to professional standards. These subjects, along with some possible strategies for dealing with them, are addressed in the section titled "Practitioners Dilemmas."

Private nonprofit accrediting organizations such as the Utilization Review Accreditation Committee (URAC) and the National Committee for Quality Assurance (NCQA) have been formed relatively recently to address service quality in the managed care industry. The chapter details national standard-setting activities by these organizations in the area of behavioral health care.

Finally, in this constantly changing managed care environment, providers are considering the advantages of associating in some form with providers from different disciplines (particularly mental health professionals with primary care physicians). Among the reasons for forming such multidisciplinary groups are to gain access to panels, to gain access to patients, and to be in a position to compete directly with the mental health management firms. The most common legal structures that groups may adopt are discussed in detail in the last section.

MANAGED CARE ARRANGEMENTS AFFECTING BEHAVIORAL HEALTH PROVIDERS

Health Maintenance Organizations

While 20 years ago the term "health maintenance organization" was relatively unknown to most patients and practitioners , now the HMO is probably the most well-known of the managed care models. For a predetermined, capitated (per member) premium, the HMO delivers or arranges for the delivery of carefully managed and controlled health care services to a set number of individual clients (Boochever, 1986).

There are two major forms of HMOs: group or staff models, which use practitioners in fully integrated group practices, and networks or independent practice associations (IPA), which use community-based practitioners in private practice (Gold, Hurley, Lake, Ensor, & Berenson, 1995). Both types or organization are typically at risk financially for the costs of care (Gold et al., 1995). This unique model, in which the insurer or arranger of health care is also the provider of health care services, creates challenges for professionals contracting to provide services for the HMO.

For example, descriptive materials developed by HMO marketers frequently stress to consumers that the care being provided by an HMO is of high quality and that the set of services is complete and comprehensive. In addition, through its coverage agreement with enrollees, the HMO basically guarantees the quality of the care provided to them.* As is becoming more and more apparent, however, the level of coverage actually provided may differ significantly from what is promised. This is not surprising given that HMOs are at risk for the cost of virtually all services and, therefore, may have a financial incentive to limit utilization (Richardson & Austad, 1991). General medical–surgical HMOs generally have been found to allocate only

*It is important to note that under breach-of-contract theory, managed care entities have been held liable for not living up to what they promised in their enrollee contracts or marketing materials. In *Boyd v. Albert Einstein Medical Center* (1988), the court ruled that an HMO might be liable for the acts of contracting physicians in part because the HMO had advertised that its providers were competent and had been evaluated by the HMO.

about 3 to 5% percent of their budgets for behavioral health services, whereas such services account for about 10% of total health care costs nationally (Iglehart, 1996).

Vague or confusing definitions of terms in managed care contracts can affect the provider–patient relationship. For example, one large managed care organization (MCO) defines an HMO as "an entity that provides, offers, or arranges for coverage of designated health services needed by plan members for a fixed and prepaid premium." What may not be clear to beneficiaries of this MCO is that those services that are "needed by plan members" are those services that are approved in advance by the HMO and that may be further limited by the HMO's utilization review (UR) process.

Preferred Provider Organizations

PPOs are broadly defined as health care financing and delivery programs that provide financial incentives to consumers to use a preselected group of providers of health care. Payment to providers is typically on a fee-for-service basis with discounts offered to the payer by the provider in exchange for guarantees of increased patient volume. Consumers are usually not locked into receiving services from these preferred providers but have financial incentives to do so (Higuchi, 1994). Higher levels of coinsurance or deductibles routinely apply to services provided by nonparticipating providers.

The PPO historically has not been considered problematic for participating providers, since in most instances benefits tend to be more generous than in the HMO model. PPOs, however, still pose significant challenges. For example, the payers designate who is "preferred," and they attempt to confine their panels to providers deemed "managed care friendly" (Zucker, 1995). In addition, practices and policies of PPOs, including UR, may restrict the delivery of mental health care. An emerging area of concern centers around provider contracting issues, where the PPO requests that participating providers sign contracts that may restrict the provider's ability to deliver what he or she considers appropriate care.

Utilization Review Programs

A survey by the Health Poll, a publication which monitors health management issues and managed care trends, revealed that 94% of the benefits managers surveyed said UR plays an important role in their company's overall health care cost management effort (Survey, 1988). Effective UR can protect patients from unnecessary care and can allow for flexible use of benefits. However, cost containment through reduction of insurance benefits and aggressive UR may increase the risk of sacrificing good care in the pursuit of financial objectives (Sederer, 1992).

UR involves the evaluation of the necessity, appropriateness, and efficiency of health care services. Typically, this process is conducted by a UR committee that periodically reviews the progress of treatment by means of written or oral communication with the provider (Richardson & Austad, 1991). The UR committee may authorize or deny reimbursement for continued treatment, or may impose limitations on the number of additional sessions or days to be paid for (Richardson & Austad, 1991). The objective of UR is to improve cost-effectiveness while reducing abuse of services. Many providers believe, however, that the imposing limits on the number of therapy sessions and eliminating covered services not considered "medically necessary" create an unworkable environment for the delivery of health services.

Another frequently expressed concern about UR relates to the qualifications and motives of UR staff. With regard to the concern about qualifications, providers have reported decisions being made by UR staff with lower levels of training, experience, or license than the provider. Futhermore, decisions may be made by unlicensed staff guided by written criteria. With regard to the concern about motives, providers sometimes perceive decisions being made by UR staff primarily for cost-saving rather than quality of care reasons.

One of the most frequent and serious complaints raised in the UR arena pertains to what providers regard as unreasonable requests for information by UR companies. Ethical and practice dilemmas arise when UR staff request clinical data, progress notes, and other information beyond what is considered reasonable by the provider.

UR practices have been challenged in the courts. The decision in *Wickline v. State of California*, regarded as a landmark case in UR, created a potential cause of action against third-party payers for cost containment mechanisms that negligently cause injury to patients. The court also discussed the role of the provider during the UR process as well as the potential liability for the service provider in the event of an injury due to negligent UR. The *Wickline* decision makes clear that even a finding of negligence on the part of the third party does not absolve the provider from liability. In effect, the *Wickline* case allows for holding the insurer liable, but only if the provider has fully pursued all available avenues for appeal. This is clearly a practice guideline for providers rendering care and encountering denial of insurance coverage (Sederer, 1992).

Employee Assistance Programs

An EAP is a program established to give employees easy access to help for personal or work-related problems that may have a negative impact on their capacity to carry out their jobs. An EAP provider may be an employee of an external corporation that offers a counseling and referral service or may work directly for the company purchasing the EAP services for its employees. Under either model, conflicts may emerge when the provider feels he or she owes a duty to both the employer (corporation) and to the patient, but the interests of these two parties differ.

Consistent with the ethical responsibilities of the provider and the law, as part of the informed consent process, the provider should review with the patient the proposed treatment and any procedures contractually agreed on by the provider in the managed care arrangement or the EAP. For example, the American Psychological Association (APA) Ethics Code (1992), Ethical Principle 1.21, states:

> when a psychologist agrees to provide services to a person or entity at the request of a third party, the psychologist clarifies to the extent feasible, at the outset of the service, the nature of the relationship with each party. This clarification includes the role of the psychologist ... the probable uses of the services provided ... and the fact that there may be limits to confidentiality (APA, 1992, p. 6).

PRACTITIONER DILEMMAS AND POSSIBLE RESOLUTIONS

This section explores some common dilemmas faced by providers operating under a managed care arrangement, and suggests some possible resolutions to these dilemmas.

Provider Contracting Issues

Many provisions in managed care provider contracts potentially have an adverse impact on the provider–patient relationship and consequently on the quality of services provided. In light of this, practitioners are faced with the challenge of deciding whether they should sign such contracts or complain about the provisions and potentially risk being rejected as a panel provider. It is important to note that to *legally* challenge a managed care contract the provider needs to execute the contract with the MCO, a contract provision must be breached, and the MCO must seek to enforce it. Only then can that provision be challenged in a court of law. Moreover, as a practical matter, if the provider is unhappy with a particular contract, the provider can always sign the contract and later terminate without cause by giving the required notice to the MCO. However, many providers hesitate to sign a contract with such provisions, since they are unaware what ethical or legal implications exist.

"No-Cause" Termination Provisions

This type of provision is standard in the industry, and historically has been part of the provider contract. A typical provision states that either party is entitled to terminate the agreement by giving the other party 30 days written notice. While such a provision may appear appealing, immediate termination of a provider for any reason may be disruptive to the provider–patient relationship.

There is concern that managed care companies could use the no-cause termination provision as a means of eliminating those providers who frequently contest decisions (e.g., concerning continued authorizations for treatment) made by the managed care company. This issue increasingly will be critical as the coverage of managed care plans expands and providers become increasingly dependent on managed care for obtaining clients. Nonetheless, challenging no-cause termination provisions appears to be gaining support as the managed care industry evolves.* It is important to keep in mind, however, that this issue has not been extensively litigated and, therefore, the information presented here represents only prospective theories upon which a claim may be successfully pursued.

There are several arguments that might be used by a provider to challenge termination without cause. First, certain due process rights currently afforded to providers in a hospital setting also may be applicable to managed care providers. For example, it is well established that hospitals sustain liability for failing to obtain and evaluate information regarding the training and experience of medical staff members and applicants before granting privileges. This liability may also apply to managed care companies and their credentialing procedures. Recent experience has made clear that managed care companies will have to intensify their credentialing procedures or face potential liability similar to that of hospitals (Curtis, 1990). Accordingly, it can be argued that managed care companies, like hospitals, should be required to provide basic due process appeal rights to a provider who is terminated.

*For example, the New Jersey Psychological Association and seven named plaintiffs recently filed a complaint against MCC Behavioral Care Inc., contesting the termination of the psychologists from MCC's provider network without cause. In addition, as discussed in more detail below, the New Hampshire Supreme Court in *Harper v. Healthsource New Hampshire, Inc.* (1996) ruled that a managed care provider who was terminated without cause was entitled to a review of that decision.

Several court cases (e.g., *Hackenthal v. California Medical Association*, 1982; *Pinsker v. Pacific Coast Society of Orthodontists*, 1969; *Salkin v. California Dental Association*, 1986) can be used to strengthen the argument for the right to appeal a no-cause termination. Courts have recognized that medical professional associations and other entities related to the provision of health care are of "quasi-public" significance (Curtis, 1990). Entities having quasi-public significance cannot expel or discipline members, so as to adversely affect their substantial property, contract, or other economic rights, without fair proceedings. Because expulsion from a managed care plan also involves judgment by one's own profession and because such plans serve the quasi-public function of providing health care, one could argue that in no-cause termination cases, certain property and economic rights are at risk.

It also can be argued that managed care companies have a duty to show good faith in terminating a contract. It appears that managed care companies believe that a contract between a health care provider and a managed care company should be treated by the courts like a standard business contract where no-cause termination provisions are prevalent. Although such provisions found in contracts have traditionally been held to be valid, courts have increasingly implied a duty of good faith that is intended to protect the "reasonable expectations of the parties" (Curtis, 1990). In effect, contracts with managed care companies should be treated as agreements to provide health services rather than as simple business arrangements.

The New Hampshire Supreme Court recently relied on both public policy concerns and the duty of good faith and fair dealing in ruling that a physician is entitled to review the decision of a managed care company to terminate him or her with or without cause. In *Harper v. Healthsource New Hampshire, Inc.*, (1996), the Supreme Court analogized the physician's relationship with the managed care company to an employer–employee relationship. In traditional employment law, a contract providing for termination by either party is an employment-at-will contract. The Court noted that "at-will" contracts are unenforceable if they contravene public policy. The Court further noted that an employer has an implied duty of good faith and fair dealing, which is violated if the employer terminates an employee "out of malice or bad faith in retaliation for action taken or refused by the employee in consonance with public policy." The Court observed that "the public has a substantial interest in the relationship between health maintenance organizations and their preferred provider physicians as well (1996, p. 11)." The Court concluded that "the public interest and fundamental fairness demand that a health maintenance organization's decision to terminate its relationship with a particular physician provider must comport with the covenant of good faith and fair dealing and may not be made for a reason that is contrary to public policy (1996, p. 13)."

Adhesion contract theory also can be used to argue against no-cause termination. According to this theory, when a contract appears to be one-sided and unfair, particular provisions will be construed against the drafter of the contract to the extent necessary to alleviate the unfairness. Adhesion contracts are commonly found where (1) a standardized agreement is prepared by one party for the other; (2) the preparer wields superior bargaining power; and (3) the contract is offered on a take-it-or-leave-it basis, with no opportunity to bargain. These elements may be applicable to the contractual relationship between a provider and a managed care entity, since a court may find the no-cause termination provision to be so unfair and one-sided that the provision would be void, and hence unenforceable.

The following are recommended steps that can be taken by a provider who is terminated without cause and who wishes to challenges that termination:

- Review the contract to determine the circumstances under which the managed care company can effectively terminate the relationship with the provider.
- If the managed care company has a basis for terminating the relationship, determine whether the company has complied with the procedures set forth in the contract.
- Upon receiving notice of termination, contact the managed care company's director of provider relations by phone to explore what alternatives for redress exist. Be as congenial as possible.
- If the telephone call is positive and feasible alternatives exist, send a written confirmation of the conversation to the managed care company.
- In the event of a negative outcome, the provider may pursue the issue further by filing an official complaint with the managed care company. Duplicate complaint letters could be sent to the state's department of insurance or other department responsible for regulating the activities of the managed care company.
- The provider's letter of appeal should cite specific reasons why he or she is uniquely qualified (e.g., cite a successful treatment history, successful working relationship with the managed care company, and specific experience and training).
- When consulting with the UR agent either to appeal a decision or to provide information to the managed care company in support of a complaint, the professional should base all communication on well-kept records and documentation of therapy.
- Be particularly sensitive to the use of the no-cause termination provision by the managed care company as an excuse to get rid of a provider whom it may view as a troublemaker.

A "good plaintiff" (one with a greater chance of success) in a no-cause termination case is one who historically has had a good relationship with the managed care company but whose relationship has changed because of the plaintiff's repeated attempts to appeal or complain about decisions made by the company. Evidence of a substantial caseload at some point during the relationship is significant, and the existence of solid documentation of the circumstances leading up to termination is essential.

No-Disparagement ("Gag") Provisions

Another provision that has created much concern in the provider industry is the no-disparagement or "gag" provision. A sample clause from US Healthcare is as follows:

> [Provider] shall agree not to take any action or make any communication which undermines or could undermine the confidence of enrollees, potential enrollees, their employers, their unions, or the public in US Healthcare or the quality of US Healthcare coverage. [Provider] shall keep the Proprietary Information [payment rates, utilization-review procedures, etc.] and this Agreement strictly confidential. (Woolhandler & Himmelstein, 1995)

While such clauses are intended to prohibit providers from "disparaging" the MCO to patients or other individuals, they may conflict with other provisions in the contract, such as requiring providers to act in accordance with their professional judgment (e.g., explaining treatment alternatives to patients). As a gag clause may be interpreted as prohibiting a provider from speaking to his or her patients about decisions by the MCO to deny benefits and the provider's attempt to appeal, such a clause may also deter providers from appealing denial of coverage decisions. Increasingly, MCOs have agreed to drop gag clauses because they did not realize that the clauses could be interpreted as prohibiting full disclosure to patients.

It is argued that attempts to limit a provider's freedom to talk about treatment options and payment policies, including discussing financial bonuses for providers who save the MCO money by withholding care ("HMO Gag Rules," 1996), interfere with the provider's ethical and legal duty to provide patients with information about the benefits, risks, and costs of various treatments. For example, the American Medical Association (AMA) Council on Ethics and Judicial Affairs (CEJA) declared that gag rules are an "unethical interference" in the doctor–patient relationship, and therefore requested that physicians strike such clauses from their contracts. According to CEJA:

> The physician's obligation to disclose treatment alternatives to patients is not altered by any limitation in the coverage provided by the patient's managed care plan. Patients cannot be subject to making decisions with inadequate information. This would be an absolute violation of the informed consent requirements. (CEJA, 1995)

CEJA's statement on gag rules follows the 1994 report, "Ethics in Managed Care," which outlined all of the ethical duties of physicians practicing in managed care plans. The report said that "the duty of patient advocacy is a fundamental element of the physician–patient relationship that should not be altered by the system of health care delivery in which physicians practice" (CEJA, 1995, p. 334).

A new Massachusetts law bars MCOs from imposing rules that limit providers' ability to speak freely with patients about all aspects of their health insurance, including alternative treatments that may or may not be covered under the patients' policies. In addition, the law seeks to protect patient confidentiality by prohibiting MCOs from demanding information about prospective patients' life histories and mental health status before covering them for state mandated mental health benefits.*

Hold-Harmless Provisions

Many managed care entities ask providers to sign contracts that contain "hold-harmless" provisions. These clauses are designed to ensure that the provider and the managed care company are viewed as separate and independent entities, each of which is solely responsible for damages resulting from its own negligence. Essentially these provisions state that liability for a provider's services is covered under the provider's own malpractice policy.

Under such a provision, the payer, managed care entity, or any of its agents or representatives shall not be held liable for any cause of action or liability arising out of

*Legislative initiatives are helpful, in that they set the stage and can be used as a model for other state and federal efforts. Any legislation, however, may have its limitations. For example, certain MCOs operating in Massachusetts may be exempted from this recent law; for example, those self-insured plans governed by the Employee Retirement Security Act (ERISA) of 1974, and those operating under Medicaid managed care. The ERISA law prohibits states from regulating the health benefit plans of companies that self insure. Medicaid managed care may have a separate set of operating guidelines from the private sector.

or in connection with services rendered by the provider. Some contracts only hold the provider liable for damages due to the provider's actions while other contracts could be interpreted in such a manner that the provider assumes *all* liability. An example of such a provision follows:

> Providers shall indemnify and hold [the MCO] harmless from any and all claims, lawsuits, settlements and liabilities incurred as a result of professional services provided or not provided by a provider with respect to any covered person. Relatedly, [the MCO] shall indemnify and hold the provider harmless from any and all claims, lawsuits, settlements, and liabilities incurred as a result of actions taken or not taken by [the MCO] in the administration of the employer's group health benefit plan.

The intent in this provision appears to be that the provider agrees to indemnify the MCO for negligence in providing or not providing services, and the company agrees to indemnify the provider for negligence or other damages in connection with administration of the plan. Requiring the provider to assume responsibility for his or her own negligent conduct, to insure him- or herself against that responsibility, and to protect the managed care company through indemnification for liability does not seem to be an unreasonable contractual arrangement. However, hold-harmless agreements need to be carefully reviewed to ensure that this appropriate intent is realized, especially in light of *Wickline v. State of California* (1987) and its progeny, which, as noted above, suggest that both the managed care company and the provider can be held liable, either separately or jointly, when a cost-containment strategy results in negligent care. Another example of a problematic clause follows:

> Liability for provider services are covered under provider's own practice liability. The payer or managed care entity or any of their agents or representatives shall not be liable for any cause of action or liability arising out of or in connection with services rendered by the provider.

This contractual provision does not appear to create a true indemnity relationship, because it disclaims liability rather than requiring the provider to indemnify against it. A court could construe the clause as an intended agreement to indemnify. However, a potential counterargument is that the agreement to indemnify was intended to cover damages that arise not only from the provider's own negligent conduct but also for damages that arise from the managed care company's negligent conduct, so long as that liability arises "in connection with services rendered by the provider."

In the foregoing examples, the hold-harmless provisions appear to be setting forth a subcontracting relationship between the managed care entity and the provider. Such a relationship would limit each party's liabilities to its own respective actions. Other provisions are even more ambiguous. For instance, one MCO's plan contained a provision that stated:

> The specialist–provider will hold the managed care organization harmless due to any malpractice litigation and will have a minimum of one million dollars worth of professional liability insurance. Providers shall notify the managed care organization within 48 hours of loss of insurance.

If one were to read this provision literally, any malpractice claim that arose could be seen to be the responsibility of the specialist–provider. In other words, the provider would be required to indemnify the managed care organization even if the organization were partially at fault. Clearly these hold-harmless provisions would be unreasonable, because malpractice liability insurance typically covers only those specific acts arising out of the conduct of the provider. Typically, the provider cannot assume liability for other parties unless the provider directly arranges for such liability and agrees to take it on. The primary purpose of malpractice liability insurance is to insure against damages resulting from the provider's negligence, not from the negligence of entities with which providers is engaged in business.

Release of Records Provisions

Another problematic provision in managed care contracts is the requirement for a broad release of records in exchange for payment. In the absence of state law, there is little check on such requests for information. The laws of New Jersey and the District of Columbia, however, expressly restrict the release of patient information to MCOs (e.g., treatment notes, session notes).

Increasingly, MCOs are asking practitioners to open up *all* their patient records for review by the MCO. State laws, however, require that patients give informed consent to the release of their records, thereby prohibiting practitioners from releasing information of non-MCO patients. A practitioner could be subject to disciplinary proceedings by the state licensing board for allowing an MCO to have access to records of a patient with whom the MCO had no contractual arrangement. In this area, clients must give full and knowing consent to the disclosure of this information, and clearly non-MCO patients have not given such consent for the release of their information. It could be argued that any action taken by an MCO against a practitioner who refuses to release such records is unlawful because the MCO is asking the practitioner to break the law.

Other Conflicts Faced by Providers

Verifying Contractual Definitions and Provisions

Many managed care entities, through contractual arrangements, limit reimbursement to services that are deemed "medically necessary." While MCOs generally are obligated to make public their definition of medically necessary, how this definition applies in any given case is often not clear. Consequently, a provider may not have a sense in advance of what services will be covered. In cases where the MCO has the sole authority to determine medical necessity, providers may face both financial liability when services are not covered and legal exposure for not delivering adequate services (Rosenbaum et al., 1995).

Conflict of Interest

The increasing complexity of service delivery and financing arrangements sometimes results in role ambiguity for providers. This, in turn, may result in potential conflict of interest situations. For example, when a professional is working for a corporation as an EAP provider, he or she owes a duty or responsibility both to the corporation and to the client. In one reported case, a psychologist working in an EAP setting in a corporation was informed by the employer that the provision of information or referral to employees related to legal issues was appropriate except if the employee was contemplating legal action against the company or if an issue such as sexual harassment in the workplace arose.

For EAP counselors who are psychologists, their ethics code provides guidance on this matter. For example, the APA (1992) Ethics Code, Principle 1.21 states:

> (a) When a psychologist agrees to provide services to a person or entity at the request of a third party, the psychologist clarifies to the extent feasible, at the outset of the service, the nature of the relationship with each party. This clarification includes the role of the psychologist (such as therapist, organizational consultant, diagnostician, or expert witness), the probable uses of the services provided or the information obtained, and the fact that there may be limits to confidentiality.
> (b) If there is a foreseeable risk of the psychologist's being called upon to perform conflicting roles because of the involvement of a third party, the psychologist clarifies the nature and direction of his or her responsibilities, keeps all parties appropriately informed as matters develop, and resolves the situation in accordance with this Ethics Code. (p. 6)

The APA Ethics Code clearly indicates that in this situation the psychologist has an obligation to approach the corporation and seek clarification on what his or her obligations are to the corporation and to the client. Furthermore, it appears that the psychologist has a duty to discuss with the patient, at the beginning of the relationship, the potential conflicts or compromising situations that can or will arise.

Limitations on Treatment

As part of their cost containment strategies, mental health management firms typically establish limited "preferred provider" panels and offer beneficiaries very strong incentives to select a therapist from those panels.* In addition, in order to control costs, employers often purchase benefit plans with a limited number of inpatient days or outpatient sessions, and the utilization of these sessions is tightly controlled by the management firms (Iglehart, 1996). For example, a typical HMO plan limits an enrollee's outpatient psychotherapy sessions to 20 sessions per year with annual and lifetime cost caps (Haas & Cummings, 1991). These limitations may create both clinical and ethical issues for providers. Clinically, short-term, limited psychotherapy may not be appropriate for all types of cases, and patients in need of longer-term treatment may be denied necessary care if it extends beyond their benefit limits. In addition, the limited number of session may impede the provider's ability to establish an effective treatment plan (Haas & Cummings, 1991).

Ethically, providers may be constrained from abandoning their clients before treatment is completed. Therefore, in cases where the client may need more sessions, a provider may be forced to provide services pro bono unless a referral can be made. At a minimum, providers are required to make responsible referrals to alternative modes of treatment (i.e., to a community mental health center).

Misleading Advertising

As noted previously, a pressing issue in dealing with MCOs is the divergence between the benefit plan the services actually approved for reimbursement. An example of this may be seen in the following case. It was alleged that an MCO had reduced the patient's benefits based on its determination that the current treatment provided by the attending psychologist did not constitute a covered benefit under the

*These incentives typically take the form of patient coinsurance obligations that are significantly lower for services of in-network providers than for services of nonnetwork providers. Indeed, it is not uncommon for patients to have no coverage at all for services of non-network providers.

plan. Although the psychologist appealed the MCO's original decision, a second denial was issued after the MCO ordered a second opinion to be conducted by a certified psychiatrist chosen by the MCO. Based on the second opinion review, the MCO determined that there was not sufficient information to support the medical necessity of care at a frequency of three visits per week. Based on its predetermined criteria, the MCO concluded that the benefits would continue for two visits per week and would be reduced to a 1-hour session per week within a couple weeks. Subsequent to this reduction, the MCO would perform a follow-up review.

The MCO stated in a letter to the provider that services that are recommended by a physician only and are essential for the necessary care and treatment of any illness or injuries would be covered. Unfortunately, this policy was not found in the benefit documents. It is important, therefore, that providers and their patients carefully review the written benefits plan and not rely solely on the payer's interpretation. In addition to advertising and marketing materials, benefit summary plans provided to the patient or insured constitute a contract between the patient or insured and the insurance company. It may need to be brought to the MCO's attention by the provider that essentially any deviation from these contractual obligations could constitute a breach of contract between the patient or insured and the MCO.

Consumer Protection Legislation

State legislatures have introduced "patient protection" legislation that generally regulates MCOs, particularly by establishing consumer protection standards designed to regulate or prohibit certain managed care practices. Presently, six states* have enacted patient protection legislation or regulations that affect behavioral health services, either by amending state HMO and PPO laws, or by enacting "free-standing" legislation† It is expected that more states will pass consumer protection laws in the near future.

Until recently, state regulation of managed care concentrated primarily on what benefits were being provided (e.g., parity between physical and mental health benefits guarantees) and who provided them (e.g., antidiscrimination provider laws). A new generation of consumer protection initiatives is evolving, however, focusing on the *manner* in which services are being provided. These new measures seek to: (1) mandate disclosure to consumers of financial arrangements between MCOs and providers, (2) prohibit interference by MCOs with communications between providers and their patients, (3) protect the confidentiality of patient records, (4) prohibit the termination of providers from managed care panels for appealing treatment decisions made by MCOs, and (5) prohibit MCOs from imposing their own financial and legal risks upon providers.

NATIONAL ACCREDITATION STANDARDS

As the marketplace for behavioral health care services continues to evolve, both established and new organizations are moving to position themselves in a leadership position in the establishment of standards for managed care organizations. Several national organizations have developed accreditation standards in order to ensure that

*California, Connecticut, Maryland, Massachusetts, New Hampshire, and New Jersey.

†For example, Maryland's Patient Access Act is a *free-standing* managed care law, while New Hampshire's law amends an existing managed care law, the state's HMO law.

health plans are able to provide uniform and quality health care. Although participation in such accreditation processes is voluntary for health care organizations, the market forces provide incentive to participate, since many large corporations will not contract with organizations that do not meet nationally recognized standards.

The Utilization Review Accreditation Committee (URAC) and the National Committee for Quality Assurance (NCQA) are two organizations that have developed national standards relevant to the provision of behavioral health services. These standards will affect providers, payers, and consumers of health care services as states increasingly substitute them for state laws.

URAC's National Utilization Review Standards

In 1989, the American Managed Care and Review Association (AMCRA) recognized the need to formulate a comprehensive approach to achieving greater uniformity in UR policies and procedures throughout the United States. The UR industry representatives sought to address providers' concern and frustration with the diversity of UR procedures and with the increasing impact of managed care on physicians and hospitals. AMCRA cofounded URAC because "it was clear that utilization management needed to be managed—whether through state regulation or federal regulation or voluntary accreditation." (Bengen, 1992, p. 4).

URAC is a Washington, DC-based, not-for-profit corporation that represents UR firms, employers, insurers, physicians and hospitals, and has been established to encourage efficient and effective UR processes and to provide a method of evaluating and accrediting UR programs. URAC's national standards were developed as guidelines for the evolving UR industry, and are used to evaluate firms seeking voluntary accreditation. Since its inception, URAC has accredited 155 UR firms that, in turn serve over 180 million people in the United States (Bender, 1995). By developing minimum industry standards to serve as a basis for a voluntary credentialing process, URAC's mission is to continually improve the quality and efficiency of the interaction between the UR industry and the providers, payers, and purchasers of health care.

URAC approved revised National Utilization Review Standards in 1994. URAC lists five objectives that the standards are designed to achieve:

- Encourage consistency in the procedures for interaction between UR organizations and providers, payers, and consumers of health care.
- Establish UR processes that cause minimal disruption to the health care delivery system.
- Establish standards for the procedures used to certify health care services and to process appeals of UR determinations.
- Provide the basis for an efficient process of credentialing and accrediting UR organizations.
- Provide consistent standards and an accreditation mechanism that can be applied efficiently nationwide for those states that choose to regulate UR organizations.

The standards can be applied to all organizations offering UR services. Managed care systems and governmental programs may vary from the standards only to the extent that the variance is addressed in the provider contract or is required by regulations, provided that the system remains consistent with the goals of the standards.

The standards cover eight areas. Section I addresses the scope of the standards and provides that they apply to UR for both "inpatient admission" and "outpatient procedures and services." Section II addresses confidentiality of patient and provider information. Section III addresses the responsibility for obtaining a certification for health care services. Section IV governs the UR staff and program qualifications. Section V deals with accessibility and on-site review procedures. Section VI limits intrusive UR practices. Section VII governs procedures for review of determinations and second opinions. Section VIII addresses appeals of decisions not to certify the procedures.

On the whole, the 1994 URAC standards appear to be superior to most current legislation that regulates utilization review programs. URAC continues to play a significant role in ensuring consistency in the procedures guiding interactions among providers, payers, and consumers during the UR process (Bender, 1995).

NCQA's Accreditation Standards for Managed Behavioral Health Care Organizations

NCQA is an independent, not-for-profit organization that accredits and reports on MCOs. NCQA has recently launched a Behavioral Health Accreditation Program. This program aims to assess the quality of managed behavioral health service delivery.

Given the size of the behavioral health market and the absence of widely accepted measures of quality and accountability, there is widespread support for behavioral health accreditation standards. These standards are important to assuring the provision of high quality services by managed behavioral health care organizations (MBHOs). It is critical to psychologists and other allied health professionals providing behavioral health care that these standards include favorable language governing how and when behavioral health services are to be provided and by whom.

Unless benefits for behavioral health and substance abuse disorders are properly recognized as essential and on par with general medical benefits, the care of patients with these disorders will be undermined and progressively diminished. (Sederer, 1992). Behavioral health care benefits must be protected from elimination as employers seek low-cost policies.

As noted above, there are more than 300 MBHOs in operation today, serving over 100 million people. NCQA's recent publication of the proposed national standards for MBHOs represents the entity's first attempt to accredit these companies. The new proposed standards represent minimum standards for services provided by MBHOs. They will help provide a mechanism with which to assess and differentiate the quality of the managed behavioral health care services available in the market today. For the first time, using the standards, employers will be able to compare behavioral health plans against each other. The proposed standards parallel earlier accreditation guidelines that NCQA developed for general medical MCOs.

Through the implementation of the Proposed Standards, the NCQA intends to:

- Provide consumers, employers, public purchasers, and the managed behavioral health care industry with a comprehensive set of accreditation standards to assess the quality of managed behavioral health care plans.
- Foster accountability among MBHOs for the quality of service their members receive.
- Encourage effectiveness in the provision of behavioral health care, through integration with general medical care, prevention, and early intervention.

NCQA's proposed standards measure managed behavioral health plan performances in seven areas: (1) quality management and improvement, which includes practitioner availability, member satisfaction, and practice guideline utilization; (2) accessibility, availability, referral, and triage; (3) utilization management; (4) credentialing; (5) members' rights and responsibilities, which includes power of patients to make decisions affecting their treatment; (6) preventive behavioral health care services; and (7) clinical evaluation and treatment records, which requires MBHOs to maintain adequate patient records.

Several concerns have been raised with regard to the proposed standards. First, some critics believe they contain insufficient safeguards for the confidentiality of patient records maintained by the MBHO. The standards are inconsistent with professional ethics codes, URAC's UR Standards, and many state laws.

Second, although the proposed standards seek to evaluate whether an MBHO truly provides sufficient access to care, they do not provide clear definitions of sufficient access. NCQA does not itself establish minimum standards for the availability of a certain number of behavioral health care practitioners. Rather, it allows the MBHO to establish its own standards. Such an approach does not assure consumers that a minimal level of coverage is being provided. Critics argue that NCQA should develop a range of standards for the ratio of practitioners to patients, considering geographic factors, delivery settings and professional mix. This would benefit consumers by extending their freedom of choice, and benefit providers by expanding their access to panels.

Third, it is argued that the standards improperly restrict the performance of certain tasks to psychiatrists. For example, the proposed standards require the triage function to be supervised by a board-certified psychiatrist with an active license and a minimum of 5 years clinical experience. Advocates would like the statute to be amended to include other health care professionals with 5 years clinical experience, who can perform this function equally as well.

Fourth, it is argued that the proposed standards do not provide adequate due process for consumers and providers facing adverse treatment or credentialing decisions. They do not, for example, prohibit MBHOs from taking action against members who complain or from terminating contracts with providers on the basis of utilization. The proposed standards should also reference practitioners' ethical codes to ensure that MBHOs recognize the importance of a professional's obligations to patients.

The establishment of MBHO accreditation standards is an important step forward in assuring that adequate quality services are provided through these delivery systems. The NCQA plans to pilot test its standards in two MBHOs—Green Spring Health Services of Columbia, Maryland and US Behavioral Health of San Francisco, California—and one MCO—Community Health Plan of Albany—New York, later this year. Accreditation of individual MBHOs will begin early in 1997. It is anticipated that these standards will soon be mandatory for behavioral healthcare services offered through other types of managed care arrangements as well.

FORMING MULTIDISCIPLINARY GROUP PRACTICES

In response to the challenges presented by managed care, mental health providers are increasingly considering forming multidisciplinary group practices.* They

*This section is excerpted from an APA publication that was researched and drafted primarily by the law firm of McDermott, Will, and Emery, under the direction of Wendy L. Krasner, JD, and Bryan Puterbaugh.

are doing so for several reasons. First, some payers (or mental health management firms), in assembling their mental health provider networks, are more interested in contracting with a relatively small number of provider groups than signing individual contracts with a large number of solo practitioners. Becoming part of a group thus increases the likelihood that an individual professional can become part of these provider networks.

Second, in many parts of the country, primary care physicians are increasingly being asked (and, in some cases, are actively seeking) to assume more of the financial risk for the total cost of health care services, including mental health services. As primary care physicians take on this financial responsibility, they tend to be much more restrictive in their referrals for mental health services than they would be under a fee-for-service structure. Consequently, mental health professionals who are closely allied with those physicians are likely to have greater access to their patients.

Finally, a large alliance of practitioners may ultimately be in a position to compete directly with the mental health management firms, by entering into carve-out arrangements directly with employers or other payers. Obviously, such an alliance will need to be competitive economically with the existing firms if it expects to capture contracts. Further, even if such an alliance is able to secure contracts, it will need substantial information and management resources in order to administer those contracts. Nonetheless, it may be possible for an alliance of professionals that is owned and controlled by the providers themselves to deliver cost-effective care, free of the types of utilization controls imposed by existing MBHOs.

There are a number of different types of arrangements through which mental health care professionals, such as psychologists, social workers, marriage/family therapists, and professional counselors, may join together with physicians (including both psychiatrists and primary care physicians). The options are limited by state law, that must be consulted before any arrangement is chosen.

It is important to realize that the choice of a legal structure does not resolve the numerous operational and governance issues that arise in connection with the formation of an integrated group. Practitioners who wish to integrate their practices must agree in advance on who will make operational decisions and how they will be made. These decisions can range from the relatively mundane (e.g., what the name of the group will be) to decisions with potentially very significant consequences (e.g., how profits of the group will be allocated, whether to bring other practitioners into the group, and whether to enter into a particular managed care contract). All member practitioners may retain an equal voice in virtually every management decision or they can delegate most decisions to a manager or management committee, reserving key decisions for a vote of all the practitioners. Within the constraints imposed by state law, each of the legal vehicles addressed here is flexible enough to accommodate the choices and preferences of group members regarding these organizational and operational issues.

It is also important to recognize that the entity which bills for the practitioners' services need not own all of the assets used in the practice. It is quite common for a separate entity (which can be owned by all, or only some, of the same practitioners) to be established to hold title to the group's office space and equipment; such an entity is often termed a management services organization (MSO). Similarly,ing several formerly independent practices, it is not uncommon for group members to remain in their own offices rather than moving to a shared space. In such arrangements, often called "group practices without walls," the individual practitioners often continue to own the assets of their former practices; they then rent those assets to the combined group based on some mutually acceptable formula. Whether one of these variations is desirable depends primarily on the tax and financial situations of the participating practitioners.

Partnerships

A multidisciplinary partnership may be formed, unless prohibited by statute, by partners that include any combination of psychologists, psychiatrists, primary care physicians, and other practitioners. Such a partnership can bill for the services of the practitioners who are its partners and any practitioners who are employees of the partnership.

Operating as a partnership has tax advantages over operating as a corporation, because only the partners, not the partnership itself, are taxed. That is, if the partnership has been properly structured, it does not pay taxes directly; rather, each partner is taxed on his or her share of the partnership's net income or losses. In contrast, a corporation itself is taxed when it makes a profit and then its shareholders are also taxed when they receive dividends from the corporation. (However, as discussed below, the problem of double taxation of corporations can often be reduced through the use of "S corporations.")

When deciding on a legal structure for an integrated group, an important consideration is the extent to which group members may be held personally liable for the negligence of other practitioners in the group.* A health care professional who is a partner in a general partnership can be held personally liable for all obligations of the partnership. These may include damages caused by actions of other partners, damages caused by actions of employees of the partnership, and business debts of the partnership.† Of course, a partnership can purchase malpractice insurance to limit the potential liability of its partners. However, the partners will be personally liable for any amount not covered by insurance. Potentially unlimited personal liability makes a general partnership much less attractive than a corporation for health practitioners.

In some states, practitioners may organize themselves as a limited liability partnership (LLP). The distinction between an LLP and a general partnership is that if one partner in an LLP negligently injures a patient, the patient is entitled to be compensated only from the assets of the LLP itself and the personal assets of the partner who treated the patient. The patient may not force the other partners of the LLP to contribute their personal assets. The partners of an LLP, however, typically remain personally liable for the LLP's business debts.

While a general partnership may operate without filing any application to the state in which it operates, an LLP must file the appropriate application form with the state and be registered. Periodic filings may be required to maintain the liability protection of the LLP structure.

*A health care professional is personally liable for damages caused by his or her own malpractice, regardless of whether he or she is a sole practitioner or an owner or employee of a partnership, corporation, or limited liability company.

†In contrast, a health care professional who is an employee of a partnership may not be held liable for the malpractice of other practitioners who practice through the partnership.

It is important to distinguish LLPs from two types of entities having similar names: limited liability companies (LLCs) and limited partnerships. LLCs are discussed below. A limited partnership is a special type of partnership in which a small number of "general partners" accept complete personal liability for the debts of the partnership, while the other investors—known as "limited partners,"—are insulated from personal liability. By law, limited partners are not permitted to play an active role in the management of the limited partnership. Limited partnerships are generally not a suitable structure for professional practices, because practitioners who have an ownership interest in the practice usually want to have an active voice in its management. Moreover, few practitioners are willing to assume responsibility as general partners for the malpractice liability of all the limited partners.

Corporations: For-profit, Nonprofit, and PCs

Corporations have several features that distinguish them from partnerships. An owner of a corporation is liable for the debts of the corporation, regardless of how they arise, only up to the amount of his or her investment in the corporation.

Corporations typically centralize their management in a board of directors and elected officers. Only the officers of the corporation, acting under authority granted by the board, may sign contracts for the corporation. A corporation continues to exist even when one or more shareholder sells his or her shares.

As discussed above, a corporations' profits are usually taxed twice: once when the corporation earns them and a second time when it distributes them to its shareholders in the form of dividends. However, corporations often can escape federal income taxes by electing to be treated as an "S" corporation. An S corporation must have 35 or fewer shareholders, all of whom are individuals (i.e., not corporations or LLCs), and only one class of voting stock. S corporations are taxed like partnerships; that is, the net income and losses of the corporation are "passed through" for tax purposes to the corporation's shareholders, who pay taxes in their individual capacity on their share of the corporation's earnings or losses. Depending on state law, S corporations also may be exempt from state income taxes. Moreover, even if a professional service entity does not qualify as an S corporation, it can often "zero out" its books, and thereby avoid taxation, by distributing excess earnings to shareholders in the form of year-end bonuses.

Relatively few states permit ordinary corporations (commonly termed "business corporations") to employ physicians and psychologists and to bill in the name of the corporation for their professional services. In those states that permit business corporations to engage in such activities, such entities provide a straightforward vehicle for assembling a multidisciplinary practice.

A few states (e.g., Michigan) that prohibit for-profit business corporations from hiring psychologists, physicians, and other health professionals nonetheless permit nonprofit corporations (sometimes known as "nonstock corporations") to engage in such activities. A nonprofit corporation may not pay dividends to its members, but it may pay reasonable salaries to its employees, even when those employees are also members or officers of the corporation. It can thus be a viable vehicle for professional practices, despite the "nonprofit" label.

A nonprofit corporation is managed by officers under the direction of a board of directors. The persons with ultimate control over the activities of a nonprofit corporation are typically knows as "members" of the corporation rather than "shareholders."

The fact that a corporation is denominated "nonprofit" does not mean that it is exempt from income taxes. Such corporations will be taxed if they earn a profit, unless they meet the stringent requirements for tax exemption (e.g., provision of charity care and limited control by practitioners); few if any entities that are dominated by practitioners will be able to qualify for tax exemption.

In many states, the "corporation practice of medicine" doctrine bars both for-profit business corporations and nonprofit corporations from employing and billing for the services of psychologists and physicians. In these states, the only type of corporation that may engage in these practices is a professional corporation.

The PC laws of each state govern the ownership, management, and operation of these corporations.* These laws vary substantially among the states. For example, some states explicitly allow, while other states explicitly forbid, PCs to have shareholders who are licensed in different professions. In states that require a PC's shareholders all to be licensed in the same profession, a PC that has physician shareholders may not have shareholders who are psychologists or other nonphysician health care professional. Some states require that a PC's officers, directors, and professional employees hold the same type of license as the PC's shareholders; other states do not. Where a psychologist or other nonphysician health care professional may be a director or officer of a physician-owned PC, the professional may be able to influence the operations of the PC by voting as a director or acting as an officer even if he or she may not be able to have a direct ownership interest in the corporation.

The PC framework allows but does not require tight integration of practices. Typically, each practitioner signs a full-time (or, if the practitioner wishes to maintain a separate practice outside of the PC structure, a part-time) employment agreement with the PC. The practitioner's compensation may be a fixed salary or may include bonus payments for productivity.

Limited Liability Companies

Statutes authorizing LLCs have been enacted in nearly all states over the last several years. LLCs are hybrids with some of the best characteristics of both corporations and partnerships. LLCs have "members" who are analogous to the shareholders of a corporation or the partners of a partnership. Members of an LLC have limited liability for the liabilities of the LLC, including both ordinary business obligations and liabilities arising out of the professional malpractice of other members or employees of the LLC. At the same time, a properly structured LLC is taxed as a partnership under federal law and the laws of the great majority of states (but not Florida or Texas).

An LLC is typically formed by filing articles of organization with the appropriate state authorities. An LLC must have an operating agreement, which serves essentially as its constitution. The operating agreement specifies how the LLC will be governed, how profits and losses will be allocated, and similar issues. All LLC members may take an active role in its management or the LLC may centralize management in "managers" who function like the officers of a corporation.

*It is not uncommon even for solo practitioners to practice in the form of a PC. Practitioners who are already incorporated and who wish to combine their practices into a larger PC have several options. They can, for example, merge their existing PCs into a new PC. They can transfer their practices into a new PC, leaving their existing PCs in place to collect accounts receivable. Alternatively, in many states, they can establish a structure in which their existing PCs become subsidiaries of a newly created "parent" PC. The choice among these approaches will generally depend on the practitioners' individual financial situations.

In some states, it is clear that LLCs may employ psychologists, physicians, and other professionals, and that it can bill in its own name for the service of those practitioners.* In other states, however, the authority of LLCs to engage in such activities remains unsettled. Where it is clear that an LLC can engage in these activities, the LLC may be the best vehicle for multidisciplinary practices.

Contractual Affiliations

As suggested above, it is not necessary for providers to actually integrate their practices into a single legal entity in order to be able to contract jointly with third-party payers. Rather, it is possible for psychologists, physicians, and other practitioners to form an entity that serves as a contracting vehicle, but that allows them to retain their separate practices. A contracting vehicle of this nature is known by a number of different names, but to minimize confusion, the term we will employ here is, simply, "network."†

Networks do not employ practitioners, but instead enter into contracts with practitioners. (Such practitioners may practice as individuals or be organized as partnerships, corporations, or LLCs). These agreements typically obligate the network to negotiate with third-party payers on behalf of the practitioners. Once the network signs a contract with a payer, the network notifies all of the practitioners with whom the network has agreements, specifying the payment terms agreed to by the payer and any unique requirements imposed by the payer (e.g., its referral procedures).

Depending on state law, networks may enter into a number of different financial arrangements with payers. In most states, networks may contract on a capitated basis (i.e., accept a fixed amount per month for each person covered by the network, regardless of the actual quantity or kind of services that the member requires); however, as discussed below, acceptance of capitation will often trigger additional regulatory requirements. When a network enters into a capitated arrangement, it is up to the network to determine how to allocate the capitated payment among network members. More commonly, a network will negotiate a fee-for-service arrangement, in which network members are paid, at rates specified by the payer, for each individual service they provide. In such cases, practitioners generally bill the payer directly, although the network may handle billing and collection functions as the agent of the individual practitioners. The ongoing expenses of operating the network can be funded by charging an "administrative fee" to the member, a "network access fee" to payers, or both.

A network typically negotiates with only some of the payers in a community. Practitioners who are members of the network are typically free to sign contracts with other payers outside of the network's arrangements, although it may be possible to design a network that restricts a member's ability to enter into contracts indepen-

*In some states, for example, New York, standard LLCs are prohibited from providing professional services, but the statute has specific provisions for professional LLCs (PLLCs).

†The term "independent practice association," or "IPA," is generally applied to a type of network that receives capitated payments from payers. The discussion in this section applies to IPAs (although IPAs may be subject to particular state regulation). This section also applies to provider hospital organizations (PHOs), provider organizations (POs), MSOs, and any other organization that does not provide professional services in its own name, but instead contracts with independent practitioners.

dently of the network or that requires the members to give the best (i.e., lowest) price to the network.

It is usually most appropriate to organize a practitioner-sponsored network as a nonprofit corporation. The founding practitioners become the members of the network, contribute its start-up capital, and are empowered to vote on key decisions and elect the network's officers. A network can be established with multiple classes of members, and the network's bylaws may require all classes of members to consent to certain decisions, in order to protect the interests of each group. For example, psychologists could make up one class of members and physicians could make up a second class. While networks can be established as for-profit corporations, state and federal laws regarding the issuance of securities may make the process more expensive and burdensome. Moreover, networks generally are structured to return any available funds in the form of provider payments rather than dividends.

Despite its status as a nonprofit corporation, a network formed for the purpose of contracting with third-party payers almost certainly will be unable to meet the standards for exemption from income taxes. Thus, to the extent the network has taxable income, it will be subject to federal and state income tax.

Networks are usually not licensed or directly regulated by states. In New York, however, networks are subject to very substantial restrictions.

The liability of a network for claims arising out of service provided by network members is somewhat uncertain. In the current environment, no entity is ever entirely insulated from lawsuits. However, to the extent the network acts solely as a contracting vehicle and does not attempt to review either the professional qualifications of network members or the quality or quantity of the services they render, the network's exposure should be limited. On the other hand, the more involved the network becomes in provider credentialing, utilization review, quality assurance, and similar activities, the greater the risks it will face and the more important it is for the network to secure appropriate insurance coverage.

The network model of provider contracting has advantages for health care professionals, who are less likely to encounter interference with their professional autonomy than those who are part of a more tightly integrated group practice. Also important is the fact that, if a professional decides the arrangement is not beneficial, it is likely to be much easier to leave a network than to leave an integrated group. Termination of a contract with a network is usually effective between 30 to 90 days after notice is given, although the health care professional may be bound for a longer period by the payer agreements negotiated by the network that he or she accepted prior to giving notice of termination.

Forming a network, however, has drawbacks as well. The flexibility afforded by the network structure also makes it harder to ensure that the entity will operate in a coordinated manner. The fact that a network with relative ease means that decisions effectively must be made by consensus, which can prevent the group from making difficult choices. Moreover, and of greater significance, payers may not be interested in contracting with networks, preferring instead to deal with more tightly integrated groups.

The antitrust laws present a particularly important constraint for network-type organizations. While a full-scale treatment of the antitrust laws is beyond the scope of this chapter, the basic concept is that the antitrust laws prohibit competitors from making collective decisions regarding with whom they will deal and what they will charge for their services. For purposes of the antitrust laws, persons or entities are considered to be "competitors" if they are engaged in the same general line of business within a single geographic area.

As a rule, members of a truly integrated group are permitted to make collective contracting decisions because they are seen in the eyes of the law as coventurers rather than competitors. Similarly, when a network enters into a capitated arrangement, network members will likely be viewed as coventurers (and not competitors) to the extent they share the risk that the cost of services required by patients will exceed what was originally anticipated.

However, when competing practitioners form a network-type organization and when that network enters into fee-for-service arrangements, the law continues to view network members as competitors. Accordingly, the network must be structured so that each member of the network is given the opportunity to make an *independent* decision about the rates he or she is willing to accept. Typically, this is accomplished by having the network develop a base fee schedule and presenting that model fee schedule to each network member for his or her consideration. A network member who accepts the base schedule agrees to participate in all payer contracts where the payment rates are at least as high as the rates contained in the base schedule. This process allows the network to promise payers who accept the base fee schedule a guaranteed level of participation from network members.*

A second key issue that networks must take into account involves state insurance regulations. Some states take the position that, when a network accepts capitation or enters into another arrangement in which the network assumes substantial financial risk, the network is engaging in the business of insurance and must obtain a state insurance license. Virtually all states permit networks to accept capitation from HMOs and some states permit networks to accept capitation from licensed insurers as well. However, it is rare for a state to permit a network to enter into a capitated arrangement directly with a self-insured employer. Practitioners interested in forming a network that will assume risk to any degree must give careful consideration to those issues before proceeding with their plans.

Employment Arrangements

It is important to note that alliances with other practitioners often can be accomplished more simply and directly through an arrangement in which a nonphysician health care professional acts as an *employee* of a physician or physician group. Obviously, this arrangement may afford the professional less control than an arrangement in which he or she is also an owner of the practice. However, it is frequently possible to negotiate a long-term employment contract that provides a substantial degree of job security. Such a contract also can include provisions responsive to concerns with respect to professional autonomy, working conditions, or other areas of importance. Further, as noted above, some state laws governing PCs permit nonshareholders to act as corporate officers or directors. In those states, an agreement might be negotiated

*An alternative approach is what is commonly known as the "messenger model." In this model, each network member is given the opportunity to accept or reject every proposal received by the Network. Because this model is cumbersome operationally and because payers are unwilling to negotiate with networks that cannot speak definitively on behalf of their members, networks that have relied on the messenger model have generally been unsuccessful in attracting contracts.

that guarantees the nonphysician a seat on the employer's board of directors even though he or she may not be a shareholder in the practice.

CONCLUSION

It is clear that the dramatic changes in the health care industry pose significant challenges to the health care community. All providers, including behavioral health care providers, must be cognizant of these changes and be prepared to offer their services through vehicles that were unknown 10 to 20 years ago. Providers should educate themselves about the pros and cons of participating in managed care, so that at a minimum they will be aware of the obligations that are associated with entering into a legally binding relationship with an MCO. Furthermore, they should have an awareness of those governmental entities and accreditation bodies that may be responsible for regulating the MCOs and setting standards for quality of care for MCO arrangements. Last, for those providers who desire a more entrepreneurial approach to their practices, it pays to access the marketplace and consider forming new arrangements to deliver their services.

REFERENCES

American Psychological Association. (1992). *Ethical principles of psychologists and code of conduct.* Washington, DC: Author.

Bender, L., (1995, March 30). UR accreditation group seeks new markets. *Medical Utilization Management, 23*(7), 1–2.

Bengen, B. (1992, September 17). Mental health experts examine industry accreditation issues. *Health Care Information Center-Utilization Review,* 4.

Boochever, S. (1986). Health maintenance organizations. In J.M. Johnson (Ed.), *Introduction to alternative delivery mechanisms: HMOs, PPOs, & CMPs* (pp. 5–10). Washington, DC: National Health Lawyers Association.

Boyd v. Albert Einstein Medical Center, 377 Pa, Super 609, 547 A.2d 1229 (Pa. Super Ct. 1988).

Council on Ethical and Judicial Affairs (CEJA),American Medical Association (1995, January 25). Ethical issues in managed care. *The Journal of American Medical Association, 273*(4), 330–335.

Curtis, T. (1990). Fair hearings for physicians denied participation in managed care plans. *Medical Staff Counselor, 4,* 45–47.

DeLeon, P. H., VandenBos, G. R., & Bulatao, E. Q. (1991). Managed mental health care: A history of the federal policy initiative. *Professional Psychology: Research and Practice, 22,* 15–25.

Freeman, M. A., & Trabin, T. (1995, September). The policies and challenges of managed behavioral healthcare. *Policy in Perspective,* 1–4.

Gold, M. R., Hurley, R., Lake, T., Ensor, T., & Berenson, R. (1995). A national survey of the arrangements managed-care plans make with physicians. *New England Journal of Medicine, 333,* 1678–1683.

Haas, L. J., & Cummings, N. A. (1991). Managed outpatient mental health plans: Clinical, ethical, and practical guidelines for participation. *Professional Psychology: Research and Practice, 22,* 45–51.

Hackenthal v. California Medical Association, 187 Cal. Rptr. 811 (Ct. App. 1982).

Harper v. Healthsource of New Hampshire, Inc., 674 A.2d 962 (N.H. 1996).

Higuchi, S. (1994). Recent managed care legislative and legal issues. *The mental health professional's guide to managed care* (pp. 86–87), Washington, DC: American Psychological Association.

HMO gag rules. (1996, January 6). *New York Times,* A 18.

Iglehart, J. K. (1996). Managed care and mental health. *New England Journal of Medicine, 334,* 131–135.

Managed care plans feel patient, provider backlash. (1996, March 18). *State Health Notes,* 1–3.

Pinsker v. Pacific Coast Society of Orthodontists, 460 P.2d 495 (Cal. 1969).

Richardson, L.M., & Austad, C.S. (1991). Realities of mental health practice in managed-care settings. *Professional Psychology: Research and Practice, 22*, 52–59.
Rosenbaum, S., Serrano, R., Wehr, E., & Spernak, S. (1995). *Negotiating the new health system: An analysis of provider contracts between managed care organizations and primary care group practices*. Washington, DC: The George Washington University, Center for Health Policy Research.
Salkin v. California Dental Association. 224 Cal. Rptr. 352 (Ct. App. 1986).
Sederer, L. (1992, September). Judicial and legislative responses to cost containment. *American Journal of Psychiatry, 149*(9), 1157–1161.
Sipkoff, M. Z. (1995, March). Managed mental health care. *Open Minds, 8*, 8.
Survey finds widespread and growing use of utilization review practices. (1988, Fall). *The Health Poll*, 1–4.
Wickline v. State of California. 239 Cal. Rptr. 805, 741 P.2d 613 (1987).
Woolhandler, S., & Himmelstein, D. U. (1995). Extreme risk: The new corporate proposition for physicians. *New England Journal of Medicine, 333*, 1706–1708.
Zucker, M. (1995, July). Evolving behavioral health group practice models. *Open Minds*, 4–5.

19

Role of Professional Organizations in Advancing Quality of Care within the Behavioral Health Professions

WILLIAM L. CLAIBORN

OVERVIEW

Most mental health professionals claim membership in at least one professional organization. The reasons for joining are no doubt many, but they are likely to include one or more of the following: desire for collegial relationships, opportunities for continuing education, support for advocacy on behalf of the professional members, opportunity for enhanced status, professional "networking," and availability of resources for marketing.

This chapter examines the role played by professional associations in shaping the quality of care provided by those of their members who are licensed behavioral health professionals. The definition of quality used here includes inferences from input, such as education and training; inferences from process, such as examination of case work and supervision; and inferences from outputs, such as report cards, ethical investigations, and health status changes for consumers resulting from clinical services. Included in the analysis are organizations that deal with quality through their admission procedures, through the participation of members, and through a sanctioning process. The chapter reviews the following professions: psychiatric nursing, psychology, psychiatry, social work, marriage and family therapy, and substance abuse counseling.

This account examines formal credentialing organizations that have credentialing as their primary approach and those in which affinity membership is the central purpose. Voluntary organizations are included as well as nonvoluntary (e.g., state regulatory boards) which collectively serve any of 14 discernible functions. The chapter concludes with recommendations regarding actions that might be taken by these organizations in the future to meet the challenges created by the changes in health care delivery, particularly in the form of managed care arrangements.

WILLIAM L. CLAIBORN • Alexandria Community Services Board, Alexandria, Virginia 22314.

Handbook of Quality Management in Behavioral Health, edited by Stricker *et al.* Kluwer Academic / Plenum Publishers, New York, 2000.

DEFINITION OF QUALITY OF CARE

In taking one's car in for repair, it is likely that the primary judgment about the quality of the work comes from your determination, as you drive away, that the vehicle works well and that the problem that caused you to seek service seems to be gone. Upon reflection, however, assessing the quality of the repair is more complex than this. For example, the overall judgment of quality might appropriately include whether the car was repaired in a timely way; that proper parts were used; that the repair lasts an appropriate period of time; that nothing else was damaged; that the specific problem was diagnosed correctly the first time; that you, the customer were, fully informed; that you were treated pleasantly; that, irrespective of the outcome of the repair, you were happy; that the cost was as expected (or was the most economical possible, given fair labor rates); that the vehicle was clean when returned; that you were kept informed of the progress of the repair and consented; that the repair agent behaved ethically; that the repair technicians were properly trained and certified; that the repair shop had its requisite permits and necessary licenses; and that the repair was fully warranted.

This list of possible indicators of quality in the auto repair industry has parallels in health services. As can be seen from examination of the above list of quality elements, there are some that are closest to an outcome (the car works properly; the customer is satisfied), some that are closer to process (proper repair procedures were undertaken and proper parts used), and some that are closer to inputs (technicians were properly trained and certified). Depending on the perspective of the observer, some of these indicators of quality are more important than others. Further, the perspective of the observer is a significant determiner of how quality is defined or judged in any given case.

Professional organizations may approach quality from both an acknowledged and an unacknowledged basis. For example, a professional credentialing organization, such as the American Board of Psychiatry and Neurology (ABPN), explicitly asserts that it seeks to measure quality of applicants in its examination process. Other organizations (e.g., a membership organization such as the National Association of Social Workers) may imply quality improvement or enhancement as an indirect benefit of activities they support, such as educational programs that grant continuing education credits. The organization might never explicitly mention quality, but the implied intent of offering educational programs is to improve the skill or knowledge of the practitioner and presumably the quality of his or her work.

Because of the difference in approaches to quality within organizations, the assessment of the role of a professional organization might legitimately be based, in part at least, on its publicly defined role. It seems fairer, for example, to hold the ABPN or the National Register of Health Service Providers in Psychology (National Register) accountable for the quality of their members' work than to hold the Virginia Psychological Association accountable in this way. The first two organizations, by intent, represent themselves as having lists of formally qualified (credentialed) health service practitioners, while the latter entity would likely not make a representation to that effect.

Types of Organizations

Professional organizations are typically of three types: (1) regulatory or mandatory, (2) voluntary credentialing, and (3) the membership. These types may be defined as follows.

The Regulatory Organization

This type of organization, normally established by legislation, certifies persons who meet statutory or regulatory tests for credentials and who pass some form of examination, usually purporting to evidence professional knowledge and skills. An example of such an organization is a state licensing board for physicians. Most often, the right to engage in a trade or profession, such as psychology or medicine, is contingent on earning such certification. Removal from membership in such an entity (i.e., loss of license or certification) can be the result of failure to pay fees, failure to meet continuing education requirements, or adverse findings by an ethical review group, a criminal or civil proceeding, or the body's own review board.

The Voluntary Credentialing Organization

The second type of organization, represented by specialty boards such as the American Board of Professional Psychology (ABPP) and the ABPN, seeks to certify persons who volunteer to have themselves evaluated as to their professional competencies. These certifying bodies usually require credentials beyond the minimum required for state licensing or certification, and the examinations they administer focus on the process of work in the profession (usually involving a review of "work samples"). In general, cause for removal from such an organization's membership may be the result of failure to pay fees or an adverse finding resulting from an ethical review or criminal conviction. Both mandatory and voluntary certifying organizations assert, explicitly or implicitly, that membership is associated with the (external) acknowledgment of some enhanced level of quality.

The Membership Organization

The third type of organization defines membership by affinity. Typical examples include national associations, such as the American Psychiatric Association, state associations, such as the Maryland Psychological Association, and regional associations, such as the Northern Virginia Association of Marriage and Family Therapists. Membership is usually based on the professional credentials of the applicant and removal from the organization is based on factors such as failure to pay dues, failure to maintain a required credential (e.g., a license), and adverse findings from an ethical or criminal proceeding.

The Survey

Twenty-one professional organizations, representing the three types described above, were surveyed about their respective roles vis-à-vis a variety of quality related activities. The groups represent marriage and family therapists, psychiatrists, psychiatric nurses, psychologists, social workers, and substance abuse counselors. They include those with national, statewide, and regional membership. Each organization was given a list of 14 functions that might be engaged in by a professional organization and asked to indicate which of those functions were part of its formal mission.

Sixteen of the 21 (76%) organizations returned completed surveys. Table 1 lists these organizations and defines the type (credentialing, regulatory, membership) and

TABLE 1. Type of Organization and Jurisdiction

Organization name	Jurisdiction	Type
American Board of Professional Psychology	National	Certification
American Board of Psychiatry and Neurology	National	Certification
American Psychiatric Association	National	Membership
American Psychiatric Nurses Association	National	Membership
American Psychological Association	State	Membership
DC Psychological Association	State	Membership
Maryland Psychological Association	State	Membership
Mid-Atlantic Association of Marriage and Family Therapy	Regional	Membership
National Association of Alcoholism and Drug Abuse	National	Certification/ membership
National Association of Social Workers (MD)	State	Membership
Natioanl Association of Social Workers (VA)	State	Membership
National Register of Health Service Providers in Psychology	National	Certification
Professional Alcoholism and Drug Abuse Counselors of DC	State	Membership
VA Association of Marriage and Family Therapy	National	Membership
VA Psychological Association	State	Membership

level of operation (national, state, regional) of each.* The results of the survey are integrated into the following discussion of quality. Some caveats: The reader is reminded that the survey responses (1) were provided by staff representing these organizations; (2) the views expressed may have been idiosyncratic; and (3) respondents were not informed about the organizing themes discussed in this chapter.

DEFINING STANDARDS

Typically, there is substantial overlap in the membership of professional organizations that share a discipline base. For example, members of the Virginia Association of Marriage and Family Therapists are required to be members of the national association. Likewise, persons listed in the National Register are required to be licensed for the independent practice of psychology in the states where they work. In addition, a very large percentage of psychologists listed in the Register hold membership in the American Psychological Association. Many of the organizations, therefore, base decisions about membership on similar types of credentials (the most common probably being academic degree and supervised experience in particular types of service delivery settings). Moreover, they may hold members to similar professional standards: for example, most state psychological associations require members to uphold the American Psychological Association's ethics code). In this sense, then, there is a discernible commonality of criteria defining quality across organizations.

Licensing authorities typically maintain the basic standards for recognition: a minimum set of academic qualifications and supervised experience. The registry type of organizations, which offer credentialing (e.g., National Register), typically have higher standards, although they reflect only an applicant's education, training, and

*NOTE: No responses were received from the mandatory regulatory agencies surveyed.

experience. In theory, specialty boards (e.g., ABPP, ABPN) have the highest standards, since they include in their evaluation process some objective examination of the actual skills required in the practice of the profession. These latter two types of organizations, then, might be viewed as offering a "value added" kind of product—a formally credentialed practitioner. In contrast, state and regional professional associations typically offer no more than access to training and a community of professionals for peer support.

Dealing with Misconduct

Most professional associations provide to external sanctioners at least implicit assurance that their members have not been guilty of serious malpractice or misconduct. The trigger for review of professional conduct is likely to be a complaint to either the state regulatory board or a state or national professional association. Decisions from the reviews of these complaints may or may not be reported to other organizations. As a result, the voluntary certification bodies may be considered as upholding the highest quality standards, may be the last to know of serious breaches of professional standards. This apparent paradox is explained by the way in which sanctioning occurs and how information moves within a professional community. For example, a regulatory review, such as by a state licensing board, may take many months or years to complete. Negative findings from such a review, if reported at all to a national professional organization, will most likely result in an independent review of the same incident by the professional association with independent determination of results and sanctions. Negative findings by one body, however, may never be reported to other organizations having shared membership.

Professional sanctions may include removal from membership in an organization, restrictions in the circumstances of practice (e.g., a requirement to practice under supervision), revocation of the right to practice for a specified period of time, public reprimands, or requirements to seek additional training or personal counseling. Given this, the consumer who is interested in knowing whether a professional has been subject to an adverse quality finding is best advised to consult with the state regulatory authority. On the other hand, a consumer most interested in knowing whether the professional is well trained might wish to survey the voluntary certification organizations. Those wishing to adopt a broader perspective might want to check both types of organizations.

PERSPECTIVES ON QUALITY

For purposes of this discussion, quality in mental health is defined as having three major dimensions: outcome, process, and credentials. (The last is sometimes referred to as a *structural* aspect of quality.)

Outcomes as Quality Indicator

Most behavioral health professionals would probably accept that outcome criteria occupy a place on the highest plane in quality of care determinations. After all, what could be more important than service results, and why else do consumers seek service other than to have a good outcome (i.e., get better)? At the same time, the familiar epigram, "the surgery was a success, but the patient died," suggests that the relationship between what a professional does (process) and its result (outcome) may not be simple, and that a perfect (high quality) technical process may result in an adverse (low quality) outcome. One could argue, therefore, that the focus for the primary determination of quality should be the execution of the process as well as any unique attendant outcomes, rather than the more global outcome of patient improvement.

In the event of a patient's condition being so grave that a procedure, even one judged to be perfectly executed, has little chance of resulting in improvement or cure, it would be unfair to consider the failure of the process to result in a cure as an indicator of poor quality.* For example, if a condition such as schizophrenia is not cured by psychotherapy and medication, does it follow that the treatments were of poor quality or inappropriate? It is more likely that a more appropriate standard for quality in this case should be symptom control and improvement in patient functioning across a variety of contexts. This example highlights the importance of defining the nature of the outcome sought from the particular procedure. Such specification is essential to an evaluation of whether the intervention was a success and produced an outcome of acceptable quality. Consensus on the expected outcome is a necessary precondition for the assessment of the quality of the outcome, since retroactive determination of the anticipated outcome can be little more than self-serving.

The Use of Report Cards

The federal government, through the Health Care Financing Administration, has been experimenting with assessment of mechanisms such as report cards for hospitals, attempting thereby to find ways to help consumers evaluate the quality of these (to consumers, arcane) institutions. Report cards typically include statistics such as the mortality rate associated with a particular procedure. Adjusted for the number of these procedures occurring in a hospital, such data provide a gross basis for comparison across institutions. Examination of data such as these generally reveals that in settings where procedures are performed more frequently, outcomes tend to be better.

There have been major criticisms of the report card methodology. A common criticism is that comparison of factors such as gross mortality rates masks differences that may be related to preexisting conditions or acuity of persons receiving such procedures in different hospitals. For example, a nationally known center for heart surgery may attract the most seriously ill patients and this difference may account for a higher mortality rate. Similarly, inner-city hospitals may attract sicker populations, which would be expected to have higher morbidity and therefore subsequent higher mortality rates.† Without the means to measure all relevant factors reliably, report cards are best used only as relatively user-friendly starting points rather than as definitive guides to quality. Similar challenges are present in any effort to assess the quality of mental health practitioners.

*The quality might be poor, however, if the application of the procedure was inappropriate, given the fact that the condition could not be treated.

†Adjustments can be made statistically for situations such as these where characteristics of the patient population are likely to affect outcomes. The technique is referred to as "risk adjustment".

Patient Satisfaction

How does the patient's satisfaction fit into the evaluation of quality? One can easily imagine a patient who is fully satisfied with a treatment that had no material effect on his or her condition and that would be judged by independent professionals to be of poor quality. One can also easily imagine a patient who is dissatisfied with the results of a treatment even though the treatment had the effect of "fixing" what it was intended to fix.

It is likely that the test for quality given by the consumer not only is broader than the specific outcome of the procedures, but also includes less tangible aspects such as the provider's interpersonal style (bedside manner), the extent to which the service satisfied the patient's original expectations, and the patient's judgment of the professional–patient relationship. Such aspects have been seen as part of the "art" of health care. If a serious attempt is to be made to include patient perceptions in the evaluation of quality, how can this dilemma to be resolved? One resolution is to accept the realities of the possible disparity between the patient's judgment and more objective assessments of outcomes and to select one or the other (or both) as the criterion. Another solution is to accept the reality of the inconsistencies but to assume that, over a long period of time and with many patients, measures of patient satisfaction will ultimately converge with the more objective measures.

It is fair to conclude, then, that while outcome measures do not represent the simple solution to the definition of quality of care, they can and should be an important part of any sustained effort to assess that construct. As is discussed below, the primary way that professional organizations deal with outcomes as a quality measure is through sanctions for unusually outrageous, unacceptable outcomes judged to be caused by malpractice.

The survey reported in this chapter provided no evidence of any general use of outcomes as a quality measure by any of the professional organizations. In addition, no such references were found in the literature.

Process as a Quality Indicator

Training for professionals focuses on processes presumed to be associated with high quality of professional performance. The use of supervision as a training mainstay is based on the premise that the use of a professional exemplar in observing the work of trainees and offering advice and guidance regarding the process of professional services planing and delivery will result in valued outcomes. Behavioral health professionals have developed many belief systems regarding what processes are of high quality and by implication what processes result in high-quality outcomes.

The research literature yields some empirical justification for associating modes of care with clinical outcomes, that is, the process–outcome link. The best-practices literature on, for example, depression or phobias offers convincing evidence that the use of particular forms of psychotherapy and pharmacotherapy are more likely than others to produce reduction in symptoms. At the same time, however, many of the process–outcome links assumed by trainers to exist have not been substantiated by empirical research. Despite this, it is clear that most trainers and trainees believe they are teaching and learning, respectively, best practices that are, by definition, indicative of quality. The fact that the literature may not support this belief does not mean, of course, that the assertion is false. Entire professions have developed around unsubstantiated assertions of good practice or process.

National certifying boards, such as the ABPP and the ABPN, base their existence in part on their presumed ability to validly assess the quality of care through the examination of clinical process. While the literature published by these boards is reasonably circumspect about the meaning of certification, the natural justification for the process of examination lies in the belief that those who pass produce higher-quality work (better process) than those who fail. The official position of the American Board of Medical Specialties (the parent organization of the ABPN) is that the primary objective of the specialty boards is the "improvement of the quality of medical education and medical care."

The process aspects of service delivery result in quality determinations in two primary ways, one positive and one negative. As an example of the positive, the evidence of competence, as assessed by the examination of process, can lead to the award of a credential that renders the practitioner eligible for reimbursement or participation in a panel of providers. (For example, some managed care companies only employ ABPN-certified psychiatrists.) With regard to the negative, evidence of gross process irregularities can result in sanctions, through regulatory investigations or through ethical proceedings that result in removal from membership or other sanction by the professional organization.

Credentials as a Quality Indicator

The term "credentials" is used broadly to refer not only to a formal certification representing a particular status, but also to the full range of educational, training, and other benchmarks used to gain admission to a professional organization, sit for licensure, or obtain other kinds of certification. All regulated mental health professions are required to have some basic credentials. For example, states typically require applicants for certification or licensure at the independent practice level to have a generally recognized professional degree representing a certain number of years of education, a defined range of course content, and additional supervised experience from appropriate credentialed professional role models. These credentials are prerequisites for an applicant to be eligible to take an examination.

Many membership-oriented professional associations require that their members hold the license for practice or possess certain other credentials. Most of these organizations have either an informal or a formal credentialing process for reviewing prospective members. The credentials required for membership are often included in the mission of the organization that defines itself as representing or otherwise serving those who possess the required credential.

One rationale for the use of credentialing is that credentials constitute a minimum level of quality for a practitioner. Conversely, it is implicitly asserted that the lack of these credentials makes it likely that the person does not possess the requisite skills, knowledge, and abilities to carry out quality work. As with the assertion relating to process discussed above, such causal connection has not been supported by empirical research.

A second basis for the use of credentials lies in the utility of credentials for creating market cartels. The history of guilds shows that they have worked not only to establish some indices of quality but also to restrict markets. A restricted market may work to the benefit of guild members because the demand for services in a restricted market tends to increase the price people will pay for those services. Most licensing laws regulate professions by proscribing unlicensed persons from performing the tasks permitted to those who hold the license. This, in essence, limits supply, which in turn typically leads to increased prices. Professions also have routinely used changes in licensing and credentialing criteria to decrease (or hold steady) competition from potential peers by restricting their entry into practice.

One way to measure the relative power of a profession is to examine the scope of practice included in the definition of its license. More powerful professions (i.e., medicine) have few restrictions, while others (e.g., marriage and family therapy) have some restrictions to keep licensees from practicing in the domain of the more powerful.

Virtually every professional organization uses credentials to determine eligibility for membership. Some, such as state licensing and voluntary specialty boards, assert that these credentials relate to quality, while others, such as state and local associations, appear to use credentials more as a test of affinity.

When credentialing criteria change, it is almost always the case that there is a "grandparenting period" in which previously credentialed practitioners are allowed to maintain their credentialed status, and in essence remain "equal" to the new higher-standard practitioners. For example, when the National Register raised its credentialing standards, the new standards were applied only to new applicants. Similarly, tightened credential rules imposed by state licensing authorities are applied only prospectively. There is an obvious reason for this: to do otherwise risks disenfranchising the substantial number (perhaps even a majority) of current members or listees, something that is usually politically unpopular and, in the case of membership organizations, self-defeating. As a consequence, however, over time the credential standards of membership (licensing, listing, or simple membership) tend to overstate the actual qualifications of the professionals who are members. To the degree that these credentials are indices of quality of care, the inference to be drawn from credentials should be limited. (It would be a surprise to see on a practitioner's wall not only evidence of membership in a credentialing organization but also a disclaimer saying that the particular professional did not meet the current standards of the organization!)

The credentialing process constitutes an examination of inputs; the use of examinations and demonstrations is a process approach to standards; and the use of outcomes assessment defines standards through outputs. As noted above, the inputs standards are typically used to determine eligibility for membership for both affinity and certifying organizations. Process standards are used by specialty boards or certification groups that seek explicitly to represent listees as meeting quality standards. Outcome standards are used to remove persons from membership, listing, or credentialed status. In other words, in the current world of professional organizations, credentials (or input standards) are used to include applicants, assessments of process are used for inclusion and exclusion, while assessments of outcome are only used for exclusion.

FUNCTIONS OF ASSOCIATIONS THAT MAY CONTRIBUTE TO ADVANCEMENT OF QUALITY

Professional organizations of the types surveyed here claim a range of functions that potentially have an impact on the quality of services provided by their members. We now turn again to the organizations surveyed for this chapter that were asked

TABLE 2. Self-Identified Functions of Organizations[a]

Organization name	1	2	3	4	5	6	7	8	9	10	11	12	13	14
American Board of Professional Psychology	×		×										×	
American Board of Psychiatry and Neurology	×		×								×	×		
American Psychiatric Association	×		×			×	×	×	×	×	×	×		×
American Psychiatric Nurses Association						×				×	×	×		×
American Psychological Association	×					×			×					
DC Psychological Association	×					×		×	×		×	×		×
Maryland Psychological Association	×					×	×		×		×	×	×	×
Mid-Atlantic Association of Marriage and Family Therapy	×	×	×	×	×	×		×	×	×	×	×	×	×
National Association of Alcoholism and Drug Abuse					×	×	×		×	×	×	×		×
National Association of Social Workers	×					×	×		×	×	×	×		×
National Association of Social Workers (MD)	×	×		×	×	×	×		×	×	×	×		×
National Association of Social Workers (VA)	×			×		×		×	×	×	×			×
National Register of Health Service Providers in Psychology	×	×	×	×		×		×			×	×		×
Professional Alcoholism and Drug Abuse Counselors		×		×	×	×	×		×	×		×		×
VA Association of Marriage and Family Therapy	×	×	×	×	×	×	×	×	×	×	×	×	×	×
VA Psychological Association	×					×			×					

[a]Key to organizational functions: 1. Education; 2. Accrediting educational programs; 3. Training standards; 4. Recognize training programs; 5. Accredit training programs; 6. Conferences, journals, etc.; 7. General public meetings; 8. Sponsor research; 9. Ethical training; 10. Protocols, standards; 11. Revoke membership for quality; 12. Public representatives; 13. Quality is standard for membership; 14. Advocate with authority Re: standards of quality.

whether or not they were involved in any of 14 specific functions. Table 2 lists the respondent organizations and summarizes their responses to the survey. The functions are defined as follows.

1. *Establishing educational standards.* Educational standards in this context refer to the requirement for completion of a curriculum or specified set of courses in identified content areas, or a requirement for a specified period of time that a candidate must be enrolled in an educational program. Virtually every organization representing mental health professions uses educational standards as part of its membership or certification process. All but two of the organizations responding to the survey identified education as one of the requirements for membership or listing. The minimum education standards are generally the same as those used by universities and other training institutions for the terminal professional degrees.*

Factors that affect educational standards include whether the educational institution is itself regionally accredited or otherwise recognized as a legitimate educational institution and whether the specific educational program is recognized by the profession, by state regulators, or by third-party payers. Each of these factors may be considered by an organization when making a decision as to whether an applicant's education or training represents a content and skill base that is reasonably comparable to what is minimally expected of a professional.

*There may be some variation in this, especially where there are several educational levels which are recognized in the professional marketplace or by regulatory authorities (e.g., masters and doctoral level psychologists).

It is well known that there is no generally accepted means for ascertaining the relative quality of academic programs and their graduates. The closest approximations of an assessment of relative quality would be polls of knowledgeable professionals and ability or achievement scores of the students admitted to the program. Higher Graduate Record Examination scores, for example, might be seen as evidence of a higher-quality student body. Other indicators might be the number of faculty publications that have been accepted by refereed journals, the number of such publications cited in the literature, or the individual professional recognition achieved by faculty members. This last indicator may be reflected in board certification, professional memberships, or offices in professional associations. There is a circularity in using this last type of indicator as one of quality: While the awarding of board certification or other memberships may have been based partly on the judged quality of the educational program, the quality of the educational program is partly determined by board certification or other characteristics of faculty membership.

In summary, to the extent we accept the premise that education to minimum standards is an important contributor to quality of care, then almost all professional agencies support this quality criterion.

2. *Accreditation of educational programs*. Respondents from national organizations were most likely to indicate that their association engages in accrediting activities that certify that discipline-specific educational programs meet certain standards. Such activities are typically focused on the qualifications of the institution (such as regional accreditation), the history of the program's production of graduates, the core curriculum, the characteristics of the students, and the characteristics and accomplishments of the faculty. These elements provide inferential evidence that the graduates of a program have knowledge, attitude, values, and skills necessary to provide quality service.

The organizations that report accrediting educational programs are, as might be expected, national organizations such as the American Psychological Association. Accreditation rarely occurs at a local or state level, or by the specialty boards (although a state organization affiliated with a national association may honor the parent organization's accreditation process and findings. Individual state organizations, including the regulatory bodies, are unlikely to have the resources necessary or the need to administer statewide accreditation programs.

As with educational standards, there is no "proof" that the standards for the accreditation process are at all related to quality. It seems intuitively correct, however, that such efforts should enhance the quality of the professionals trained by the program.

3. *Establishing training standards*. Most of the respondents whose organizations use minimum educational standards for admission or listing also set minimum standards for training. This means they require applicants to have a certain number of hours or years and a specific type of training to be eligible for membership, to be listed, or to sit for the relevant examination. For example, the National Register requires applicants to have a minimum number of hours of supervised experience in an organized health service training program, internship, or postdoctoral traineeship.

While in some ways, these types of requirements are similar to those for educational program completion, there are far fewer institutional controls and protections applied to training than to education. College and university educational programs are usually regulated by states and well-established regional accrediting bodies. There is, however, no parallel regulation for training programs. Any individual or organization can establish a training program with minimal regulatory intrusion. As a consequence, groups that rely on training standards often must delegate to some other organization the accreditation of training.

The use of accredited training as a minimum requirement is not well established in the regulatory area. Thus, while it might be permissible to refuse licensure to a person who was educated in a university program that was not regionally accredited, it is not likely that similar rules could be applied with regard to internship or other training experiences. Regulatory and membership bodies may offer "deemed status" to educational and training programs that are accredited by professional associations, but they still consider each individual training resume submitted by an applicant. This suggests there is significant variation in the quality of training evidenced by members in many membership organizations, and thus, variation in the value added by training to the quality of the professionals within those organizations.

4. *Accrediting training programs.* As is true with educational programs, accreditation of training programs is a function reserved primarily for national organizations. In the present survey six organizations indicated that they accredit training programs. Few organizations possess both the mandate and the resources to conduct such accreditation. In addition, these organizations do not make completion of an accredited training program a requirement for membership.

5. *Recognizing training programs.* This concept constitutes a low level of endorsement of the quality of a training program, and is often applied to programs offering continuing education activities. For example, many organizations have means to accept continuing education or professional development credits, and they "recognize" training organizations as being qualified to offer educational or professional development programs to their members. Often the organizations do not formally accept continuing education credits offered by programs that they have not recognized—particularly if the accumulation of credits within a specified time frame is mandated for (say) the relicensure of members. Usually recognition is dependent upon the training organization meeting standards related to the structure of the program, the use of formal measurement techniques for participants to evaluate the outcome of training activities, and sometimes the credentials of the trainers themselves. While many training programs formally evaluate their training activities, few use posttraining tests of competence or knowledge acquisition to assess the effectiveness of the training. The failure to assess these aspects of the training weakens the quality value of these programs.

6. *Sponsorship of meetings, journals, and other professional activities.* All the organizations responding to the survey, except the national specialty boards, reported having active programs that include sponsorship of meetings, support of journals, and other activities aimed at professional development. National conferences by the major organizations occur annually, with statewide conferences often occurring once or twice a year. Relatively resource-rich national organizations are more likely to produce journals, while statewide and local organizations are more likely to have newsletters (with information about members and local political happenings of interest). None of the organizations requires that its members participate in its conferences or subscribe to its journals. Further, there is no attempt by organizations to monitor outcomes of their members' participation in any of these activities, for example, to answer the question, "Do members learn anything at the conferences or by reading the

journals?" These activities are more appropriately viewed as professional development opportunities provided by these organizations in the interest of their members than as proof of quality enhancement. Most organizations permit nonmembers to attend their conferences and subscribe to their journals; in theory at least, the benefits are available to all. Typically, the great majority of attendees at conferences are members, although only a small percentage of members (e.g., 10–15%) usually attend any one conference.

7. *Public meetings.* One way a professional organization might contribute to the commonweal would be to offer programs to the general public that would increase public understanding of the profession, increase the ability of the public to judge the competence of a professional, and improve the ability of the public knowledgeably to "shop" for quality services. Seven of the survey respondents indicated that they offered such public opportunities. Such meetings tend to be infrequent, poorly publicized, and relatively few members of the public ever benefit from them. As a consequence, these types of activities probably have very little impact on quality.

8. *Sponsorship of research.* Within the organizations surveyed, sponsored research tends to be focused on research questions that have public policy implications. Three of the respondents, all national organizations, indicated that they support research and similar projects. While the survey did not include questions about the number or type of projects sponsored by the individual organizations, it seems fair to conclude that these efforts are relatively infrequent, small in scale, and focused. While a research project offers no direct contribution to the quality of members of an organization, its results may be shared by the sponsoring organization, either publicly or in context of specific attempts to influence public policy. Sharing of information from studies seems to have the potential for no more than a minor contribution to quality among professionals, unless the study focuses on some specific aspect of practice. This is relatively infrequent.

9. *Training in ethics.* Most of the membership organizations responding to the survey indicated that they support training in professional ethics. While there is no direct relationship between ethical practice and quality of care, a professional's ethical behavior may significantly affect other people's perceptions of that professional and the quality of care he or she provides. Professional associations typically represent adherence to ethical principles as an indicator of the quality of their members. In addition, both the associations and their members cite the existence of ethical standards in their marketing efforts. Ethics codes also constitute the primary basis for self-policing by these organizations. No data were available on the number or percentage of members who participate in ethics training. Organizations may present case examples in newsletters or other publications; they may offer workshops dealing with applications of ethical principles; or they may provide self-study opportunities for their members. These activities are likely to contribute to the overall quality of the professional activity, if not to the quality of individual episodes of care.

10. *Development and promulgation of protocols or standards of care.* Almost two thirds of the responding organizations indicated that they endorse protocols or standards of practice. Interestingly, this area seems to be largely the domain of the federal government, through its review committees, and of scholars who review the literature and conclude what is best practice. Managed care providers also are promulgating service protocols, both to obtain best practices and to control costs. In the latter case, the focus may be on limiting payment for services beyond a "best practice standard," or to

avoid paying for treatments beyond those recognized as usual and customary. While it seems easier to develop best practice standards for simple medical conditions, we can expect increased effort in the behavioral health area by both government payers and private purchasers of care. This would seem a fertile area for professional organizations that presumably seek to retain and control the scope of practice. Assuming the initiative in defining the parameters of appropriate, effective, and cost-effective would advance the quality of practice. Protocols and standards of practice seem to have great potential, at least theoretically, for influencing and improving care, but the influence will be no better than the actual standards of care. To the degree these standards can deal with individual differences and to the degree they are empirically supported, they are likely to have a positive impact on quality of care. Regardless of the form, they are likely to improve care by eliminating or reducing deviant or very unusual treatments.

11. *Revocation of membership or listing for quality concerns.* Most national organizations responding to this survey indicated that they have procedures for revoking the membership or listing of professionals who seriously violate professional standards of care. These events usually occur in response to formal complaints from the public or other professionals. A complaint usually leads to a review and determination, which then results in a finding. Based on the finding, the organization makes a decision on the appropriate action to be taken against the professional. This may include a range of sanctions such as removal from membership or listing, limitations on practice, or required supervision.

Other professional organizations may make subsequent decisions about a sanctioned professional based on the findings of the original review entity. For example, the National Register may revoke the listing of a professional who has been found guilty of a serious offense by a state licensing authority. In most cases, however, a separate due process must occur before subsequent actions are taken, although local or regional chapters of national organizations may rely on the findings of their parent organization as a basis for sanctions of their own.

The findings of this survey suggest that formal sanctioning is an unusual occurrence. This finding is supported by information received from the Department of Health Professions in Virginia which regulates health professionals, including mental health providers. In fiscal year 1994, this department processed 751 complaints related to professional standards of care, 784 related to professional conduct, and an additional 500 relating to other issues. A total of 588 (28%) of these complaints resulted in sanctions to professionals. The most common sanction was a reprimand or warning, followed by probation, suspension of license or certificate, and revocation of license or certificate. Physicians had the highest rate of complaints, at 19.58 per 1000 licenses (this was the rate for all physicians, not only psychiatrists). The next highest complaint rate was among professional counselors (11.34 per 1000 licenses), followed by psychologists (11.31 per 1000), and social workers (9.18 per 1000). In contrast, professional counselors had the highest rate of sanctions (3.44 per 1000 licenses), followed by physicians (2.08 per 1000), and social workers (1.06 per 1000). Psychologists licensed in Virginia received no sanctions in fiscal year 1994.

Given the very small numbers of sanctions, significant variation would be expected in rates within professions across years. This is, indeed, what is observed. For example, while psychologists were subject to no sanctions in Virginia in fiscal year

1994, their rate in fiscal year 1993 was the highest among mental health professionals (3.2 per 1000 licenses).

Sanctions by nonregulatory entities are also rare events. For example, during fiscal year 1994, the National Register reported a removal rate of 0.001, while the American Psychological Association reported a rate of only 0.0005.

12. *Public representations*. The results of this survey suggest that most organizations make some public representation that affiliation with their organization is an indication of quality. This is an interesting finding given that these same organizations may support few of the quality related functions reviewed in this discussion.

13 *Quality is membership standard*. Professional specialty boards (i.e., ABPN; ABPP) are the only entities that define the judged (by peers) quality of a provider's work as their standard for membership. Successful completion of an examination, including work samples evaluated by other senior professionals, is the criterion for quality within these two organizations. They alone attempt to assess directly the capacity of a professional to deliver high-quality services as a part of the process to obtain membership.

14. *Advocacy with authorities regarding standards of quality*. With the exception of the specialty boards, nearly all the respondents claimed that they advocated with public authorities for improvement in the quality of health care. Such advocacy occurs primarily through the provision of information and education to targets such as legislators, regulatory authorities, third-party payers, and funders. The advocate's message typically is that professional credentials (i.e., those possessed by its members) are the appropriate means to ensure protection of consumers and (presumably) assure high quality of care. Reference is usually made to the educational standards and the other functions undertaken by the organization to ensure the quality of its members.

CONCLUSION

Most of the professional organizations responding to this survey use minimum professional education standards as a prerequisite for membership or listing and most also directly offer or support continuing education programs. These organizations typically maintain processes for making judgments about and applying sanctions to members who have committed serious breaches of professional ethics or standards, although, as has been noted, very small numbers of professionals are ever sanctioned. Some accredit education and training programs and approximately half endorse or promulgate treatment standards. At the same time, most of these organizations make representations regarding the quality of professionals who are accepted for membership or listing. Only a few organizations, that is, the specialty boards, try to assess quality in a direct manner, by examination of work samples. There is a communality among the professional organizations in that they rely to a great extent on the same criteria, primarily education and training, for membership or listing.

While the initial credentialing process is presumed to ensure some minimum level of quality of professionals, the respondent organizations have few requirements for continuing quality enhancement, except as represented by continuing education requirements. Overall, there is little research evidence to support the conclusion that any of these activities actually contributes to an improved quality of care. At the same time, even with the absence of proof it is probably worth retaining these activities because of the dearth of reasonable alternatives and the possibility that these elements do contribute, at least marginally, to quality of care.

Development of Best Practice Standards

The area having perhaps the most potential for improving quality is the development and promulgation of empirically based protocols and standards of care reflecting best practice. These types of tools* could be used for both educating and credentialing professionals as well as for postlicensure continuing educaiton. While it is very difficult to evaluate directly the outcomes of the clinical interventions of individual providers, it might be possible to have select professionals commit to follow best practices as defined by their professional organization through its practice guidelines or standards of care. The organizations could support training in these standards and the credentialing of trainees in particular areas of practice. Currently, professionals declare their own areas of competence but can rarely offer empirical evidence to support their declarations. With the development of minimum standards of care for various conditions (e.g., depression; obsessive–compulsive disorder) could come specialty certification managed by national organizations that would evaluate providers' mastery of best practices by examining their work samples (such as is done by ABPP and ABPN).

Provider Report Cards

Another area with potential high return for quality improvement is the development of a report card for individual providers within particular disciplines. Under such a model, a professional organization would maintain a database for each of its practitioner members, reflecting patient satisfaction and patient reported outcomes (as well as other clinical indicators as they become available). These data would be translated into a summary report card for each practitioner and this report card would be made available to the public.

The validity of such a report card, of course, would be limited by the absence of more objective clinical outcome data, and the limitations as well as the significance of the report would need to be carefully explained to potential consumers. At the same time, following the model of local consumer ratings services, it could serve as a simple but (to the potential consumer) valuable check for quality based on consumer feedback. If this reporting system were administered by a local professional organization, the potential for abuse could be minimized.

Clearly, the successful development of such a system must be predicated on members having a high level of trust in their professional association and the profession itself having a strong commitment to self-regulation. While such a high level of professional trust and commitment would be difficult to achieve, it would be in the finest tradition of public accountability. The increasing pressures to publish data on the performance of health care organizations and hospitals may soon be accompanied

*A more recent development is in the area of "clinical pathways"—optimal procedures for the delivery of care to target groups within integrated service systems.

by similar pressure for data on group practices and possibly individual providers. The professions may choose to wait and subsequently be forced into a reporting system developed and controlled by others, or they may take the initiative and develop their own systems.

As we have seen, professional associations serve many functions, some of which may be associated with improvements in the quality of care. More importantly, all these organizations are in a position to significantly increase their contributions to quality well within the usual exercise of their mission. For example, while local organizations might best address comparison of quality across individual practitioners, national groups might most usefully develop standards of practice. At the same time, certification organizations are in a position to encourage the development of criteria, including those for outcomes and client satisfaction, which may more meaningfully represent the "essence" of quality. Membership organizations can support efforts to improve quality by making quality enhancement one component of membership expectations. One way this might be done is through the support of programs that certify proficiency by assessing skills mastered in sponsored training activities.

In the context of managed care, which is rapidly becoming the normative health services delivery system in America, the economic survival of professionals will be determined by membership on panels of providers and integrated practice groups increasingly accepting risk from managed care organizations. Criteria for membership will continue to be determined both by the policies and procedures of the managed care companies and by legislation. A public display of willingness to be accountable would place professionals in a relatively strong position for influencing the development of public laws related to the delivery of health services. For example, a stronger case could be made for "any willing provider" legislation if, for example, professionals supported publicly useful, operational definitions of the "quality" of providers.

If professional organizations are not willing to deal with the issues of quality, then others will, possibly in ways that professionals find objectionable. An example of the latter is to be found in the history of peer review projects, which were implemented by the American Psychological Association and the American Psychiatric Association, both under contract to CHAMPUS (Civilian Health and Medical Plan of the Uniformed Services) (Shueman & Penner, 1988). These projects created national rosters of professional reviewers who were charged with assisting in the determination of the quality of care provided to CHAMPUS beneficiaries. This strategy was implemented to avoid, among other things, arbitrary reductions in funding of mental health services under the CHAMPUS program. For a variety of reasons, the project was abandoned by both professional associations following 7 years of contentious operation. One lesson from the projects, however, was that there was a significant lack in common definitions for standards of practice, making it exceedingly difficult to discern good care from bad, reasonable from excessive. The prime consequence (probably inevitable) was the shifting of responsibility for the development of standards of care and related mechanisms for quality assessment and management away from the national associations and to proprietary companies. The response of the professional membership to the project was overwhelmingly negative, driven by the hope of eradication of the (admittedly flawed) review system, rather than commitment to the task of improving its validity.

For the purposes of this chapter, then, perhaps the clearest lesson to be drawn from the history of these particular projects is that if professional associations ever seek to regain a central participatory role in the development of the complex policy agenda surrounding quality of care issues and mechanisms, manifest acceptance of responsibility for this role is essential. In other words, key stakeholders (external regulators and sanctioners alike) will need to be convinced that the associations are indeed willing to put their respective houses in order. Grudging guild-oriented postulations alone will not suffice. For the public interest to be served, rather than that of the membership, there must be a sustained commitment to the acquisition and expenditure of significant resources in the service of this goal. Absent this, professionals will have forfeited any right to a place at the policy table. Worse, blunt, poorly targeted external regulation will have replaced the disinterested, scientifically driven and highly focused process of operationalizing the assessment and management of health services quality. The very real socioeconomic benefits associated with professional status are based on the trust of sanctioners. As such, benefits must be earned.

REFERENCE

Shueman, S. A., & Penner, N. R. (1988). Administering a national peer review program. In G. Stricker & A. Rodriguez (Eds.), *Handbook of quality assurance in mental health* (pp. 441–453). New York: Plenum Press.

20

The Consumer's Role in Assessing Quality

BARRY BLACKWELL, KATHLEEN EILERS, AND DON ROBINSON, JR.

INTRODUCTION

The evaluation of consumer satisfaction is an idea whose time has finally come. It is 30-plus years since Donabedian (1966) suggested that satisfaction was the "ultimate validator" of quality care. Skeptics expressed concern that it was too general a measure and of questionable validity based on reservations about psychiatric patients' ability to make rational judgments (Sheppard, 1993).

In the last decade philosophical, pragmatic, and scientific forces in both the public and private behavioral health sectors have created a resurgence of interest in consumer–client–patient involvement and in satisfaction as a quality indicator. During this time period, an increase in homelessness and the second wave of deinstitutionalization reinforced the importance of community outreach and engagement strategies. The passive construct of "compliance" has evolved into an active interest in the "therapeutic alliance," empowering consumers to participate in treatment choices (Tower, 1994; Blackwell, 1997).

Simultaneously, success in business increasingly has been equated with coming "close to the customer" (Peters & Waterman, 1982). Meanwhile, managed care has moved beyond cost containment to quality concerns, including how to ensure consumer satisfaction (Gilbert, Lumpkin, & Dent, 1992).

Accompanying this renaissance are three separate but interrelated themes: how to directly measure consumer satisfaction; how to assess it by other means; and perhaps more importantly, how to ensure consumer involvement in program planning, implementation, and evaluation. This chapter deals with each of these themes and provides examples of contemporary initiatives from the private, public and managed care sectors.

BARRY BLACKWELL • Department of Psychiatry, University of Wisconsin Medical School, Milwaukee, Wisconsin 53211. KATHLEEN EILERS • Milwaukee County Mental Health Division, Milwaukee, Wisconsin 53226. DON ROBINSON, JR. • Merck-Medco Managed Care, Montvale, New Jersey 07645.

Handbook of Quality Management in Behavioral Health, edited by Stricker *et al.* Kluwer Academic / Plenum Publishers, New York, 2000.

CONSUMER SATISFACTION AS AN OUTCOME MEASURE

Why Measure Consumer Satisfaction?

Measuring satisfaction is not just politically correct in today's sociopolitical *Zeitgeist*, but may have other practical implications as well. Satisfied consumers are more likely to follow recommendations and treatment plans (Korsh, Gozzi, & Francis, 1968; Sherbourne, Hays, Ordway, DiMatteo, & Kravitz, 1992; Nguyen, Attkisson, & Stegner, 1983). Those who are dissatisfied tend to drop out or disenroll and are more likely to be litigious (Vaccarino, 1977; Ware & Davies, 1983). Satisfaction may influence an individual's personal decision to access treatment or select a particular provider as well as any recommendation to others about how and where to seek help (Marquis, Davies, & Ware, 1983). The more competitive the health care environment, the more satisfaction becomes significant in capturing market share.

The Scope and Significance of Satisfaction Measures

Disease-related outcomes, while useful in traditional double-blind studies of selected patient samples, are too time consuming, narrowly defined, and impractical for large population bases. Consumer satisfaction, in contrast, is simpler to measure, universally applicable, motivates people to respond and has public relations appeal. Not surprisingly, the Health Outcomes Institute has documented the increasing use of consumer satisfaction surveys in all health-related areas (Olnhausen & Werni, 1995). A recent government and academic task force on outcomes assessment in mental health and substance abuse strongly recommends the inclusion of consumer satisfaction (Smith, Manderscheid, Steinwachs, & Flynn, 1995). The American Managed Behavioral Health Association (AMBHA) includes a measure of consumer satisfaction in its report card for use by all participant behavioral health care organizations.

Several excellent reviews have documented the measurement of patient satisfaction in the behavioral, psychiatric, or mental health field (Attkisson & Pascoe, 1983; Ruggeri, 1994; Williams & Wilkinson, 1995). One of these (Ruggeri, 1994) provides details of 16 studies published between 1982 and 1993, involving populations in Britain, Canada, Italy, Sweden, Chile, Australia, and the United States. These efforts in the behavioral health field are parallel to those that document similar interests in general medicine (Lewis, 1994) and nursing (Larrabee, 1995).

The Concept of Consumer Satisfaction—What Is Being Measured?

While seemingly simple, the concept of patient satisfaction is quite elusive, difficult to define, and modified by several contingencies (Pascoe, 1983). For example, being satisfied may depend on whether or not expectations exist, and if so, whether they are met. Expectations may be related to cultural norms as well as to previous experience with the health care system or lack of it. People with long-term psychiatric disorders and extensive experience with treatment systems tend to express more dissatisfaction than those who have brief contact; but it is unclear if this is due simply to illness itself or to greater exposure to systems of care.

Satisfaction is not a unitary construct. Surveys of satisfaction often fail to specify what aspect of care is being assessed. Consumers may evaluate the provider, the clinic, or the insurer and they may express short- or long-term dissatisfaction (Ruggeri, 1994). Within a particular episode of care, consumers may focus more on the personal than the technical or medical components, even though the latter are often more powerful determinants of outcome (Marshall, Hays, Sherbourne, & Wells, 1993). At least five dimensions of satisfaction have been defined (Ware, 1981), including quality, convenience, finance, physical environment, and availability.

Also fundamental is the question of whether the person evaluating care views him- or herself as an active consumer judging quality or a passive recipient who is simply expressing some level of confidence in the provider. The fact that overall satisfaction rates tend to be high especially among the elderly (Pascoe, 1983) suggests that consumers often assume a passive role. In a review of over 50 studies, Lebow (1983) found an average satisfaction rate of 77.5%.

Williams (1994) has pointed out that aggregate data on a satisfaction item may subsume at least three subsets; active assessment of quality, passive confidence in the provider, or reluctance to express negative viewpoints because of discomfort with criticism. "Satisfaction" also may be modified by preexisting attitudinal sets. For example, Woodside, Nielsen, Walters, and Muller (1988) distinguished four customer subtypes, which they labeled "old-fashioned," "value-conscious," "affluent," and "professional want-it-alls."

To the extent that an instrument is not constructed with these considerations in mind, its validity will be in question. Finally, it is clear that quality and satisfaction are not synonymous, a distinction to bear in mind when developing marketing strategies that use the results from satisfaction surveys (Taylor, 1994).

Problems in Measurement

Ruggeri (1994) lists three types of problems in the development and use of satisfaction measures: study design, construction of the instrument, and its psychometric properties.

Study Design and Sampling Issues

Although satisfaction may appear simple and appealing to measure, the low response rates often make results less meaningful (Lebow, 1983). Mail surveys are typically the least successful (40%), followed by the telephone (43%) and home interviews (64%). Response rates may be even lower in some government-funded programs such as Medicaid where consumers often lack telephones or are more mobile. Economic incentives in such populations for returning forms appear to have little or no effect, although the amounts paid were small (Nelson, Hartman, Ojemann, & Wilcox, 1995). Obtaining data without anonymity may incur socially desirable responses that can artificially inflate satisfaction ratings (Le Vois, Nguyen, & Attkisson, 1981; Soelling & Newell, 1983).

Samples also may not be representative of the population depending on whether satisfied or dissatisfied consumers are more likely to respond (a question still not answered). At least one managed care company (K. Hoover, personal communication) has consistently achieved response rates in excess of 80% in commercial populations by the use of professional telephone survey interviewers, introductory letters announcing the phone survey, and modest efforts to trace new addresses.

Instrument Construction

Items on a survey instrument often reflect the concerns of the investigator rather than the consumer and may be based on assumptions that are not valid (Williams & Wilkinson, 1995). Hevey (1995) recently presented data at a national meeting where items developed by the Mental Health Corporation of America (MHCA) were based on focus interviews in which consumers were asked to identify positive and negative service encounters (critical incidents), which were then condensed into items or dimensions and subjected to feedback from consumers with regard to format, burden, and appropriateness. Such a strategy helps ensure the relevance of items to respondents.

Ruggeri (1994) has noted an increasing sophistication over time in instrument design. There is a notable trend toward multidimensional scales, although there is little agreement on the particular dimensions to study in the behavioral health field. When data from the Medical Outcomes Study were analyzed (Marshall et al., 1993), they revealed that patient satisfaction could be considered both as an overarching, unidimensional construction (general satisfaction) and as a set of discrete dimensions that tapped into six unique aspects: time, technical, interpersonal, communication, financial, and access. All these domains except financial satisfaction correlated highly with general satisfaction (0.83 to 0.98). Financial satisfaction had a correlation of only 0.4 with general satisfaction. Visit specific satisfaction correlated only modestly with general satisfaction (0.35). High covariance between multiple dimensions poses a content and statistical validity challenge, because it suggests that measures are not independent.

The generalizability of these findings is limited because the studies were confined to outpatients with four chronic physical health problems and depression. Pooled data from AMBHA hopefully soon will allow similar assessments in the behavioral health field across many conditions. When this occurs, it may be possible to correlate domain or visit specific scales with patient behaviors including utilization, compliance with treatment, disenrollment, or provider preferences (Sherbourne et al., 1992).

Psychometric Properties

Very little research has ben conducted on the basic psychometric properties of satisfaction survey instruments (Ruggeri, 1994). One exception is Hevey (1995) who reports an attempt to define the respondent burden or acceptability of the MHCA instrument in terms of time taken to complete, as well as the relevance and difficulty of questions and the scales used.

Concerns about high satisfaction rates and low sensitivity of scales have been partly addressed by widening the response range (beyond a dichotomous satisfied–dissatisfied), assuring anonymity, and involving relatives who tend sometimes (but not always) to be more critical in their evaluation of services (Grella & Grusky, 1989).

The validity of the content of surveys has been addressed in a number of ways such as involving consumers in selecting items (Eisen & Grob, 1978; Elbeck & Fecteau, 1990), widening the number of dimensions studied, combining structured scales with unstructured interviews, and obtaining data on both setting specific and across setting concerns.

While previously fewer than 14% of satisfaction studies reported reliability data

(Ware & Davies, 1983), a more recent survey of peer-reviewed articles suggests a test–retest agreement of around 70% (Ruggeri, 1994).

Available Instruments

As managed care organizations struggle to demonstrate consumer satisfaction, the search for valid and reliable instruments will intensify. Whether or not these will remain proprietary or will enter the public domain is unknown, but Table 1 provides a list of some of the instruments on which published data are available.

The Proper Use of Satisfaction Surveys

Satisfaction surveys are psychometrically challenged by twin handicaps. People appear hesitant to express criticism, and the extent they wish to do so may influence their willingness to fill out forms. This may bias the sample but can be addressed by attention to sample size and response rates. Consultants to the AMBHA report card process (see below) suggest that sample sizes around 500 and return rates above 70% are necessary to derive significant and generalizable conclusions. Below this, there is a risk that real differences between programs may be missed (type I error) and aggregate data may be misinterpreted. The latter is particularly possible, because consumer satisfaction is an appealing contemporary concept subject to cosmetic use for public relations or marketing purposes. The most appropriate use of such data will occur when valid and reliable findings are employed to produce program change that results in improved consumer satisfaction. This has yet to happen, at least on any widespread scale. The sad fact is that satisfaction is often measured, but the results are seldom used. Williams (1994) remarked that satisfaction surveys merely endorse the status quo while fostering an illusion of consumerism.

THREE CONTEMPORARY INITIATIVES IN THE MANAGED CARE, PUBLIC, AND PRIVATE SECTORS

Development of a Consumer Satisfaction Report Card by the Managed Care Industry

The Process of Development

In 1993, toward the end of the first decade of managed behavioral health care, the 19 largest organizations formed a consortium: the American Managed Behavioral Health Association. A major goal of this consortium was to collect and disseminate information about the beneficial impact of managed care on reducing costs and improving access to and quality of health care. It was initially hoped that these data would influence the direction of National Health Care Reform, with particular regard to the preservation of mental health benefits and the role of managed care organizations in delivering them.

In January 1994, these goals led to a perceived need to develop reliable outcome measures that would be used industrywide to measure utilization, quality of care, and consumer satisfaction. From the outset, the purpose was to design a report card that

TABLE 1. Patient Self-report Treatment Satisfaction Measures[a]

Name	Publication date	Source	Contact	Notes
Consumer Satisfaction Questionnaire (CSQ)	1975	University of California at San Francisco	Clifford Attkisson 415-476-9690 (fx) Thomas Greenfield 510-642-7175 (fx)	Proprietary instrument available in 8, 18, and 31 question formats. Applicable to both visit-specific and across-visit evaluation. Permission and fees required. Contact by fax only.
Consumer Satisfaction Survey (CSS 2nd ed.)	1991	American Association of Health Plans	Aron Carlson 202-778-3249 (ph)	Public domain instrument, with notification. Selection format, with a choice of 63 questions. Applicable to visit-specific and across-visit evaluation.
Medical Outcomes Study (MOS-9)	1986	Medical Outcomes Trust	617-426-4046 (ph)	Public domain instrument with one-time minimal fee. Nine question format for visit-specific evaluation.
Patient Satisfaction Questionnaire (PSQ)	1976	RAND	Ron Hays 310-393-0411 (ph) 310-393-4818 (fx)	Public domain instrument, available in 80, 50, and 18 question formats for visit-specific and across-visit evaluation.
Reid-Gundlach Social Service Satisfaction Scale (R-GSSSS)	1983	North Carolina State University	Nelson Reid 919-515-2492 (ph)	Proprietary instrument originally developed for the social services, has been used in behavioral health by adaptation; 34-item scale for across-visit satisfaction. Released on condition of data sharing.
Service Satisfaction Survey (SSS-30)	1989	University of California at San Francisco	Clifford Attkisson 415-476-9690 (fx) Thomas Greenfield 510-642-7175 (fx)	Developed out of the CSQ (see above) in a 30 question format for across-visit evaluation. Permission and fees required. Contact by fax only.
Treatment Satisfaction/Process-Patient (TSP-P)	1994	William J. Filstead and Associates, Inc.	William Filstead 847-255-8214 (ph) 847-255-8215 (fx)	Proprietary instrument requring fees and permission. Uses a 14-question format for visit-specific evaluation.

[a]NOTE: All instruments have some measurement reliability and validity documentation. Contact the appropriate listed party for details on content and statistical validity.

would be useful, practical, and cost effective. This was intended as a minimum data set to foster cross-company comparisons. It was not to be an exclusive instrument but rather to be used in conjunction with any other company specific measures.

As a first stage in this process, AMBHA retained the services of Foster-Higgins, a commercial consulting firm, to gather information on selected practices from each of the constituent managed care companies. The results revealed a wide diversity of methods, response rates, and motivations concerning the measurement of consumer satisfaction. Respondents also expressed natural concerns about relinquishing proprietary information, sacrificing the individual effort expended toward a shared purpose as well as the potential that more objective and reliable measures might result in lower satisfaction ratings.

All these understandable misgivings were overcome and a year later, in January 1995, technical assistance was sought from the Kennedy School of Government at Harvard University to develop a core set of questions that would measure consumer satisfaction. In May 1995, AMBHA sponsored a national symposium at which the proposed instrument was offered for discussion and input by the National Alliance for the Mentally Ill and the Substance Abuse and Mental Health Services Administration. The following month, in June 1995, the agreed upon document was presented at the National Press Club for further comment and input by consumer organizations and government agencies.

Following these steps, a final version was approved and data collection was begun by each of the managed care companies. Another national conference is planned for later in 1996, at which aggregate data will be reviewed and further input sought.

The Consumer Satisfaction Report Card

The instrument is designed for use in a random sample of adults with language at the eighth grade level (English only). There are a total of six questions that measure access (amount of time to first appointment), intake (caring, knowledgeable, and prompt), clinical care (rating of the therapist and willingness to refer others to them), outcome (perceived benefit in presenting problems), and global satisfaction (services received).

In addition to standardized content, AMBHA agreed on guidelines for conducting telephone or mail surveys. These stipulate a minimum response rate of 70% and a minimum sample size of 500 per company. Respondents must be contacted between 2 and 6 months after intake and must have attended at least one visit. Data are to be presented in raw numbers and percentages with the sample size and response rates stipulated.

A Consumer Satisfaction Team in the Public Mental Health Sector

In 1994, Milwaukee County began implementation of a 5-year plan for public mental health services of which one author (KE) is the administrator. The vision of this plan clearly stated that: "Persons with mental illness were full and equal members of the community." It was also the responsibility of the system "To provide consumers with support in the ways they choose to live, learn, love, work, and play." Essential to the accomplishment of this vision is giving consumers a voice in system changes and development. Simply put, the plan sets a goal of having a community-based, consumer-driven mental health system in Milwaukee County.

The issue of consumer satisfaction has been slow to develop in public mental health systems. This has been rationalized by beliefs that persons with serious mental illness who were dependent on the public sector for care and treatment are incapable of expressing valid opinions and in any event are a captive audience who often have no options for choosing providers. Since the public sector providers already saw themselves as overwhelmed by the number of people needing service and diminishing resources, there was little need to "cater" to people's wants or to be in competition for clients.

Slowly these attitudes are changing; as consumers demand voice in decision making, not only about their own treatment but about the system of care that is provided, professionals are looking for new ways to listen and respond. With these populations the usual patient satisfaction questionnaire, mailed or handed to a person, is of limited value. Often the consumers are unable to attend to the paper-and-pencil task or are reluctant to voice their dissatisfaction in this format. The responses to these tools are almost always strongly positive, even though we know from other comments that consumers are not that satisfied.

One idea that is growing in popularity is the use of consumer satisfaction teams. Based on a model developed in the Philadelphia public mental health system, Milwaukee County has created and funded a separate agency that is directed and staffed by consumers of mental health services or their family members. In response to a request for a proposal, a sponsoring agency was chosen to begin development of the team. The sponsoring agency hired the executive director, who then advertised, interviewed, and hired staff. All employees of the team and the executive director must have had experience as a consumer of inpatient and community-based services. The staff of this agency operate independently and are not beholden to any other provider of services.

The consumer satisfaction team has as its goal to interview consumers in every place where public mental health services are delivered. This includes crisis settings, inpatient facilities, residential, day treatment, community support programs, and traditional outpatient clinics. Before beginning the process, all staff in these programs need to be aware of the mission of the consumer satisfaction team and understand that they are empowered by division administration to gather information directly from consumers and to report their findings. It must be clear that this is a serious commitment on the part of the funding source to value what consumers have to say and to act on their input.

The focus of the interviews is to ask the consumers in an informal setting what in the particular program contributes to their recovery and what impedes it. In addition to client comments, team staff make their own observations about the services delivered and the interactions between clients and agency personnel.

Findings from the team interviews are presented in written format to the agency–program executive director and the administrator of the Mental Health Division. A monthly meeting is held with the division administrator to hear the team's assessment of visited programs and to receive recommendations. Following this meeting, recommendations are shared with the agencies, with the expectation that the consumer satisfaction team's recommendations will be implemented or a response as to why this is not feasible will be provided to the division administration. Compliance with the team recommendations is a factor in continuing a contractual relationship with an agency.

Initially, consumers are surprised to be asked their opinions in this open and informal format. Knowing that those asking the questions also are consumers of mental health services allows for rapport building and more trust than would occur if those asking for information were seen as part of the "system." In addition, this method provides a way for the division to hold agencies accountable for consumer satisfaction. It is easy to track what suggestions or concerns were voiced by consumers and whether or not any action was taken.

Information from the consumer satisfaction team identifies systemwide needs as well as individual concerns. For example, the team recognized that persons living in group homes had concern about moving to more independent settings, such as supervised apartments. This led to the idea of establishing a buddy system where a group home resident could spend the day with a person successfully living in a supervised apartment to see what it was like.

Another finding has been the need for the continuing education of staff in community programs. Although institutional staff receive mandated in-services, often those in community or residential programs are not kept abreast of changes in the treatment of mental illness or new ways of helping the person with mental illness direct their own recovery. With specific information and observations, educational programs can be targeted to a specific need.

There are many ways to ensure consumer satisfaction. The consumer satisfaction team is one model that is developing credibility with both consumers and providers. It has the advantage that data are fed back to produce program change.

A Professional Organization Assesses Consumer Satisfaction

The Wisconsin Psychiatric Association (WPA) is a peer organization representing a majority of psychiatrists practicing in the State. In mid-1994, the president and council of the WPA requested that one of the authors (BB) make an attempt to evaluate the consumers' view of psychiatric services.

To date, this has involved conducting focus groups with all seven consumer advocacy organizations in Milwaukee, the major metropolitan area of the state (population 800,000). Each meeting lasted about an hour and was completely unstructured and open-ended. Meetings took place at a time and place convenient to consumers who were invited to share their experiences and concerns about relationships and interactions with psychiatrists. Altogether, a total of 73 consumers and family members provided a total of 156 concerns. These are listed in Table 2 under 11 categories. Forty percent (62 comments) concerned unsatisfying personal interactions and another 40% were in the four categories failure to educate, unsatisfactory medication checks, stigma, and lack of access to medical doctors.

These data were presented to the WPA council and then to the semiannual meeting of the organization in order to stimulate a dialogue with invited representatives from several consumer organizations. In addition, each of the seven focus groups was provided with tabulated concerns and a second follow-up focus group was held to discuss ways in which these concerns could be addressed and resolved by psychiatrists.

TABLE 2. Nature and Number of Consumer Concerns

	No. of comments
Unsatisfying personal interactions	62
Failure to educate patients and families	19
Unsatisfactory medication checks	17
Lack of access to MDs	13
Stigma	12
Insurance concerns	10
Poor integration of care	8
Inadequate care	5
Ethical violations	5
Inattention to social support	3
Return to work	2
Total	156

This is an ongoing process and any actions are yet to be determined. Some of the creative suggestions to date include the following:

- Identifying exemplary psychiatrists selected by consumers as role models at state meetings.
- Role playing of interactions with consumer participation.
- Inviting psychiatrists who are consumers or family members to share their experiences.
- Initiating a hot line to provide quick access to information most often sought by consumers and family members.
- Developing and teaching empathic ways to conduct a brief interview ("med" check).
- Joint ventures between psychiatrists and consumers to modify legislation, influence insurance companies, and reduce stigma.

CONCLUSION

How to ensure and measure consumer satisfaction has become a major component of behavioral health care in the final decade of this millennium. The assumption that people with mental illness could not express their opinions, were not worth asking, or were too sick to participate has been replaced by the recognition that consumer involvement and satisfaction should be a central focus in planning programs and measuring outcome.

The managed care and private and public sectors are exploring innovative methods to accomplish these goals. These efforts are still in their infancy and their influence remains to be assessed. Clearly, no single method will be sufficient; satisfaction surveys may prove helpful, but to the extent they are insensitive and produce high global scores, they should not be allowed to breed complacency or justify inaction. They should not be used solely for marketing purposes. More costly but cumbersome alternatives need to be explored, including consumer focus groups, analysis of critical incidents, and most importantly involvement of consumers in program planning and implementation.

Attempts to ensure consumer satisfaction are works in progress. Future editions of this volume will reveal whether our accomplishments match our aspirations.

REFERENCES

Attkisson, C. C., & Pascoe, G. C. (Eds.). (1983). Patient satisfaction in health and mental health services. In *Evaluation and program planning 6. Special issues*. New York: Pergamon Press.

Blackwell, B. (1997). From compliance to alliance: A quarter century of research. In B. Blackwell (Ed.), *Treatment compliance and the therapeutic alliance* (Chap. 1, pp. 1–17). Harwood Academic Publishers.

Donabedian, A. (1966). Evaluating the quality of medical care. *Mildbank Memorial Fund Quarterly, 44,* 166–203.

Eisen, S. V., & Grob, M. C. (1978). Assessing consumer satisfaction from letters to the hospital. *Hospital and Community Psychiatry, 30,* 344–346.

Elbeck, M., & Fecteau, G. (1990). Improving the validity of measures of patient satisfaction with psychiatric care and treatment. *Hospital and Community Psychiatry, 9,* 998–1001.

Gilbert, F. W., Lumpkin, J. R., & Dant, R. P. (1992). Adaptation and customer expectations of health care options. *Journal of Health Care Marketing, 12*(3), 46–55.

Grella, C. E., & Grusky, O. (1989). Families of the seriously mentally ill and their satisfaction with services. *Hospital and Community Psychiatry, 40,* 831–835.

Hevey, D. J. (1995). Quality function deployment. Symposium: Behavioral Health Care Tomorrow, Dallas, September 21, 1995.

Korsch, B. M., Gozzi, E. K., & Francis, V. (1968). Gaps in doctor–patient communication: I. Doctor–patient interaction and patient satisfaction. *Pediatrics, 42,* 855–871.

Larrabee, J. H. (1995). The changing role of the consumer in health care quality. *Journal of Nursing Care Quality, 9*(2), 8–15.

Lebow, J. L. (1983). Client satisfaction with mental health treatment: Methodological considerations in assessment. *Evaluation Review, 7,* 729–752.

Le Vois, M., Nguyen, T. D., & Attkisson, C. C. (1981). Artifact in client satisfaction assessment: Experience in community health settings. *Evaluation and Program Planning, 4,* 139–150.

Lewis, R. J. (1994). Patient views on quality care in general practice: Literature review. *Social Science and Medicine, 39,* 655–670.

Marquis, M. S., Davies, A. R., & Ware, J. E. (1983). Patient satisfaction and change in medical care provider: A longitudinal study. *Medical Care, 21,* 821–829.

Marshall, G. N., Hays, R. D., Sherbourne, C. D., & Wells, K. B. (1993). The structure of patient satisfaction with outpatient medical care. *Psychological Assessment, 5,* 477–483.

Nelson, D. C., Hartman, E., Ojemann, P. G., & Wilcox, M. (1995). Outcomes measurement and management with a large Medicaid population: A public/private collaboration. *Behavioral Healthcare Tomorrow, May/June,* 31–37.

Nguyen, T. D., Attkisson, C. C., & Stegner, B. L. (1983). Assessment of patient satisfaction: Development and refinement of a service evaluation questionnaire. *Evaluation and Program Planning, 6,* 299–314.

Olnhausen, J. L., & Werni, T. L. K. (1995). Interest in patient satisfaction increases. *The Newsletter of the Health Outcomes Institute, 2*(3), 2.

Pascoe, G. C. (1983). Patient satisfaction in primary health care: A literature review and analysis. *Evaluation and Program Planning, 6,* 185–210.

Peters, T. J., & Waterman, R. H. (1982). *In search of excellence: Lessons from America's best run companies.* New York: Harper & Row.

Ruggeri, M. (1994). Patients' and relatives' satisfaction with psychiatric services: The state of the art of its measurement. *Social Psychiatry and Psychiatric Epidemiology, 29,* 212–227.

Sheppard, M. (1993). Client satisfaction, extended intervention and interpersonal skills in community mental health. *Journal of Advanced Nursing, 18,* 246–259.

Sherbourne, C. D, Hays, R. D., Ordway, L., DiMatteo, M. R., & Kravitz, R. (1992). Antecedents of adherence to medical recommendations: Results from the Medical Outcomes Study. *Journal of Behavioral Medicine, 15,* 447–468.

Smith, G. R., Manderscheid, R. W., Steinwachs, D. M., & Flynn, L. M. (1995). *Principles of consumer outcomes assessment*. Arlington, VA: National Alliance for the Mentally Ill.

Soelling, M. E., & Newell, T. G. (1983). Effects of anonymity and experimenter demand on client satisfaction with mental health services. *Evaluation and Program Planning, 6*, 329–333.

Taylor, S. A. (1994). Distinguishing service quality from patient satisfaction in developing health care marketing strategies. *Hospital and Health Services Administration, 39*, 221–235.

Tower, K. D. (1994). Consumer-centered social work practice: Restoring client self-determination. *Social Work, 39*, 191–196.

Vaccarino, J. M. (1977). Malpractice: The problem in perspective. *Journal of the American Medical Association, 238*, 861–863.

Ware, J. E. (1981). How to survey patient satisfaction. *Drug Intelligence and Clinical Pharmacy, 15*, 892–899.

Ware, J. E., & Davies, A. R. (1983). Behavioural consequences of consumer dissatisfaction with medical care. *Evaluation and Program Planning, 6*, 291–298.

Williams, B. (1994). Patient satisfaction: A valid concept? *Social Science and Medicine, 38*, 509–516.

Williams, B., & Wilkinson, G. (1995). Patient satisfaction in mental health care: Evaluating an evaluative method. *British Journal of Psychiatry, 166*, 559–562.

Woodside, A. G., Nielsen, R. L., Walters, F., & Muller, G. D. (1988, June). Preference segmentation of health care services: The old-fashioneds, value conscious, affluents, and professional want-it-alls. *Journal of Health Care Marketing, 8*, 14–24.

21

Afterword

WARWICK G. TROY AND SHARON A. SHUEMAN

In this final brief chapter, we attempt to leave the reader with a sense of what we see as the main challenges facing behavioral health as the field begins to confront quality management issues at a time of profound changes in health care organization, financing, and provision. We also hazard some prognostications as to the kind of developments that must occur within behavioral health care if its practitioners are to cope effectively with the prospective changes and allow the continued development of effective quality management initiatives.

A final assignment we assume is one that smacks directly of editorial privilege. We are extremely troubled by the absence of any real signs that education and training programs across the disciplines are working with any degree of urgency to reform curriculum design and formats for practical training to enhance the preparation of accountable entrance-level providers for working within new parameters and fresh imperatives. Absent a clear commitment to professional competency development on the part of the organized professions, the single largest and longest lasting source of threats to the quality of behavioral health services will both endure and do significant damage.

THE CHALLENGES FACING HEALTH CARE

It is useful initially to identify the key elements of the matrix of imperatives within which behavioral health care delivery most likely will have to work in the decade ahead. These are summarized below.

1. *Quality of care will become the preeminent market variable.* Corporations and other service delivery organizations will be forced to make quality of care issues the primary lever in their attempts to acquire competitive advantage in the behavioral health marketplace. While the claim of some industry apologists in the behavioral health care marketplace—that competition is now on the basis of quality rather than price—is clearly inflated, it is also apparent that things have begun to change significantly. As should be obvious to readers of the preceding chapters, the continuous development

WARWICK G. TROY • Department of Family Medicine, University of Southern California, Los Angeles, California 90033. SHARON A. SHUEMAN • Shueman Troy Associates, Pasadena, California 91106.

Handbook of Quality Management in Behavioral Health, edited by Stricker *et al.* Kluwer Academic / Plenum Publishers, New York, 2000.

of technologies for services planning, delivery, monitoring, and evaluation, together with the increasing availability of expertise to implement these technologies in health care will continue to provide delivery systems with ever greater capacity to meet the accountability demands of payors, consumers and consumer representatives, and regulators. Significant development will be required in this area for years to come. Outcomes of services will increasingly need to be defined in measurable terms and assessed with regard to relative costs.

2. *Accountability to the entire stakeholder community will be emphasized.* Providers as well as the service delivery systems of which they will increasingly be a part will come to fully accept the fact that accountability has (and has always had) multiple targets: the stakeholders in health care—consumers, consumer advocates, payers both public and private, and regulators. Independent providers, as well as professional organizations, traditionally have resisted the principle of accountability to any entity other than the patient. Operational accountability to payers (whether public or private), the public (as exemplified by state and federal regulation of health services), or consumer organizations has been both imperfectly understood and poorly developed within the provider community. The increasing sophistication of stakeholders as well as the urgent social and economic pressures to demonstrate cost-effectiveness in service delivery will combine to make accountability the primary responsibility of health service providers and systems of care. Inevitably, all stakeholders will be involved, albeit in different ways, in defining how health services are delivered as well as in defining and evaluating desired outcomes and service quality.

3. *Providers will increasingly assume financial risk.* It has become apparent that the only way simultaneously to confront cost and quality concerns in (behavioral) health care is to place the ultimate responsibility for managing the resources in the hands of those who actually provide the care (and hence, are in a position to ensure its quality). Consequently, there will be continually increasing pressures on provider organizations to accept financial risk. In turn, this will necessitate that these organizations develop increased sophistication in the theory and practice of accountability, that is, its values, concepts, and technology. Smaller group practices by and large, will be unable to develop the quality management systems or maintain the capital base necessary to discharge these responsibilities and will inevitably be forced to merge with other practices or be absorbed by larger, formally integrated groups. These larger groups, in collaboration with their own networks of specialized (e.g., inpatient) services, will develop the information systems and other trappings of management infrastructure essential to the planning and delivery of a comprehensive package of behavioral health services under capitated payment conditions. The largest among these groups also will develop the capacity to contract directly with payers, thereby bypassing managed care organizations (MCOs), a development already apparent in general health care.

4. *The role of MCOs will devolve: Away from direct services management.* As provider organizations increasingly assume risk as well as the primary responsibility for ensuring the necessity, appropriateness, and quality of the services they provide, the role of the MCO as it is currently configured will surely change. The new roles, while currently unclear, will probably include providing a range of management support to provider organizations and negotiating with large (nationally based) purchasers on behalf of provider organizations. The self-redefinition challenges faced by MCOs may, dwarf in fact those faced by provider organizations. Ultimately, the role of a service

provider is clear; the prime role of the MCO, however, can evolve in one of many ways and may become a multiplicity of functionally related roles. Many see the near future as an opportunity for MCOs to involve themselves in a wider range of behavioral health services rather than the limited (psychotherapy, medication management, chemical dependency treatment) interventions that have traditionally passed as behavioral health (Cummings, 1995). For example, MCOs may become more involved in the development of specialty behavioral health programs that involve prevention and health promotion, such as disease management (of physical conditions such as diabetes as well as mental health problems such as depression); alternatively, managed care organizations may play a more significant, and urgently needed, role in educating consumers and empowering them as managers of their own behavioral health care.

5. *There will be clearer definition of services to be paid for by the health care dollar*. One of the most vexing issues from the perspective of both providers and payers has been the ambiguity about what type of behavioral health services health care purchasing is intended to acquire. Under the fee-for-service system, no effective mechanisms existed to determine whether services being provided were medically necessary. Indeed, the concept of medical necessity was poorly understood (and often not regarded as legitimate) by providers. As purchasers and providers are better able to distinguish medically necessary behavioral health services and are able to explicate that distinction within their service agreements, many of the types of psychotherapy-related services traditionally delivered by mental health providers will be relegated to a place outside the third-party payment system. In this operational vein, standardized measures of symptoms and health status, together with the formal assessment of functioning, will replace the more subjective and currently more prevalent provider assessments to determine necessity for treatment as well as quality of outcome. The essential task of quality management then becomes one of "assuring" outcomes deemed to be efficacious, outcomes that are attainable, measurable, and reliably associated with improvement in the health status of the recipient of care. This will not be possible without a central role for accountability mechanisms such as quality assessment and management within the behavioral health service planning and delivery systems.

THE NEED FOR NEW APPROACHES TO TRAINING

One of the consequences of the changes that will occur over the next decade is that the respective roles of the major mental health disciplines within the health care delivery system will become more clearly defined. Given the dearth of evidence of the relative superiority of, for example, doctoral-level over masters-level providers in the delivery of uncomplicated psychotherapy services, one could argue that the lower level and less costly professional groups will (and should) become the providers of choice for routine behavioral health problems. This will leave the more highly trained professionals to define their own roles within these new health systems. Even physicians, who until now have had a virtual monopoly on prescription privileges, are facing challenges in this practice area from nurse practitioners and psychologists.

Strategic efforts by professionals to position themselves to be able to contribute meaningfully to a professional world buffeted by change, much of it seemingly haphazard, increasingly will depend on the capacity of those individuals to draw upon a set of previously acquired, essentially *generic* competencies. These are those that transcend traditional roles and scope of practice concerns and equip the professional flexibly to accommodate to an ever changing context (see Broskowski, 1995; Troy, 1994; Troy & Shueman, 1996). Unfortunately, programs that currently purport to prepare entry-level professionals in the behavioral health disciplines only imperfectly comprehend the need for accountable training to meet the changed imperatives; indeed, nor do they possess any mandate for such radical reform. Further, programs typically lack the infrastructure necessary to envision, plan, and implement such challenging initiatives. As a result, entry-level providers routinely emerge from their training not only lacking the skills and knowledge required for the complex world of health care, but also possessing a values base antithetical both to the science of practice and to the manifest responsibility of the behavioral health care workforce routinely to acknowledge its obligation to multiple stakeholders.

This phenomenon surely is at the heart of the quite extraordinary reluctance of the behavioral health professions over the years to hold themselves accountable to sanctioners of behavioral health services for formal, designated outcomes, particularly those translated by the informed selection and use of protocols of intervention informed by empirical research. Put bluntly, it is why health services have had to be "managed" (Broskowski, 1991). Absent the manifest "owning" of accountability principles (the normative base discussed above) by the behavioral health workforce, on one hand, and the acquisition and use of formal competencies associated with mechanisms of accountability (knowing what and knowing how), on the other, health reform that is in the interests of the consumer will remain what it has always been for behavioral health in particular—an elusive goal.

The changed contingencies besetting the world of health care have not yet quite reached the world of academic training in the behavioral health professions, and until they do the preparation of entry-level providers and other professionals working in the world of health is not likely to change. The current plight of academic health centers scarcely augurs well for their counterpart institutions in behavioral health, particularly since the former have always maintained operational connections with health and medical service delivery systems, something that cannot be said of disciplines outside of the established health professions.

Absent widespread change in the nature, scope, and format of professional education and training, the capacity of the professional to transcend traditional roles and strategically create, if not new ones, then a different mix of activities, is limited. Given that one should never underestimate the power of creative, flexible, and venturesome individuals significantly to modify parts of their immediate world, the odds for enduring professional survival are not high for the majority. And, if this alone were not sufficient reason to give pause, the continuing threat to the prevailing quality of service provision in behavioral health is disturbing both in the nature of its impact and the magnitude of its scope.

It is clear that in the current world of health care, there is much that is chaotic, infelicitous, and disturbing. The curious "underworld" of behavioral health, marginalized for decades by the larger health care system and the general public alike and hitherto curiously isolated from most of the modest quality imperatives with which even the premanaged care world had to contend, is in the process of the most rapid change of its existence. Pressure by the large payers to have the rate of services cost escalation reduced, new payment mechanisms, increased prevalence of empirically based protocols and treatment guidelines, and growing demands for demonstrably cost-effective care in their various ways have all essentially remade the previously predictable and not altogether uncomfortable world of the traditional provider. Many practitioners see these changes as utterly dismaying. We maintain, nonetheless, that it is precisely these structural changes, seen as villainous by the majority of independent practitioners, that offer perhaps the best and certainly most enduring chance that activities associated with the assessment and management of services quality will become routinely incorporated within the process of health services planning and provision, rather than remaining a marginalized and formalistic addition to it.

We see nothing paradoxical in this. The role for quality management will be—is now—enhanced because the industry has (tacitly) agreed that the high road to satisfying the entire set of imperatives identified above is the creation of better integrated service delivery systems fueled by invigorated demands for accountability. Thus it is that the imperatives identified earlier are responsible for the substantial change in the ways in which (behavioral) health services are now being organized and, in turn, for what many see as a reduction in the quality of professional life of the ("independent") provider. An additional change will be workforce related: There will occur an inevitable shakeout of behavioral health providers. Those sufficiently comfortable with working within integrated systems associated with the provision of health services will remain; many providers who see working under managed arrangements as an intolerable compromise will eventually opt out of a system they no longer find recognizable, in which they find minimal reward, and for which they were never trained.

In time, the behavioral health workforce will be more homogeneous with respect to competencies—knowledge, skills, and the all important attitude–value components (Troy & Shueman, 1996). It will be this workforce that will eventually be able to contribute significantly and consistently to the quality landscape through its commitment to and preparedness for professional roles and activities associated with the armamentarium of quality management. This includes population-based planning rather than the prevailing focus on episodes of care; adoption and routine use of empirically supported intervention protocols and outcome measurement; knowledge of and sensitivity to the needs and characteristics of vulnerable and traditionally underserved populations; sharing an organizational commitment to minimizing continuity of care problems; involvement in health promotion and prevention activities; and an enhanced focus on the planning and delivery of appropriate behavioral health services via the development of alternative treatment modalities that serve to improve access to needed care.

REFERENCES

Broskowski, A (1991). Current mental health care environments: Why managed care is necessary. *Professional Psychology, 22*, 6–14.

Broskowski, A. (1995). Evolution of health care: Implications for the training and careers of psychologists. *Professional Psychology: Research and Practice, 26*(2), 156–162.

Cummings, N.A. (1995). Behavioral health after managed care: The next golden opportunity for professional psychology. *Register Reports: The Newsletter for Health Services Providers in Psychology, 20*(3) and *21*(1), 1, 30–33.

Troy, W. G. (1994). Developing and improving professional competencies. In S.A. Shueman, W. G. Troy, & S. L. Mayhugh (Eds.), *Managed behavioral health care: An industry perspective* (pp. 168–188). Springfield, IL: Charles C. Thomas

Troy, W. G., & Shueman, S. A. (1996). Program redesign for graduate training in professional psychology: The road to accountability in a changing professional world. In N. Cummings, M. Pallak, & J Cummings (Eds.), *Surviving the demise of solo practice: Mental health professionals prospering in the era of managed care.* Madison, CT: Psychosocial Press.

Index

ISBN 0-306-46149-8
90000
9 780306 461491